INTRODUCTION TO THE THERAPEUTIC PROCESS

JACK E. HOKANSON
Florida State University

▲ ADDISON-WESLEY PUBLISHING COMPANY

Reading, Massachusetts • Menlo Park, California
London • Amsterdam • Don Mills, Ontario • Sydney

*To my parents: loving, supportive, and
eternally searching for a better way of life*

Library of Congress Cataloging in Publication Data

Hokanson, Jack E.
    Introduction to the therapeutic process.

    Includes bibliographical references and index.
    1. Psychotherapy.   I.   Title.
RC480.H59   616.89'14   81-20623
ISBN 0-201-10525-X   AACR2

ISBN 0-201-10525-X
ABCDEFGHIJ-MA-898765432

PREFACE

My favorite undergraduate psychology course, taken some thirty years ago at CCNY, was entitled Human Motivation. It was taught by Professor Max Hertzman, a learned and inspiring teacher. The course was captivating because the whole semester was devoted to reading great works of literature—by Ibsen, D. H. Lawrence, Chekhov, Tolstoy, and many others. Professor Hertzman guided our class discussions into analyses of the characters portrayed in these works. We came to understand their emotions, conflicts, and relationships and the social forces operating in their lives. We also gained an appreciation of how change comes about in someone's personality.

As I now reflect back on that course I admire Profesor Hertzman's scholarship even more. In virtuoso fashion he would frequently relate our class discussions to formal personality and clinical theories, never pushing one theory over another. He apparently had no favorite point of view. Rather, he insisted that the class examine the theories in terms of their logic, internal consistency, and conformity to existing data. His nondogmatic approach to psychology, I believe, imbued the whole class with a basic eclecticism which many of us have tried to maintain in later careers.

This learned instructor seemed to have one overriding purpose in his teaching. By combining great works of literature with psychological theory the class gained an awareness of, trite as it may sound, the real-life processes which underlie theory. We were not just learning abstract concepts or memorizing definitions. At a rudimentary level, at least, we were beginning to learn how psychological problems come about and by what processes they may be overcome in the everyday lives of people.

In the years since I took that course theory and research have expanded dramatically in the field. Current-day students who are interested in the mental health area have to contend with a vast array of theoretical orientations, varied philosophies about psychological adjustment, and many competing systems of psychotherapy. Textbooks often present these diverse points of view in smorgasbord fashion, having, for example, one chapter on Freudian therapy, another on Carl Rogers, yet another on transactional analysis, and so forth. To the beginning student such diversity may appear chaotic.

Having now taught graduate and undergraduate courses in therapy for quite a long time, I have come to appreciate the distress experienced by students. Many undergraduates feel that they have dutifully learned all the theories and have carefully studied the various therapy orientations. Yet they sense a critical gap in their preparation for a career in the helping professions. As best I can discern, they seem to feel deficient in understanding the actual *processes* of therapy. How does one get started with a client? What kinds of decisions are made early in the therapeutic process? How are these decisions arrived at? Where is one going with a client, and what are the intervening steps? Students express difficulty in translating the many concepts they have learned into an awareness of the practical business of conducting psychotherapy. They may not necessarily want to engage in treatment, but they would like to know what it is about.

Writing an introductory textbook which attempts to fill this gap is a difficult and somewhat risky task. A major problem is the fact that considerable controversy and difference of opinion still exist in the mental health field. Taken as a whole, there is little agreement within the profession as to "standard" therapy processes. While a great deal of psychotherapy research has been published in the last twenty years, relatively few definitive conclusions can yet be drawn. Thus the textbook writer has to use a combination of clinical theory, incomplete research results, and a certain degree of chutzpah in attempting to describe therapeutic processes.

This book admittedly represents my own interpretations and judgments about many aspects of clinical practice. I have tried to do justice to a wide variety of theories and therapy traditions, and to rely on empirical data where possible. Nevertheless, in view of our incomplete knowledge in this area, the final product can only be viewed as one person's model of therapy processes. Perhaps the book can be seen as a first approximation to providing some order and structure to a very ambiguous field of study.

I am deeply indebted to Stephen O'Hagan, Eugene Levitt, Lee Sechrest, and William Sacco for their help and commentary on this material. Thanks also to Rose Boccio for her untiring efforts in preparing the manuscript. Finally, a strong sense of appreciation is felt toward my students, whose frank discussion and encouragement made this book possible.

Tallahassee, Florida   J. E. H.
June 1982

CONTENTS

PART ONE

THEORETICAL AND PROFESSIONAL ISSUES

CHAPTER ONE

AN APPROACH
TO THERAPY

INTRODUCTION

Helping a fellow human is a cherished value. Whether it involves the complex medical practice of a surgeon, the community-oriented work of social planners, the intricate process of psychoanalysis, or just the everyday assistance one might give a neighbor, such an endeavor strikes chords deep within us.

In the field of mental health, humanitarian motives seem to account to a large degree for the growth and attractiveness of professions in this area. Clinical psychology, psychiatry, social work, counseling, psychiatric nursing, vocational rehabilitation, and special education, to name a few, are professions that have undergone dramatic expansion since World War II. Quite obviously these fields have grown in response to needs for such services in an increasingly complex society and as a result of enhanced public conscience with regard to troubled individuals. But in addition, a strong push also comes from the deeper and personal motives of those—young people in particular—who are seeking careers in one of the "helping professions."

These professions have grown in three general directions during the 1960s and 1970s. The first direction is based on the growing recognition that the application of psychological principles to helping others goes far beyond the realms of the traditional mental hospital or psychological clinic. Today it would not be unusual to see these principles actively and purposefully applied in such diverse settings as the family doctor's office, a fifth-grade classroom, a meeting of corporate executives, or a spontaneously formed neighborhood self-help group. The second direction of growth is reflected in the trend toward *paraprofessional* involvement. Quite clearly, the needs for mental health services have outstripped the availability of Ph.D. psychologists and psychiatrists or graduate social workers. Thus critically important technical positions are evolving that will provide a considerable proportion of the day-to-day psychological help needed by people. Mental health workers in these positions

3

require extensive training, of course, but not to the degree involved in obtaining an M.D. or Ph.D. The third direction of growth is toward a scientific, research-based approach to mental health problems. This approach involves data-based evaluations of the success of different treatments, the development of improved diagnostic methods, and basic experimentation on the very concepts that mental health workers utilize. For these reasons the term *applied behavioral science* seems to be an appropriate emerging title for the field. Thus the entire mental health field is undergoing growth, in terms of its *breadth* of application, the *depth* of personnel involved, and its scientific basis.

The variety of fields devoted to mental health, each with its own terminology, presents difficulties for the writer. To avoid confusion and jargon, I will try to use a minimum of specialized terms in this book. Rather, limited and conventional usages that will hopefully be appropriate for most specialties will be adopted. To this end, the term *psychotherapy* will be used in its broadest meaning, to refer to the use of interpersonal, behavioral, and psychological techniques to improve the human condition of another person. The individual receiving this help will be referred to as the *client;* the individual providing the help will be called the *therapist.* Hopefully these generalized labels will not offend definitional purists and will be viewed as conveniences by which to communicate to a diverse audience.

HISTORICAL TRENDS

The field of psychotherapy is emerging from its adolescence into a vigorous maturity. However, in order to achieve this status it has had to overcome some growing pains. Many of the early "schools" of psychotherapy were based on very casual observations of limited numbers of clinic patients. In addition, these approaches were to a large extent developed from the personal philosophical views of the various theorists involved. Thus philosophical assumptions about the "nature" of people and value judgments concerning the meaning of individual adjustment and happiness, coupled with a few generalizations about the structure of personality, formed the cornerstones for early theories of psychotherapy. Since philosophical views are virtually impossible to verify by scientific methods, an unfortunate trend toward cultism and dogmatism has been part of the history of psychotherapy. Many students and professionals, as late as the 1960s, became ardent disciples of a "master," becoming, for example, exclusive Freudians, Rogerians, or Skinnerians, and so forth. Competing theorists and therapy techniques were frequently dismissed as philosophically alien and not worthy of serious study. This trend in some instances reached the point where considerable numbers of university departments of psychiatry, psychology, counseling, and social work taught only their "preferred" theory to students, thus perpetuating an unscientific, narrow, and basically untenable approach for yet another generation of therapists.

These historical factors operated to influence the training of therapists into relatively narrow molds. If an individual happened to attend a school in which, for example, an orthodox Freudian approach was preferred, then the "successful" student mastered the "party line," espousing acceptable concepts and therapy procedures. Such effects on training, and ultimately the practice of psychotherapy, had several unfortunate consequences. As later research has suggested (see Parloff, Waskow, and Wolfe, 1978), therapists with these rigidities are not exceptionally successful with a wide range of clients; further, such dogmatism seemed to impede the development of psychotherapy as a profession based on scientific principles. Since many of the early therapists already "knew" the correct theory, attempts at critical examination of basic concepts and therapy effectiveness were far from rigorous. Faulty research designs, biased measures, and self-serving conclusions seemed to be rampant among these early research projects (Eysenck, 1960).

In recent years this doctrinaire allegiance to a narrow point of view seems to be less pervasive among mental health workers. Although philosophical and theoretical differences still exist (see Strupp, 1978), many contemporary theorists (e.g., Bergin and Lambert, 1978; Korchin, 1976) have fostered the notion that a flexible and multidimensional approach to therapy is professionally and scientifically sound.

This broadening of the field in our present era confronts students of psychotherapy with many new problems. They usually must gain an understanding of a far wider range of theories and technical skills than their counterparts of a generation ago. They are also faced with a continual influx of new research results that bear upon therapy and assessment. Furthermore, current students have to contend with well over one hundred different kinds of psychotherapy that exist in the field (Report of the Research Task Force of the National Institute of Mental Health, 1975). This vast array of theories and therapy systems can be confusing to experienced professionals and can sometimes be overwhelming to individuals who are just beginning in the field. This confusion often becomes highlighted when one considers the practical application of therapy with clients. How does a clinician make the appropriate selection from among the welter of existing therapies? What criteria are used in attempting to match a treatment approach with a particular client's problems? What kinds of information are needed to make such decisions? How is the information weighted and conceptualized in arriving at a choice of treatment?

As one reviews the contemporary literature on psychotherapy (see Garfield and Bergin, 1978), several trends and generalizations may be cautiously noted. First, most investigators agree that the questions mentioned above are centrally important. Second, most would probably agree that with few exceptions the answers to these questions are not yet availale on the basis of existing research. Finally, there appears to be a consensus that until an empirically based framework for treatment decisions is arrived at, practicing therapists will have to use a combination of clinical theory, personal judgment, and partial research results to guide their work with clients.

THE PURPOSE OF THIS BOOK

As stated earlier, one of the principal aims of therapy research is ultimately to provide a set of guidelines for determining which therapy approach will be most effective for a particular problem. Several component problems are associated with this long-range endeavor. One is the need to describe the techniques and the sequencing of procedures that are involved in each therapy approach. Another is a specification of the goals that each treatment is designed to achieve. Yet a third is the development of a system by which to describe and categorize various problems so that they can eventually be matched to recommended treatments. Making progress on all these dimensions is obviously a slow and complicated process, and one can speculate that several decades of further research will be required.

It seems possible, however, to make some first approximations of a framework for organizing treatment approaches and problems, and this is the purpose of this book. Given our present state of knowledge, such a set of guidelines would obviously be rough and tentative. Furthermore, it would be based on the author's interpretation of present-day trends in research, theory development, and clinical practice. Nevertheless, it is felt that proposing an overall model may serve a twofold purpose: to assist beginning students in gaining a more organized perspective on this complex, multidimensional field and to put forth a middle-of-the-road therapy system that can be refined and modified as new research findings become available.

Naturally, any attempt to impose a structure on such a diverse area runs multiple risks. Complex issues will occasionally be oversimplified. Personal bias will undoubtedly be conveyed, or a particular point of view will be overstated. In several instances, the descriptions of some of the therapy processes will reflect the author's opinion of how they should function, rather than how they probably operate under the pressures of actual practice. Thus the reader should be cautioned on several counts. The material that follows in this book cannot possibly capture the richness and subtlety that occurs in clinical practice, nor can all points of view be represented with total fairness. It is hoped, however, that the student of psychotherapy will come away with several important gains: (1) a workable but tentative system for matching some broad classes of client problems with some equally broad treatment strategies; (2) an appreciation of the various stages of therapy that are likely to occur within each treatment strategy; and (3) an awareness of the major unresolved issues and research questions still to be answered in the field.

ORGANIZATIONAL PLAN

In this section, and indeed for the remainder of this chapter, an outline of a multidimensional approach to therapy will be provided. This will serve both as a general orientation to present-day approaches and as a framework for the more detailed technical material in subsequent chapters. Therefore it is hoped that the reader will pay particular attention to this organizational structure and will continue to refer to it throughout the course of this book.

Two types of overview will be provided. The first is a general description of a proposed *sequence* of events that occur in therapy, starting with a client's first contact with a therapist or agency and continuing all the way through to the conclusion of treatment. Hopefully such an outline will offer a broad perspective on the various stages of the therapeutic process and how one stage follows another in an orderly fashion. The second overview takes a *cross-sectional* view of the process, focusing on the different types of problems that clients display and how these various problems dictate different treatment goals and different therapy approaches. This material lays the groundwork for decision making regarding the recommended treatment strategy for each client.

The Sequence of the Therapeutic Process

Let us first take an overview of the various steps involved in the process of therapy. Some of these steps will appear to be self-evident; nevertheless, it seems advisable to explicitly state them in this introductory section. This sequence of steps can be outlined as follows:

I. First contact with the client
   A. Introductions and outline of services
   B. Explanation of procedures
   C. Review of professional-ethical issues
   D. Preliminary agreement to proceed

II. Assessment of the client's problems
   A. Intake interview
   B. Psychological tests
   C. Information from others
   D. Self-observation techniques
   E. Conceptualization of client's problems

III. Therapist-client negotiations regarding goals of treatment
   A. Crisis management
   B. Behavior change
   C. Corrective emotional experience
   D. Self-exploration and change

IV. Implementation of treatment
   A. Explanation and structuring for client
   B. The processes of therapy
      1. Supportive therapy
      2. Behavioral approaches
      3. Relationship therapy
      4. Insight and change techniques
   C. Evaluation of success

Each of these stages of the therapeutic procedure will be reviewed in the remainder of this section. As will be seen, the overall process requires interpersonal sensitivity, abilities to understand many complexities of human behavior, and extensive knowledge of a wide variety of therapy skills.

First contact with the client Most clients make their first contact with a therapist or agency not really knowing what to expect or how they should behave. Furthermore, all clients bring a unique set of anxieties and hesitancies to the therapeutic situation that may hamper full and open discussion of their problems. For these reasons the first person with whom they make contact (whether it be a private practicing therapist, the intake worker at a mental health agency, etc.) should be prepared to deal with these initial difficulties. To accomplish this, several basic areas need to be covered with the client at the outset. A general introduction that identifies the therapist (or agency) as to professional credentials and areas of practice is an appropriate beginning. As part of such an introductory discussion, a brief review of the general services that can be provided may also serve as a preliminary orientation for the client.

Naturally, clients are also asked to summarize the reasons for their seeking of help. If it appears that the therapist (or agency) is appropriate to deal with such problems, then a description of the intake procedures may be given to the client, which should provide some structure and help clarify any misapprehensions as to what may be expected in the beginning phase of treatment.

As part of this first contact, discussion of ethical and professional issues may also be necessary. For example, a client who is in legal difficulties may be concerned with issues of confidentiality. Another client with medical complications may require clarification of the professional liaison between the therapist and the client's physician. Finally, a brief discussion of the client's problems in relation to the professional services offered by the agency or therapist should result in a preliminary agreement to proceed or referral to a more appropriate agency. A detailed discussion of this introductory stage of therapy will be provided in Chapter 3.

Assessment of the client's problems After the initial agreement between the agency and client to enter into the intake procedures, the next stage of the process is a careful analysis and assessment of the client's problems. Arrangements are make for an *intake interview*, an information-gathering session in which the details of the client's problems, their history, their effects on current life processes, and the sources of the problems are reviewed. The gathering of this intake information may require several interviews, depending on the complexity of the material and the readiness of the client to disclose personal information.

Several other sources of information may be utilized as part of this assessment stage. *Psychological tests* can provide an evaluation of intellectual achievement, behavioral and emotional patterns of reaction, indications of inner and environmental areas of stress, and attitude-value issues, all of which may be pertinent to the client's problems. Arrangements may be made to interview family members and other concerned individuals in the client's life with regard to their perceptions and evaluations of the problems. Finally, *self-observation procedures* may be initiated, in which the client is told how to keep accurate records of the occurrence of the relevant problems and symptoms, what events seem to precipitate them, how they cope with stressful situations, and so forth.

In addition to the information obtained through these procedures, consultation with professionals in other fields is frequently necessary. Evidence of the involvement of physical symptoms may require general medical, neurological, or nutritional assessment by appropriate professionals. Likewise, legal or economic complications, for example, may necessitate contact with a lawyer or community social agency.

Following this gathering of information from a variety of sources, the therapist is faced with the task of evaluating and combining the data into a meaningful and consistent *conceptualization of the client*. If done properly, psychological problems and environmental stressors are seen in the context of the client's total life-style and personality, rather than just as reflections of a particular diagnosis or other stereotyped label. Details regarding these various assessment procedures and a conceptual framework by which to integrate this information will be provided in Chapters 3 and 4.

The assessment stage is of critical importance in the overall process of therapy. Although the information obtained is rarely complete, at least a preliminary formulation of the client's difficulties is arrived at, which permits the subsequent stages of therapy to be tailored to the particular needs of each individual. Upon completion of these procedures, the therapist and client are in a realistic position to meet again to consider what the *goals* of therapy should be and ultimately to review what treatment strategy may be used to reach those goals.

Therapist-client negotiations regarding goals of treatment Naturally, all clients do not bring the same sets of problems into therapy; neither will the goals of treatment be similar for each individual. Thus two general areas of the client's difficulties may be considered: (1) the behavioral-emotional-attitudinal patterns that seem to be producing the problems and (2) the life circumstances and external stress that contribute to these problems. While not always easily discerned, identification of these problem-producing factors will define those areas of living that require change.

At this important point of the therapy process, then, the client and therapist are in a position to discuss and negotiate which changes can appropriately and realistically be worked toward. These agreed-upon changes thereby represent the *goals* of therapy.

Several possible limitations of this process require discussion. First, the assessment procedures may not have resulted in sufficiently detailed information by which to clearly identify areas to be changed. Second, the client may be in disagreement with the therapist as to the factors that are producing problems. Third, the client may be too anxious or defensive to engage in realistic discussion of these issues. And finally, the client may not feel sufficiently familiar with the therapist to trust his or her judgment on personal matters of such magnitude. Any one or a combination of these possibilities might well occur at this early stage of the therapy process—and it is these sorts of difficulties that represent many of the challenges of carrying out successful therapy.

It is evident that the therapist must meet these challenges in a patient, supportive, and sensitive manner. It may indeed require numerous sessions of further discussion and analysis for some clients to develop enough trust and confidence in the therapist to openly and honestly reveal themselves. Similarly, some problem areas may be enormously complex and subtle and therefore necessitate a relatively great amount of work in their analysis and clarification. The main point here, then, is that, while client-therapist negotiations regarding therapeutic goals is a central part of the overall treatment process, at times this can be a relatively long and delicate process. The initial goals may even change as therapy progresses and new perspectives are gained. One of the case illustrations to be presented below will exemplify such a situation, and more detailed descriptions of these procedures are given in Chapter 4.

Implementation of treatment Following the setting of treatment goals, the therapist must determine the appropriate therapy methods by which to achieve these goals. For some types of goals (for example, helping a client overcome a specific phobia) the choice for the therapist is reasonably clear, in that considerable research has been published regarding the most efficient therapy. For others, however, the relative paucity of empirical evidence requires that the therapist use professional judgment (and common sense) in arriving at such therapy decisions.

Once arrived at, however, an appropriate description of the treatment procedures is presented to the client. This usually includes an explanation of the procedures themselves, they way in which they are related to the treatment goals, the anticipated length of time involved, and points in the procedures that may prove to be difficult and trying for the client. As part of this structuring, definition of the client's tasks is also given, with instructions regarding in-session work, activities to be engaged in between sessions, record keeping, and so forth. In this fashion, the actual therapy procedures are structured as a mutual effort, with both participants aware of techniques and goals of the entire process.

The actual treatment procedures to be utilized with each particular client are selected from a wide array of techniques that exist in the profession. These techniques have frequently been historically identified with particular schools of therapy. However, research evidence again suggests that most practitioners in the field utilize these procedures in a flexible and eclectic fashion, as is appropriate to each client. This is the approach put forth in this book, and descriptions of a wide range of techniques are presented in Chapters 5 through 10.

At the conclusion of therapy, and after an appropriate follow-up period, evaluations of the effectiveness of the treatment in meeting the goals are conducted. To the extent that it is possible, this evaluation should be preplanned such that the goals have been clearly specified and the measures to be used are objective and unbiased. In this fashion systematic information can be collected regarding the services provided to each client, as well as scientific data necessary for the continued maturation of the profession. Specifics on such evaluation procedures are presented in Chapter 11.

A Cross-Sectional View of the Therapeutic Process

The *cross-sectional* perspective of the therapeutic process given here is a proposed way of conceptualizing therapy goals and their associated treatment strategies. This perspective should help the reader develop a framework upon which to organize the varieties of problems for which clients are seeking help and also to acquire a basis for decisions regarding the choice of treatment for each type of problem.

Four types of goals It is a truism to state that each client brings a unique set of problems into therapy. Indeed, it is important that the therapist continually appreciates that uniqueness throughout the entire therapeutic process so that an open and empathic relationship with the client is maintained. However, it is frequently helpful for the practitioner to utilize some broad and flexible categories regarding both the types of problems encountered and the treatment goals that are logically related to each of those problem classes. I have found four classes of goals to be a workable system during the beginning stages of treatment. At this early phase, when information about clients' problems is necessarily general and incomplete, these goals represent first approximations. More detailed and specific therapy aims should be developed for each client as the treatment process unfolds. Phrased in another way, these general goals provide guidelines for the initial directions to be taken in therapy, and as such, they provide some criteria for decision making during the intake stage. This four-category system is not a radical departure from generally accepted clinical practice. Rather, it is an attempt to describe and formalize an approach used by many practicing clinicians.

In this light, then, four brief case sketches designed to exemplify the four major categories of client problems and treatment goals will be described. Each sketch is oversimplified and stereotyped in order to highlight the different goals involved. Hence the reader is urged not to become overly involved with the details of each case but rather to focus on the differences between them and to note how each seems to dictate different aims at the start of therapy.

Case 1. Consider first the case of a seventeen-year-old girl with an essentially "normal" background—a wide range of social relations, an adequate academic record, good rapport with her family, and so on. Within a matter of days in her life, a convergence of several unexpected and tragic circumstances occur that bring about a psychological crisis. A cold-blooded admission by her boyfriend that he has been courting her only because of sexual favors and the death of her mother in an automobile accident bring her to a point bordering on a "nervous breakdown." Overwhelmed by grief, guilt, anger, and waves of cynicism about the stability of her world, she is faced with emotions and circumstances that are completely foreign to her and for which she has never had to develop coping mechanisms. In this highly disturbed emotional state there are frequent occasions when she does not think logically, when she contemplates suicide, and when she experiences the uncanny sensation that her personality is shattering.

The goals of therapy in this case seem rather direct. The therapist does not have the luxury of time, but must intervene quickly and decisively in helping to stabilize a dangerous and potentially explosive situation. The specific aims here are: (1) helping the client to gain control over her intense and debilitating feelings; (2) reestablishing logical, reality-oriented thought processes and behaviors; and (3) mobilizing friends and family to provide emotional support and guidance during this crisis. These represent a set of limited, crisis-oriented goals that do not fit the usual romanticized image of "depth therapy"; yet clearly they can be of critical importance in the subsequent adjustment of this individual.

Case 2. Consider next the case of a forty-year-old man whose elevated blood pressure (signaling the possibility of future cardiac difficulties) is aggravated by a long-term smoking habit, a tendency to overeat, and a hard-driving, relentless approach to his business. Aside from this burgeoning medical problem and its associated behavioral components, he seems to be free of psychological or social deficits. He is vocationally successful, is a contented and involved family man, has a good perspective on his life, and so on. It can be reasonably argued that this man is not in need of long-term depth psycho-therapy, which attempts to uncover hidden conflicts and unconscious motiva-tional systems. However, he could certainly profit from therapy that will assist him to discard some clearly harmful behavioral patterns (smoking and over-eating) and will help him to gain control over the pace and intensity with which he approaches his business activities. Again, such specific and limited behavior-change goals may not be as exotic and captivating as those usually associated with deep psychoanalysis, and yet they could well represent the difference between a healthy and vigorous middle age versus invalidism or even death for this client.

Case 3. This case portrays yet another set of goals—ones that principally involve the relationship between client and therapist. A thirteen-year-old boy has grown up in an environment in which virtually all encounters with adults have resulted in negative experiences. Parents, teachers, and other adults have been uniformly rejecting, punitive, or exploitive. As might be expected, this teenager has thus developed strong and generalized anxieties, anger, and a pervasive sense of vulnerability. To protect himself he has developed a tough, independent exterior, which meets the environment with attitudes of "I don't need anyone" and "I'll take advantage of others before they get me." Although understandable, a continuation of this adjustment into the later teenage and adult years holds the promise of a wide range of possible problems: difficulties in school and on the job; delinquency; isolation from others; and a generally bleak, suspicious view of the world.

The problems are compounded by the fact that the very coping mechanisms by which he emotionally survives (toughness, exploitation) will likely sour future relationships with others—even those that are potentially positive and affectionate—thus perpetuating his debilitating view of the world.

The principal therapeutic goal with this client could be simply stated as the development of a healthy, positive relationship with the therapist—a relation-ship in which the client can learn that not all adults are rejecting and uncaring, in which he can safely begin to discard his surly and exploitive approach to others, and in which he can learn to exchange affectionate emotions with another person. Hopefully the reader has an intuitive feel for the importance of these goals, although admittedly vague and booby trapped with many possible complications, and how profound an effect they can have on this young person if adequately accomplished.

Case 4. The last illustration provides yet a fourth vantage point regarding therapeutic goals. A twenty-eight-year-old accountant, on the advice of a friend, has applied to a community mental health clinic because he has felt progressively more dejected, unfulfilled, and alienated over a period of years. His complaints are vague and generalized but represent a considerable degree of personal agony for him—to the point where these concerns have become the predominant preoccupation in his life. He states that he is both distressed and confused by his condition, because in his estimation his life seems to be going well. He is economically successful, has a large circle of good friends, and engages in a variety of entertaining leisure activities.

Both the therapist and the client in this illustration are faced with a confusing and ill-defined problem. From the limited amount of information provided by the client, neither can point to maladaptive behaviors, inappropriate attitudes, or stressful circumstances that may be bringing about the client's long-term distress. Thus this situation very likely involves several goals, the first of which is the process of *discovery*.

The client, apparently unable to discern and specify complex patterns in his life that contribute to his emotional difficulties, could probably profit from a period of self-exploration. Because this task is ambiguous to begin with, the self-discovery process may be relatively prolonged and wide ranging, including an investigation of such areas as interpersonal relations and intimacy issues, emotional carry-overs from earlier experiences, unattended difficulties with values and morality, or indeed, unrecognized dissatisfaction with his entire life-style.

Upon achieving this first goal of insight into the complex patterns that produce the client's distress, both client and therapist are in a position to determine a second set of goals: those pertaining to bringing about *change* in maladaptive behavioral, emotional, or value-belief systems. It is apparent that the several therapeutic goals involved in this case present the clinician with a considerably more involved process than was suggested by the earlier cases, and most would agree that the requirements for the management of such a case involve extensive sensitivity, skill, and training.

Goals and treatment As stated earlier, the four cases just described were selected to illustrate four different classes of client problems and treatment goals. As such they form a convenient framework by which to organize discussion of various therapy procedures which apply to each. Although no classification system can capture all of the complexities of the field, the one to be proposed here may serve as an adequate working model by which to study this area.

Considerable controversy still exists as to the most effective treatment procedures for the different types of client problems. Some of these controversies are carry-overs from the historical cultism described earlier and are probably best ignored. However, there remain some very real and critical issues that must await careful and unbiased research before they can be resolved. In the discussion of treatment procedures that follows, the reader should keep in mind the tentative and general nature of the proposals.

The first case illustration, that of the seventeen-year-old girl who had recently lost her mother, represents a class of therapeutic goals that is termed *crisis management.* This category consists of immediate, usually short-term emergency-oriented goals that relate to helping the client stave off impending disaster. These high-risk situations may involve an incipient psychotic episode, suicide, explosive acting-out behaviors, or impulsive and ill-planned life decisions. Treatment procedures appropriate to such clients can be grouped under the general term of *supportive therapy.* This type of therapy represents an amalgam of techniques that have been developed by practitioners in a variety of settings: emergency consultations in psychiatric hospitals; crisis teams in community outpatient clinics; suicide prevention centers; drug and alcohol units; and community "hot-line" services. Principles of supportive therapy will be reviewed in Chapter 5.

The case of the forty-year-old with potential heart trouble exemplifies a situation in which goals involving *behavior change* are most salient. Habits and behavioral patterns of long standing are creating a hazardous health situation for this client and hence represent the focus of therapeutic efforts. Assuming then that client and therapist agree upon the goals of changing these maladaptive behaviors, treatment techniques stemming from the general area of *behavior modification* and self-regulation procedures seem most appropriate. As will be described in Chapter 6, this class of therapy procedures is based largely on principles derived from psychological research in the areas of operant and classical conditioning, observational learning (modeling), and cognitive processes.

The case of the thirteen-year-old boy represents a set of goals that require a major restructuring of interpersonal relationships. The psychologically damaged juvenile in the illustration does not present the psychotherapist with a specific set of symptoms or behaviors that can be profitably changed, nor is he in a crisis condition. Rather, he portrays the development of a broadly based, maladaptive "way of life" that is an outgrowth of the persistently negative interpersonal experiences in his background. This way of life thus includes not only maladaptive behavior patterns but also habitual emotional reactions, a particular style of perceiving others, rigid expectations about people's behavior, and attitudes concerning the world in general. Using the therapy relationship itself as a vehicle for a *corrective emotional experience* thus becomes the aim with such clients; that is, the goal is to develop a relatively long-term interpersonal experience that can change the client's overall negative approach to people.

Central to the treatment procedures for such clients is the development and maintenance of the client-therapist relationship; hence the term *relationship therapy* is frequently applied. The specific techniques involved are less well defined than those cited earlier, and indeed, even the theoretical bases for this approach have yet to be clearly formulated. Nevertheless, throughout the history of psychotherapy a number of theorists have referred to the importance of the client-therapist relationship per se in producing therapeutic changes. Alfred Adler (1927) suggested that it is fundamental in producing positive "social feelings" towards one's fellow man and community, in place of previously held patterns of exploitation. Carl Rogers (1951) similarly has proposed that the process of being able to fully experience oneself, and thereby also being able to authentically relate to others, is basically an outgrowth of the therapist's relationship with the client. Alexander and French (1946) have perhaps most directly incorporated these ideas in their concept of the "corrective emotional experience" as being the basic ingredient in therapeutic activities. As described here, it is recognized that the particulars of the "therapeutic relationship" and its healing qualities are left vague. Material spelling out the processes and therapy techniques pertinent to relationship goals will be presented in Chapters 7 and 8. For now, attention is drawn to the importance of the goals themselves as distinct from the others described in this section.

The case of the alienated and dejected accountant who could find no reasons for his distress presents an example of perhaps the most complex set of goals in the proposed framework. Here is an individual who is apparently unable to discern the significant forces operating in his life — inner motivational-emotional systems and environmental conditionings and pressures. The case is illustrative of clients who focus on relatively obvious aspects of their lives and can find no suitable explanation for their symptoms and distress. With these kinds of clients, we can make the reasonable assumption that there indeed are maladaptive (but unrecognized) reaction patterns or life stresses that are related to the symptoms and feelings of distress. Once uncovered and carefully analyzed, the client and therapist are in a position to actively bring about a change in these patterns or life circumstances. We have here then a sequence of at least two goals: *insight* and *change*.

The reader will no doubt recognize that the therapy techniques pertinent to the first half of these goals (the self-exploration process) have a long and complex legacy. Procedures stemming from Freudian and neo-Freudian theory, as well as client-centered, existential, transactional, and gestalt approaches, provide a rich array of self-discovery techniques. As suggested earlier, as these procedures result in the uncovering of debilitating emotional-behavior-attitudinal patterns, a second class of therapy techniques becomes appropriate — those designed to bring about change in these patterns. Here, as already discussed, the entire range of behavior modification and self-regulation procedures are relevant. In addition, therapy techniques involving cognitive-attitudinal change (e.g., rational-emotive therapy, problem-solving approaches, and social-psychological attitude change procedures) are also part of the therapist's repertory.

This linking of self-exploration procedures with subsequent efforts to help the client actively change maladaptive patterns goes a step beyond our usual conceptualizations of traditional insight therapy. However, several trends of thought in recent years seem to make this linkage feasible. Some theorists (e.g., Martin, 1977) have raised the question of whether cognitive understanding of one's problems is enough. In essence, these critics suggest that merely knowing the sources and operations of one's anxieties, for example, does not ensure their change or reduction. Coupled with such critiques has been the development of a variety of treatment approaches specifically designed to change disruptive emotional reactions (see Marks, 1978) or maladaptive thought patterns (e.g., Ellis, 1970; Beck, 1976). In light of these advances the marriage between insight procedures and active change techniques that is being proposed here seems to be a reasonable reflection of an emerging trend in the field. This complex and sequenced range of treatments will be described in Chapters 9 and 10.

Therapy Tasks

This brief outline of the multiple stages, decision points, and techniques involved in helping troubled individuals should provide the reader with an appreciation of the scope of the educational requirements to be mastered. To recapitulate, in the proposed overview, the therapist must first acquire the personal skills and sensitivities that permit clients to openly describe and discuss the psychological difficulties for which they seek help. Second, mastery of various assessment techniques must be achieved so that the therapist can more closely evaluate and analyze the factors in the client's life that underlie these problems. Third, the therapist must develop interviewing and judgmental skills by which to assist the client in formulating meaningful and appropriate treatment goals. As a first approximation to a category system by which to conceptualize various possible goals, the goals of *crisis management, behavior change, corrective emotional experience*, and *self-exploration and change* have been proposed. Finally, the broadly trained therapist must master a wide range of treatment techniques along with the judgmental abilities of when to apply them. Again, as an initial attempt to group these techniques into working categories that correspond to the four classes of goals, the following have been suggested: *supportive therapy; behavior modification and self-regulation techniques; relationship therapy;* and *insight and change techniques*.

In coming to the close of this introductory material an important caution needs to be raised. Neither the four sets of goals nor the corresponding therapy approaches should be viewed as representing rigid, mutually exclusive categories. To the contrary, when working with the clinical realities of each individual client, it is entirely possible that combinations of goals may be established. Similarly, when we review the details of each of the therapy approaches in later chapters the reader will note considerable overlap among the procedures. For example, the use of behavioral techniques undoubtedly also involves relationship issues as well as supportive components. Likewise, it is hard to conceive of insight therapy in isolation from the central role played by the relationship between client and therapist. The same kinds of overlap can be detected across all these approaches, and thus they can be more realistically viewed as therapy dimensions rather than inflexible categories. Which of these dimensions is emphasized with a client, thereby forming a conceptual corner-stone for a treatment strategy, depends of course on the needs and specific goals of that client.

As will be noted in subsequent chapters, the approach outlined here is an attempt to cut across theoretical and "school" lines and at the same time present a practical and workable framework within which to study psycho-therapy. Since much of the later material in this book is built upon this "goals-treatments" system, particular attention should be devoted to it. It is outlined in Table 1.1, and it will be presented again in more elaborate form in Chapter 4, where we will take a more detailed look at the uses of intake information and decision making.

Interpersonal Issues

I have stressed in this chapter that each client enters the therapeutic situation with a unique set of expectations, anxieties, and personal sensitivities. The ability of the therapist to become aware of these aspects of the client and to respond in a supportive, empathic, and professional manner is critical for the success of treatment. Therapists who relate to the client primarily as a diagnostic entity, or focus only on the client's problems rather than the whole person, have been found to be relatively unsuccessful (Mitchell, Bozarth, and Krauft, 1977). Similarly, poor outcomes occur with therapists who start out with preconceived ideas about the client's difficulties and therefore do not listen with sensitivity to communications from this special person (Truax and Mitchell, 1971). Problems can extend to the point where the therapist's own psychopathology can have a detrimental effect on a client's adjustment (Bergin and Lambert, 1978; Parloff, Waskow, and Wolfe, 1978).

We are touching here on a host of crucial interpersonal questions that are fundamental to successful therapy. How does one develop a trusting and mutually respecting relationship with a client? Under what interpersonal condi-tions will clients be open and candid in discussing their lives? How can the client's motivation and cooperation in the therapy process be enhanced?

These questions will be dealt with in Chapter 2, along with related professional and ethical issues. These topics will be covered early in the book because they appear to be fundamental to successful treatment, regardless of the therapy approach. Following this basic material, the remaining chapters will review intake procedures, clinical decision making, treatment strategies, and the evaluation of psychotherapy.

UNRESOLVED ISSUES AND RESEARCH QUESTIONS

One of the major tasks facing professionals in the field of psychotherapy is the ability to specify what kind of treatment clients should receive. Large-scale clinics and hospitals as well as individual practitioners encounter a wide range

Table 1.1
A proposed system of treatment goals and corresponding therapy approaches

Goal	Treatment
Crisis management	Supportive therapy
Behavior change	Behavior modification and self-regulation techniques
Corrective emotional experiences	Relationship therapy
Self-exploration and change	Insight therapy

of mental health problems, and ideally, they should be able to function in the following manner:

- Client A, who displays problem type K, should receive treatment program X.

- Client B, who displays problem type L, should receive treatment program Y; and so forth (Kiesler, 1971; Bergin and Lambert, 1978).

As can be imagined, a vast amount of research is required in order to determine the most effective treatments for different types of psychological problems. The research task is doubly complex because a great deal of preliminary work has to be done to clearly describe the specific symptoms and patterns involved in each problem type. In addition, the various treatment programs also have to be detailed as to the particular techniques to be used, their sequencing, and so forth. Finally, in such an immense research endeavor, the specific goals of each treatment need to be indicated with precision, so that clear criteria are established by which to evaluate whether or not treatment objectives have been reached.

As we will see in the remaining chapters, the field is making slow but steady progress in these areas (see Garfield and Bergin, 1978). However, the sort of research required to achieve this level of professionalization is both time-consuming and expensive. Several well-defined problem areas (for example, specific phobias and certain sexual dysfunctions) seem to have been researched enough so that specific treatments can be recommended. However, the great majority of mental health problems are still in a state of limbo, with insufficient empirical data to clearly dictate which goals and treatments will be most appropriate.

In the meantime, practicing therapists are faced with the day-to-day realities of distressed clients. Most therapists undoubtedly wish that they had a research-based manual available indicating the most effective goals and treatments for each client. Such an encyclopedia could be combined with their own sensitivities and judgments about a particular client to tailor a truly effective therapy program. Unfortunately the field is many years away from this state of affairs. Thus practitioners have to rely heavily on personal judgments, informal clinical tradition, and largely unsubstantiated theory to guide their work.

The "goals and treatments" framework outlined in this chapter comes primarily from informal clinical tradition and should be recognized as such. Later in the book, where possible, treatments based on research results will be indicated; for now the reader is faced with the same dilemma facing practicing clinicians: how to make the most effective use of therapeutic theory and tradition, while awaiting the slowly emerging research results.

CHAPTER TWO

PROFESSIONAL, ETHICAL, AND PERSONAL ISSUES

Providing adequate mental health care to the public requires far more than a repertory of therapy techniques. A variety of critical factors are involved in that complex territory between community needs and the delivery of effective services. The mere availability of clinics and hospitals is obviously one such factor. The quality of training of those who staff these facilities is another. The providing of safe and humane treatment depends both on the ethical principles that guide practitioners and on legal safeguards that regulate the mental health agencies themselves. Finally, the personal qualities of therapists play an important role in treatment. Hence, before we proceed to the chapters covering the technical aspects of psychotherapy, it is important that we review these fundamental professional, ethical, legal, and personal issues. All of these issues are related in assuring competent and ethical treatment for all who are in need.

THE DELIVERY OF MENTAL HEALTH SERVICES

Many factors determine the availability of treatment to the public. The geographical location of mental health facilities, the cost of treatment, and the length of waiting lists are some obvious issues. More subtle features also seem to play a role in whether or not clients can avail themselves of services. Such intangibles as feeling welcomed by an agency and being able to understand the nature of the services also affect clients' decisions to seek treatment. A growing body of evidence suggests that improvements are needed in these areas (Korchin, 1980; Lorion, 1978), and those in mental health professions continue to seek better and more efficient ways to serve the public. Many of the issues are controversial and are as yet unresolved, and students entering the field should be aware of the emerging trends.

To put the issues in perspective, let us first review some of the history of providing mental health services. Fifty years ago the principal mode of receiving psychotherapy was through private practice clinicians or through a few charitable and private clinics. Relatively few individuals other than the affluent received psychological care. After World War II, with the advent of Veterans Administration hospitals, both inpatient and outpatient mental health services became available to disabled service personnel through this government agency. The postwar years also saw a gradual rise in state- and community-sponsored clinics—usually as adjuncts of large hospital complexes. A major expansion of community services occurred in the 1960s, when, with the passage of the Community Mental Health Centers Act of 1963, the federal government committed itself to supporting the concept of local and neighborhood clinics as the primary means of providing services. Funds to build and staff such centers were aimed at providing quality mental health care for all who needed it.

The aims of the Community Mental Health Centers Act, however, did not seem to be fulfilled by any appreciable degree in the ensuing years. The locations of public clinics, which were largely determined by the availability of mental health personnel, were a major problem. As reported by Albee (1977), over half of all the psychiatric clinics in the nation were in the northeastern states. Furthermore, out of some 2000 surveyed clinics, only 56 were found in rural areas. And among the few that served children, only 4 percent were found in predominantly rural states (even though one-third of all children live in these states).

Problems regarding the uneven delivery of services seem to occur even in geographical areas where mental health facilities are located. Several large-scale surveys of both private and public clinics indicate rather marked variations in the percentage of clients who are accepted for treatment (Lorenzen, 1967; Kadushin, 1969). Estimates of acceptance rates vary between 20 and 85 percent, depending on the nature of the clinic. Numerous other surveys, summarized by Garfield (1971, 1978) also indicate that approximately 40 percent of clients who actually begin treatment drop out of therapy before the sixth session, even though treatment is judged not to be complete. A closer inspection of these data points to the fact that the variables of social class, educational level, and race are important in determining acceptance and premature dropping out. In general terms these research results suggest that clients at the lower end of the socioeconomic and educational scales and those who are black are least likely to be accepted for individual psychotherapy, and if accepted, most likely to terminate treatment early in the process (Garfield, 1978; Lorion, 1978; Korchin, 1980).

Concerns with these problems has led, in the last decade, to serious consideration of both private and public health insurance plans. These essentially involve prepayment of fees, either through insurance premiums paid by the individual, employers, or unions, or through taxes for a national health program. As a member of such a plan, an individual in need of mental health services could ostensibly receive help from a therapist (in private practice or in an agency), who in turn would be reimbursed for these services by the insurer (a private company or a government agency). Proponents of this approach (e.g., Cummings, 1977) argue that it would solve many of the problems of the past and make professional treatment more generally available. Critics of this approach (e.g., Albee, 1977) suggest that the problem of unfair distribution of services to the poor would not be solved and indeed might even be made worse since economically disadvantaged individuals may not avail themselves of treatment regardless of the source of payment.

Both camps in this controversy agree, however, that there are numerous other problems that insurance-based programs have highlighted. Drawing from the experiences of several private or state insurance plans already in existence (e.g., the Kaiser-Permanente Health Plan and California's Medi-Cal Program), these problems can be outlined under four categories. A review of these issues may be instructive because in many ways they seem to represent general problems faced by the profession that are likely to command great attention in the next few years (McSweeny, 1977).

1. *The program needs to be cost-effective.* Experience with private insurance plans indicates that providing unlimited and unrestricted therapy services would soon bankrupt any program. It is generally agreed that psychotherapy for "recreational" or vague "personal growth" reasons should be excluded from coverage. Rather, it is argued, only clients with specific and clearly defined problems that hamper their roles as breadwinners, parents, spouses, and so on, should receive insurable treatment. Such restrictions place many therapists in a dilemma, for there is a large gray area of disorders that are left in limbo. Such problems as mild to moderate depression or anxiety states, which do not result in loss of work, may be judged to be inappropriate for coverage. Similarly, many varieties of interpersonal problems may be too subtle or disguised to warrant insurability. Along similar lines, clients who require long-term contact with a therapist (for example, a disturbed, borderline-psychotic individual who needs frequent supportive sessions) place a financial strain on insurance programs.

Concerns about cost-effectiveness also create pressures toward providing relatively brief, symptom-oriented therapy. Extended numbers of sessions used to uncover hidden problem areas would be frowned upon by the accountants in such programs. Intensive time spent trying to establish a relationship with an alienated, predelinquent adolescent might also be viewed as too financially burdensome to the system.

The implications of cost factors in public or private mental health programs present a major challenge to therapists. To a large extent it is the responsibility of therapists themselves to help administrators and legislators in formulating policy. Such policy obviously has to take into account the financial aspects of the program; however, the helping professions have to take the lead in safeguarding the public's access to appropriate coverage and treatment. A major component of this challenge will be the necessity for the development of more specific and definable diagnostic classifications and methods of treatment. This task, it appears, will be a major focus of work in the next ten years.

2. *Treatments have to be demonstrated as effective.* Setting up a broadly based insurance program, whether public or private, carries with it the responsibility of consumer protection. In essence, this means that in order for a therapist to be reimbursed for services rendered there has to be some kind of monitoring to show that the treatment was professionally acceptable and effective.

There are many issues embedded in this priniciple. Treatments available within the program have to be specified with reasonable clarity. In addition, research justification has to be provided that indicates which type of treatment is appropriate for the various disorders that are insured. Finally, procedures for monitoring and evaluating treatment effectiveness have to be described and implemented. Here again, as we saw earlier, the profession has quite a long way to go before these tasks can be accomplished in any complete fashion.

3. *The credentials of service providers have to be established.* Therapists and their professional organizations should have a major voice in determining the appropriate training and experience requirements for practitioners within the profession. This sort of credentialing will be important in determining who will be eligible therapists within a public or private health program, that is, who will be eligible for reimbursement for services to insured clients. Because of the diversity of professions within the mental health realm (e.g., social work, clinical psychology, psychiatry, etc.) and the differences in training required for these professions (ranging all the way from a paraprofessional certificate to a Ph.D. or M.D.), there will undoubtedly be considerable controversy in this area should any large-scale health plan be instituted. A great deal of cooperative work will be required among the various professional organizations to clearly specify training requirements, the particular skills expected, and the roles to be played by mental health workers from the various disciplines.

4. *Treatment should be made available and attractive to all who need services.* This feature of mental health programs, of course, addresses the problem of currently underserved segments of our population. As we saw earlier, this serious issue will not be solved easily. Even where treatment facilities are readily available, much evidence indicates that many disadvantaged individuals do not utilize the services. It also means that various types of incentive programs that will attract clinicians to rural and other underserved areas will have to be tried and evaluated. In sum, major research and program development efforts will be required over the next decade to provide effective and attractive treatment approaches for the disadvantaged.

Without demonstrable improvement in this area Albee's contention that tax-supported mental health plans will be discriminatory (1977) probably remains true.

We can see in all these points a sort of encapsulation of many of the main problems facing the mental health field in general today. The prospects of large-scale federal or private insurance programs seem to be hastening work on these issues. Aside from the specific treatment questions involved, these developments are also prompting renewed interest in the area of evaluation and research design. The American Psychological Association, for example, has established a task force of prominent researchers whose mission is to consider all aspects of how a national health program would be monitored and evaluated. Such a task will call for many detailed and innovative techniques for measuring and assessing treatments, therapists, administrative procedures, the distribution of services and their cost-effectiveness, the response of the public, and so forth—in effect, evaluation of an immensely complex public health program. At the heart of this task is the necessity to build into the program an ongoing system of measurement and evaluation so that its effectiveness can be continuously monitored and improved.

PROFESSIONAL TRAINING

We saw in the previous section that one of the main concerns facing the mental health professions is making trained practitioners available to the public. In an area where several disciplines (psychiatry, psychology, social work, guidance and counseling, etc.) converge, there is some inevitable competition and conflict as to the roles and functions of each. Clarifying these roles will take continued analysis and negotiation among the professional organizations involved. Eventually it is hoped that responsible licensing and certification laws pertaining to each group will result in enhanced effectiveness in providing services.

Common to all the mental health professions is the basic value of assuming responsibility for the well-being of another person. A heart surgeon in the midst of a transplant operation literally holds life and death in his or her hands. Detailed knowledge of anatomy and surgical procedure as well as practiced physical skills are required before the physician can assume responsibility for another's life. Taking on the responsibility of providing psychological help may carry the same awesome burden. Although perhaps not with the same drama and immediacy of the surgical amphitheater, psychotherapy involves the possibilities of more subtle and long-term tragedies. Improper or casually administered therapy that results in years of incarceration in the back wards of a custodial hospital, or drives the addict to overdose, or relegates a shy client to a lifetime of reclusiveness and alienation are life and death issues that equal those facing the surgeon. In this context then, let us review the formal training requirements for the various professions involved in providing psychological help.

Psychiatry

A psychiatrist has completed medical school and a general medical internship. After receiving the M.D. an individual undergoes two or three years of specialized training in a *psychiatric residency*, which involves closely supervised work in diagnosis, psychotherapy, and the various somatic therapies (e.g., drug therapy), in addition to classwork and seminars. Following this period of training, the psychiatrist is eligible to take board examinations in psychiatry, which are administered by the state in which he or she will practice. Upon passing these exams, the tile psychiatrist can be appropriately claimed. The combination of intensive medical and therapy training, involving some six to eight years of postgraduate education, obviously places the psychiatrist in a unique role to treat both the psychological and physical aspects of mental illness.

Clinical Psychology

Clinical psychology involves a Ph.D. in psychology, with specialization in the clinical area. A one-year internship in a training facility approved by the American Psychological Association is also a requirement for this specialty. Most Ph.D. programs in clinical psychology require four to five years beyond the bachelor's degree and adopt what has been termed the *scientist-practitioner model* of training. The scientific emphasis is reflected in extensive course work in all of the basic areas of psychology (learning theory, developmental, physiological, social, personality, etc.) and extensive preparation in measurement theory, research design, and statistics. This phase of the Ph.D. training culminates in the doctoral dissertation, an original piece of research aimed at advancing the borders of science in this area. The practitioner side of the training encompasses extensive course work on psychological assessment, psychotherapy, and professional-ethical aspects of clinical work. Included here is also supervised practice in training clinics and hospitals, which is capped with a full-time internship toward the end of the Ph.D. program. Most states require an examination in clinical psychology before an individual who has received a Ph.D. is certified or licensed to practice independently.

As with psychiatry, clinical psychology also involves a special combination of skills, but with a thrust in a different direction. By virtue of their training, clinical psychologists not only are able to engage in the practice of assessment and therapy, but they also are in a position to provide research-based advancement of the field as a science. Indeed, as we shall see in later chapters, some of the most significant breakthroughs in the field of mental health over the past several decades have been direct outgrowths of basic psychological research.

Social Work

If one were to survey community mental health clinics, it would very likely be found that a sizable proportion of day-to-day therapeutic contact with clients is performed by social workers. The usual postgraduate degree in this specialty is the Master of Social Work (MSW), although some who are oriented towards university teaching go on for the Ph.D. The MSW is awarded after a two- to three-year period of graduate training involving course work on individual, group, and family therapy, the use of community social services, and the role of family and culture in personal development — in short, a wholistic approach to the study of the individual. A considerable part of this training involves supervised field experience in mental health clinics, hospitals, and other community agencies.

Guidance and Counseling

The field of guidance and counseling has undergone some interesting changes over the past twenty years. Several decades ago, persons with an Ed.D. degree in this area were primarily trained to provide educational and vocational counseling in school settings. A large part of such positions involved the administration of aptitude and vocational interest tests and counseling students concerning appropriate academic programs and careers. These important though limited functions have broadened considerably over the past twenty years to include counseling for psychological and social problems, individual and group therapy experiences designed to enhance personal growth, and rehabilitation counseling for clients who are emerging from relatively severe psychological disabilities. Currently these functions are carried out not only within school systems but also in such diverse settings as psychiatric hospitals, community agencies, halfway houses for former hospitalized clients, drug rehabilitation centers, and so forth.

Educational requirements for the Ed.D. (or Ph.D.) in guidance and counseling have broadened in keeping with these multiple roles. Considerable emphasis is still placed on measurement theory, assessment procedures, imparting vocational and academic information, educational organization and administration, and career development. In addition, theories and techniques of individual therapy, group processes, and rehabilitation procedures are important facets of training. As part of such four- to five-year graduate programs, students also receive considerable amounts of supervised field experience and must conduct an original piece of research for the doctoral dissertation.

Psychoanalysis

The term psychoanalyst seems to be frequently misunderstood among the general public. This is probably because the term *psychoanalyst* is often confused with the general term *psychotherapist* and because a term such as *psychoanalytic therapy* refers to a general theoretical approach to psychotherapy rather than a formal title. In actuality, a psychoanalyst is an individual who has completed training as a psychiatrist, clinical psychologist, or social worker, and who engages in further training in an accepted *psychoanalytic institute*. Such training can typically involve from two to five years of intensive education, which includes both formal course work and undergoing personal psychoanalysis. This personal therapy, conducted by a training analyst at the institute, can involve two to five sessions per week extending over several years. During this extensive therapy, which is largely insight oriented, the analyst-in-training gains a remarkably detailed and in-depth personal knowledge regarding basic motivational and emotional systems, interpersonal relations, and nuances of one's developmental history. Upon completion of the course work and personal analysis, the individual can be appropriately called a psychoanalyst.

This very extended and expensive training results, of course, in acknowledged expertise in self-exploration therapy — a status that commands ample prestige and fees. The fact that there are relatively few psychoanalysts, plus the expense of such treatment, has prompted some critics to minimize their importance and to portray psychoanalysis as the therapy for the rich. Such a one-sided evaluation, however, seems to overlook many of the important contributions made by psychoanalysts with regard to personality theory and therapy techniques.

Paraprofessional Training

Three major factors that have prompted intense interest in subdoctoral education in the mental health field have come to light over the past fifteen years. First, large-scale survey research has shown that considerable numbers of people who have psychological difficulties do not seek help from professional therapists. Rather, they principally consult clergymen, family doctors, or teachers, that is, individuals who usually are cognizant of psychological issues but who generally have had little training in psychotherapy. Of importance here is the finding that these clients report a level of satisfaction with these services that is comparable to that reported by those who go to professional therapists (Garfield, 1978). Second, a related line of research has investigated the effectiveness of nonprofessionals who have undergone short, intensive periods of training before assuming a therapeutic job. Here again the findings suggest that students, housewives, and people generally interested in helping others perform consistently and effectively in therapeutic roles (Cowen, 1973). An important qualification in these results however, is the observation that effective therapists, regardless of background or training, have personal qualities of warmth and sensitivity — a finding that will be discussed more fully below. Third, another factor of importance has been the growing national concern with the delivery of health services to the public. Recognizing that medical schools and graduate programs are not turning out sufficient doctoral-level practitioners, numerous areas in the health field have developed training at the technical level to fill this need.

In the area of mental health such paraprofessional roles encompass a wide range of activities. A partial list would include youth counselors (Big Brother or Big Sister programs), emergency or crisis workers attached to community clinics, telephone counselors on "hot line" facilities, counselors in drug and alcohol units, psychological technicians administering therapy programs in the wards of psychiatric hospitals, and applied behavioral specialists, working under physicians' supervision, who deal with behavioral-emotional components of medical illness.

This entire trend of paraprofessionalism is an integral part of a *team* approach to mental health services. An entire program of therapy, let us say, to a group of former alcoholics in a community outpatient clinic might involve: (1) a consultant psychiatrist who coordinates the entire treatment process and is also directly responsible for medical issues with each client; (2) a clinical psychologist whose concerns are psychological assessment and super-vision of individual psychotherapy; (3) a social worker who works with the families of the clients, as well as their employers; (4) a local minister with training in group work who participates in clients' weekly Alcoholics Anony-mous meetings; and (5) several paraprofessionals who have individual therapy sessions with each client on a weekly basis to discuss current adjustment problems and how best to cope with them, and to carry out longer range treatment procedures aimed at controlling drinking. As can be imagined, a closely coordinated and well-planned team effort is required for such a complex enterprise.

Emerging Training Methods

One of the more exciting prospects in the field is the development of research-based programs for the training of therapists. This area, reviewed by Matarazzo (1978), now appears to have progressed to the point where some practical applications can be made in training at both the paraprofessional and graduate levels of education (e.g., Truax and Carkhuff, 1976; Ivey, 1971; Glowgower and Sloop, 1976). Although many of these programs have been developed from different theoretical perspectives, they seem to share a common core of procedures: (1) After obtaining theoretical, classroom knowledge about ther-apy, students are exposed to experienced clinicians who demonstrate the actual treatment procedures to be learned. (2) Following this phase of "modeling," student therapists practice the techniques in situations where client behaviors are "role played" by the training assistants. (3) During these practice sessions, corrective feedback is provided, areas of personal discomfort or anxiety are discussed, "listening" skills are enhanced, and of course, therapeutic interventions are practiced and refined. (4) After extensive role-playing experience, students are gradually phased in as cotherapists with ongoing cases, where at first they serve principally as observers of an experienced clinician. As they adapt to the technical and emotional demands of actual therapy, the students gradually assume a greater role in the process. (5) When students enter the last phase of training, that is, working alone with a client, they are carefully observed (through a one-way screen) by the supervisor. Feedback is thereby available in an immediate fashion at the close of the session. (6) Such training programs have incorporated several technological advances that seem to strengthen their effectiveness. Video recording allows students to see rather dramatically their behaviors and reactions during treatment sessions—responses that they might otherwise be unaware of because of defensiveness or lack of attention. A "bug in the ear" device (similar to a hearing aid) is also a creative adjunct to training, in that supervisors from an adjoining viewing room can communicate instructions and feedback to the student while a therapy session is taking place.

As indicated earlier, such developments as these in the area of training appear to be promising, and the preliminary research results on their effectiveness are positive. However, as suggested by Matarazzo (1978), it is clear that extensive research and creative energies need to be devoted to this traditionally underexplored topic.

ETHICS

Ethical considerations are intimately related to training and professional issues. A clinician may be well trained technically and may make his or her services equitably available to the public, but if these services are provided in an exploitative or insensitive fashion the possibility for doing considerable harm to clients exists. It is important therefore that we review some of the principal ethical and legal aspects of mental health care in this early portion of the book.

The psychotherapy relationship is one of the most private ones an individual is likely to experience. This privacy is a two-edged sword. On the one hand, it permits a nonpublic setting in which a client can safely explore and openly work on problems. On the other hand, the very privacy of the relationship places the client in an extremely vulnerable position relative to the therapist. The usual safeguards and restraints imposed on public relationships are for the most part minimized in the session-to-session behavior of the therapist. This vulnerability is compounded by the usual circumstance of the therapist being viewed as an expert, or being depended upon by the client. Under these conditions then, we can ask the rather blunt question, "What prevents the therapist from taking advantage?" The answer of course is the ethical principles by which the therapist conducts his or her practice and governs the relationship with clients.

A number of years ago the American Psychological Association set up a standing committee on ethics, which was charged with the task of developing a code of standards for psychologists. The approach and guidelines developed by this group seems to be a reasonable vehicle for our general discussion of ethics. Rather than simply trying to decide on an abstract set of principles, this committee requested that psychologists from all areas of the profession submit examples of actual incidents involving ethics, with indications of how each ethical dilemma was resolved. In this way, the committee acquired a grasp of "real-life" issues in the daily working lives of practitioners. By collating and organizing these incidents into categories, the committee was able to develop a set of principles that had generality as well as relevance. Since this is a standing committee on ethics, its work continues in evaluating new and contemporary issues as they arise in a changing culture. Thus new principles and standards are continuously evolving, and they are periodically reviewed in professional journals and at meetings.

The principles that are relevant to psychotherapy were very nicely summarized by Bordin (1955). He approached the issue by suggesting that the therapist has four areas of ethical responsibility: to the client; to the agency that employs the therapist; to the profession; and to the community. In the following sections, each area of responsibility will be briefly reviewed, along with examples of some of the more frequent problems that occur.

Responsibilities to the Client

The major areas of concern here pertain to three general issues. These can be described as (1) maintaining a professional therapeutic relationship with the client, (2) problems of confidentiality, and (3) utilizing appropriate therapy procedures for which the therapist has been trained. Perhaps an example of each issue, involving some subtle aspects, will convey the processes by which ethical problems develop and will at the same time make discussion of more blatant examples unnecessary. In many ways responsibilities to the client represent the most complex ethical issues; hence most emphasis will be placed on this area.

Therapist X has a private practice that has been reasonably successful, and he enjoys a good reputation in the community. His private life, however, is not so successful. The focal point of his problems involves a marriage filled with strife—constant bickering and mutual recriminations with a wife who he perceives to be chronically hostile and nagging. These marital problems have been going on for years, and neither partner seems able or motivated to improve the relationship.

Now this therapist begins work with a client who has entered therapy to seek help for a drinking problem. Employing appropriate techniques, both therapist and client work hard, over numerous sessions, in exploring the alcoholism problem, and they are coming to the point where the client is beginning to get control over it. At this point the client spends part of one session describing how his wife has been surly and obnoxious over a period of years—even admitting that this is understandable in view of his drinking. Some vague but strong emotional stirrings are prompted within the therapist. He doesn't fully tune in on the last part of the client's statement. What strikes him emotionally is the description of the obnoxious wife. The therapist feels drawn toward having the client discuss his marriage more fully. Moreover, without fully realizing it, each time the client talks negatively about his wife, the therapist seems to convey strong interest and support—in effect, subtly guiding the patient to progressively stronger negative descriptions. The therapist rationalizes his own behavior by telling himself that exploring the client's marital difficulties will help clear up the drinking problem, while at the same time the therapist fails to recognize his own vicarious satisfaction at having the client belabor his wife. This process extends over numerous sessions, with the client becoming progressively more convinced of the hopelessness of his marriage. During this same period, productive work on the alcoholic difficulties has declined dramatically. Several months later the client decides to stop therapy, having concluded that his drinking problem is insoluble, and is also considerably more cynical and pessimistic about his marriage.

The destructive behavior of therapist X would probably never form the basis for a malpractice suit; indeed, neither therapist nor client could even clearly specify what went wrong with the treatment. And yet this therapist's behavior was unethical. He had lost his *objectivity*, allowing his own needs, rather than those of the client, to dictate the course of therapy. Even more insidious is the fact that the therapist indirectly enmeshed the client in his own unresolved difficulties, much to the detriment of the client's overall adjustment. In sum, he failed to maintain a professional, objective relationship with his client.

The case of therapist Y exemplifies ethical issues regarding confidentiality. Therapist Y is a social worker employed in a community clinic in a state that does not have a privileged communication law protecting the confidences of social workers' clients. This therapist treated a middle-aged housewife for almost a year and had considerable success in clarifying problems of low self-esteem, indecisiveness, and guilt surrounding some indiscretions earlier in her marriage.

A year after therapy was concluded, the client is in the midst of divorce proceedings that involve a strenuous court battle with her husband over custody of their child. The husband's attorney, knowing of the wife's previous therapy, has the court issue a subpoena to have the therapist testify. The intent of the attorney is to elicit information damaging to the wife's case.

The therapist is in a potential dilemma. On one hand, the ethics of preserving the client's confidences are strongly felt. On the other hand, the presiding judge, adhering to the letter of the law in this state, may rule that the information is pertinent and thereby require the therapist to testify. Under these circumstances refusal to testify, even on ethical grounds, may lead to a contempt of court citation; attempts to testify with less than complete candor run the risk of perjury.

On the surface the conflict resolves itself into a decision to follow either one's own ethical dictates or the judge's interpretation of legal statutes—a decision that may have long-term professional and personal implications for the therapist. There are, however, several more complex professional issues that underlie this incident. First, it could be argued that the therapist, being aware of the laws governing confidentiality, should have informed the client at the beginning of therapy as to possible conflicts in this area. So forewarned, the client could have exercised her own judgment as to appropriate disclosures in therapy—at the same time recognizing that important areas of therapy may thereby be closed. The ethical principle embedded here is that the client should not be left with even the implicit assumption that everything is confidential when in fact that may not be true. The second issue involved in this illustration bears on professional tactics regarding confidentiality. Although such specific incidents as therapist Y's court appearance are occasionally unavoidable, fighting the battle to protect privacy can hardly be won on a case-by-case basis. Therapists' efforts in this cause are probably better directed through their professional society, which can work with state legislatures for the enactment of fair and protective laws.

Therapist Z illustrates a third ethical responsibility to the client, that of using appropriate techniques. Problems arise in this area rarely on the basis of a therapist maliciously employing indefensible treatments, but rather as a result of unrecognized deviations from acceptable procedures and a faulty level of professionalism. Dr. Z is a clinical psychologist who was a good graduate student and psychology intern. He obtained the Ph.D., having become skilled in a wide range of standard therapy techniques and well able to apply them correctly to different types of clients. Upon graduation he decided to return to the small town in which he was raised in order to provide mental health services to this isolated area. As it turns out he is the only mental health professional in a wide geographical region, and his services are much needed.

Over the years his practice thrives to the point where he is too busy to attend professional meetings or keep up with the current writings in his area. His professional isolation is exaggerated by the fact that there are no other mental health workers with whom he can consult or exchange views. Under these conditions his techniques undergo very minor changes, as he develops his own "personalized style" of therapy. These deviations are subtle enough so that Dr. Z does not recognize them, nor is there anyone else available to provide corrective feedback.

If we project this slow drift over ten years we now find Dr. Z using some remarkably unusual treatment procedures, still unaware of their deviancy. At this point tragedy occurs. One of his clients, who had been depressed for some time without improvement, commits suicide. The client's family, having wondered about some of the techniques which the client had described to them, decide to sue Dr. Z for malpractice. Having departed from professionally acceptable therapeutic procedures, he is in an ethically and legally indefensible position.

To summarize this section, we have encountered several ethical problems that occur with some frequency with regard to clients. Note that in each of the examples, the problems did not arise because of obvious or purposeful transgressions by the therapist, although these do occur occasionally. As will happen, difficulties came about because the therapists failed to maintain first-rate professionalism. Failure at the arduous tasks of keeping up with current developments in the field, becoming knowledgeable of the laws pertaining to mental health practice, and perhaps fundamentally, maintaining an awareness of one's own inner stresses and conflicts frequently seem to be at the roots of these problems.

Responsibilities to the Employing Agency

In this brief section we shall review ethical problems that usually involve divided loyalties. Therapists have obligations to both their clients and to the agency for which they work, and at times these responsibilities come into conflict.

Consider the situation of the twenty-year-old paraprofessional who accepts a job with a municipal youth services agency in a large city. His job is vaguely described to him as going into a tough neighborhood, establishing a liaison with a particular gang of juveniles, and then working with these young people to "keep things cool." The paraprofessional interprets his function as a therapeutic one, with the juveniles as his clients. After considerable time and effort, he has started to make some inroads. A considerable number of the thirteen- to fifteen-year-olds in the group are beginning to relate to him as someone who might be trusted and with whom they can openly discuss conflicts involving school, family, drugs, crime, and so on. A substantial proportion of the older gang members, however, still view him with suspicion and occasional hostility.

During the summer months, the crime rate in the neighborhood increases considerably, with several elderly victims of robbery being seriously hurt. The city government decides that all agencies connected with the neighborhood will have to crack down hard to suppress the crime wave. This directive includes the youth services agency. Our paraprofessional is therefore told that he is to supply the agency director with a list of names of all the "hard-core" cases among these juveniles—the implication being that they will be generally questioned and watched by the neighborhood police.

The ethical conflict is a difficult one. Responsibilities to the neighborhood, protecting potential victims, and cooperating with legitimate police functions compete with the budding therapeutic role being established with the young people. If the list is provided there is a good chance that the relationship with the juveniles will be destroyed. If the request is refused, police work may be impeded, others may be victimized, and the youth worker's job may be in jeopardy.

The personal ethical decision faced by the paraprofessional here is agonizing and risky. Obviously, open and frank discussion of the implications of either choice with agency supervisors is important. It should be pointed out, however, that a major part of the dilemma can be attributed to the vague assignment that was given to the youth worker to begin with. Had it been clearly specified that the paramount aspect of the job was to assume a therapeutic role with the juveniles, the worker could reasonably assume (in the absence of knowledge of a specific crime) that privacy should be maintained. If the original job assignment was to uncover criminal activities, the decision would also be relatively clear. The general point here is that *prior* to taking a position that potentially involves such conflict, the roles, responsibilities, and ground rules governing the therapist should be clearly specified and agreed upon.

Responsibilities to the Profession

The practice of psychotherapy grows out of a fundamental tradition of providing service to others. The various professions involved in this enterprise should not have to advertise this as an image. Rather, it should be reflected at the very core of the daily lives and work of its practitioners. Ethical responsibilities to the profession therefore involve behaviors that pertain to this basic set of values.

Problems in this area frequently involve two general issues: personal notoriety of a negative sort and therapists' attempts to increase their income by means that reflect poorly on the profession as a whole. The latter area perhaps requires some elaboration and example. A therapist is attempting to get a private practice established in a community. Discrete public announcement and a notice sent to potential referral sources are accepted means informing others of one's practice. Half-page advertisements in newspapers or television commercials portray the profession with a huckster image that runs counter to the service tradition and are clearly unethical.

Perhaps more insidious is the practitioner who, in an attempt to solicit clients, gives "scare talks" to PTA groups hoping that some nervous parents will bring in their children for consultation. Equally unethical is the therapist who communicates to several major referral sources that he or she is qualified to treat a wide range of client problems, when in fact some maladies are beyond his or her competencies. Without belaboring this point, then, no one would argue with the practitioner who receives a fair salary or fees in keeping with training and skills; however, a serious breach of ethics occurs with attempts to break these boundaries.

Responsibilities to the Community

Most people would agree that one's *ultimate* responsibility is to the community. However, this general ethical statement can have many meanings. Helping a disturbed individual become a valued, productive member of the community is a large part of this responsibility. Contributing one's special skills for the betterment of the community is expected of all good citizens. Protecting the general population from social or personal dangers is also everyone's responsibility. Special ethical problems arise, however, when these various ethics come into occasional conflict. If, as part of therapy, one gains knowledge of felonious behavior on the part of the client, can this be ethically kept private? By the same token, if one becomes aware of unethical and injurious practices by a colleague, can the professional look the other way? Most would agree that the ethical individual cannot passively ignore such problems. Knowledge on the part of a therapist that a client represents a "clear and present danger" to others requires (legally and ethically) that the proper community agency be involved in the case, be this the police, the courts, or a child welfare agency. Similarly, knowledge that a colleague is, for example, taking sexual advantage of clients, as will occasionally happen in the profession (see Holroyd and Brodsky, 1977), usually calls for action by professional ethics committees. Depending on the specifics of each situation, active and appropriate measures to protect the community are an integral part of therapists' ethical standards.

In summary, Table 2.1 presents an outline of the major areas of ethical responsibility, along with a listing of problems that are frequently encountered.

LEGAL TRENDS IN MENTAL HEALTH CARE

In addition to knowing the ethical issues involved in providing treatment, students should be aware of the broad legal developments in recent years affecting mental health care. These trends occur largely through the vehicle of court decisions and for the most part pertain to individuals who are confined to institutions. The issues on which courts have rendered decisions usually involve questions in which treatment methods and institutional policies are seen to come into conflict with clients' civil liberties.

We can begin by reviewing several court actions that have had rather widespread effects on mental health institutions. First, an individual who is in enforced hospitalization because of mental illness has a *right to treatment* that is aimed at improving mental health and returning the client to the community (*Rouse* v. *Cameron*). In this very important decision the courts in effect ruled that patients could no longer be confined in hospitals simply for custodial purposes, but that the institution had to provide reasonable treatment programs for their clientele. Of course, the court could not dictate what "reasonable" or effective treatments might be; however, the decision was intended to reorient many institutions from a custodial to a treatment mission. In a related decision

Table 2.1
Summary of ethical responsibilities

Area of responsibility	Specific issues
To the client	Confidentiality; use of standard techniques; updating competencies; maintaining professional contacts; maintaining objectivity
To the employing agency	Divided allegiance between welfare of client vs. agency; possible confidentiality conflicts; specifying role and responsibilities
To the profession	Maintaining high standards of personal and professional conduct; promoting dignified image of the profession; using acceptable methods to inform public of one's services
To the community	Safeguarding the welfare of the public; possible conflicts regarding confidentiality; arranging for appropriate control over potentially dangerous clients

(*Lake* v. *Cameron*), the courts also enunciated the principle that an individual who requires confinement (for the protection of self or society) should receive the "least restrictive alternative" consistent with safety and personal liberty. Finally, at this general level, courts have also put forth the principle of *informed consent*, which in effect states that clients (or a responsible guardian) have the right to make decisions regarding the acceptability of a proposed treatment (*New York City Health and Hospital Corporation* v. *Stein*; *Haynes* v. *Harris*; *Kaimowitz* v. *Michigan Department of Mental Health*). The notion of informed consent involves several components. First, the individual giving consent must be capable of making a careful, rational decision and must have the competence to weigh the various alternatives that are presented. Second, the consent must be given in the light of full knowledge of the treatment procedures involved, the likelihood of success, the risks, and the availability of other treatments. Finally, the decision to accept treatment must be a free one, without direct or indirect coercion entering in.

Beyond the general principles espoused thus far, the courts have also ruled on a number of more specific treatment issues and institutional procedures. To put these in some perspective, let us first review the treatments themselves. Many mental hospitals, in efforts to rehabilitate patients (particularly chronic, long-term patients) have had these individuals engage in hospital work. Such jobs within the institution could involve custodial tasks, clerical work, assisting the nursing staff, helping to run the library, and so forth. As part of such programs, institutions frequently "paid" for the work with hospital scrip or "tokens" that could be used by patients to purchase various amenities and privileges in the PX, cafeteria, and wards.

The purposes of such programs were, of course, to teach clients money management, to motivate more adjustive behavior, and to prepare the client for eventual independent living outside the hospital. Such a "token economy" system, however, also involves the withholding of amenities until they are, in effect, earned by the client. A central ethical-legal issue in this realm involves the definition of the term *amenities*.

Many treatment programs have used such "privileges" as private rooms, grounds or PX privileges, recreational activities, food treats, and so on, as the amenities to be earned. The restriction of such facilities has raised the question of which of them represent basic rights of patients versus which are privileges that can be properly withheld. In an important decision pertaining to hospitalized psychiatric patients and the mentally retarded (*Wyatt* v. *Stickney*) the courts ruled that institutionalized individuals have inherent rights to comfortable sleeping quarters, healthy meals, access to the out-of-doors, visitors, religious services, and a number of similar basic services. The implications for treatment programs that involve the withholding of amenities are quite definite. Careful selection of those that are clearly privileges and not basic rights is required of such programs. While therapists therefore have to give up the use of many powerful inducements as tools in fostering productive behaviors, the courts have argued that this loss is counterbalanced by the protection of fundamental rights of institutionalized clients.

The *Wyatt* v. *Stickney* decision also bears upon another issue in treatments involving hospital work. The court ruled that such hospital work may also be of benefit to employees, and therefore the staff could well be in a *conflict of interest* between meeting institutional needs as opposed to producing therapeutic benefits for the client. As in any complex organization, there is a risk of exploitation under these conditions. The court ruling bears on this issue by stating that patients should be paid wages for hospital work even though therapeutic effects are apparent and that other amenities, such as institutional privileges, could not be based on the work performed. The implications of this decision are important in that treatments involving the development of productive vocational behaviors must be carefully arranged to be independent of institutional maintenance or to incorporate a pay scale commensurate with clients' work.

Treatments Involving Aversive Procedures

Perhaps no other area of therapy is more controversial on legal-ethical grounds than the use of punishing electric shock, nausea-producing drugs, or isolation. Treatments using such methods have been used with some success with clients suffering from alcoholism and sexual deviations. Such clients are usually able to give informed consent and are therefore willing to undergo the aversive procedures in order to reduce these undesirable behavior patterns. Problems arise, however, when electric shock treatments or drugs are used as punishers to suppress maladaptive behaviors with incompetent or incarcerated individuals where informed consent may not be reasonably obtained. In some instances such stimuli have been utilized in attempts to curb severely self-destructive behaviors in mental retardates or strong aggression among prison inmates. The courts have placed stringent restrictions in such cases, including requirements for a thorough investigation of alternative treatment modes, used only as a "last resort" intervention to prevent serious physical injury, the obtaining of informed consent by client or relative, close medical supervision, approval by human rights committees, and so forth. Considering the occasional abuses in this area that come to light, such legal restrictions seem to be timely and judicious (see Friedman, 1975).

Institutional Safeguards

Espousing general principles and the rendering of court decisions does not guarantee ethical and judicious practice on a day-to-day basis in institutions, clinics, and private consulting rooms. Unfortunately, even the best-intentioned therapists at times grow impatient, become overzealous, or exercise faulty judgment. Some mechanisms for regulating treatment programs so as to protect clients' civil liberties on a regular basis have therefore been recommended (Friedman, 1975). These can be viewed as a sort of first line of defense in avoiding abuses. First is the development and publication of clear guidelines based on both psychological and ethical principles for the administration of treatment programs. These guidelines need to be specific, well-exemplified, and tailored to the particular clientele, therapeutic approach, and type of setting in which they will be applied. Second, staff at all levels should undergo thorough training and frequent updating on the guidelines, with an emphasis on the practical, everyday ramifications of these standards. Third, dedicated review committees should be instituted, composed of practitioners, civil libertarians, and concerned laypeople, who can continuously monitor, evaluate, and guide treatment programs through the sometimes thorny patch of providing both effective and principled therapy.

THERAPIST PERSONALITY

The topics dealt with in this chapter pertaining to the availability of services, consumer protection, training, ethics, and legal safeguards seem to form a common core of issues that are fundamental to providing competent and humane treatment to the public. We need to review one last area in this regard, one that is perhaps the most difficult to define and document. This concerns the role of the therapist's personality in the treatment process.

Those who have read Ken Kesey's *One Flew over the Cuckoo's Nest*, or who have seen the movie, can hardly forget Nurse Ratchet, an apparently competent and diligent nurse. Only as the story unfolds do we get a deeper view of her personality and how destructive she is to her patients. Kesey has captured in beautiful dramatic form what most mental health workers have informally recognized for many years. Some individuals have personal characteristics that make them first-rate therapists, while others consistently bring about no improvement in their clients, or even make them worse.

The past twenty years have seen several important lines of research that take these personal issues out of the realm of casual observation and into the light of scientific investigation. To begin with some background statistics, Bergin (1971) and Bergin and Lambert (1978) compiled impressive data to suggest that about 13 percent of clients who go into therapy actually get *worse*. Of these we can reasonably assume that some would have deteriorated anyway. However, the real impact of Bergin's findings is his estimate that about 8 percent got worse *as a result of therapy*. Technically poor assessment procedures or inappropriate therapy decisions? Perhaps. But one cannot help worrying about how many Nurse Ratchets there are among us.

Investigations that bear directly on this problem began with Whitehorn and Betz (1954) and were followed by the work of Carl Rogers and his students (Rogers, 1967). In an early review of this literature Truax and Mitchell (1971) suggested that successful therapists generally have qualities of *nonpossessive warmth*, *empathic understanding*, and *personal authenticity*. These qualities seem to be related to success regardless of the level of training or the theoretical orientation of the therapist. *Nonpossessive warmth* refers to the quality of relating to clients as worthwhile human beings, with unconditional acceptance of them as persons (although not necessarily condoning all their behavior). Relating to a client as simply a member of a diagnostic category, or in an overly judgmental fashion, or essentially as a nonperson who happens to display certain problems, all run counter to this principle. *Empathic understanding* pertains to qualities of how one gets to know another person. A therapist can gain an understanding of a client by tests, observation, and good listening and then intellectually organize this information in an interpretative framework. This is apparently not enough, for what seems to be required here is to understand what the client is living through, *from the client's frame of reference*. To an extent, this getting inside the other individual and acquiring a sense of how he or she experiences and perceives the world almost calls for a novelist's sensitivities and abilities to extend oneself. Finally, the principle of *authenticity* calls for a consistently open and honest personal approach to the client. The therapist cannot hide behind a disguise, whatever it may be—a practiced professional demeanor, rigid adherence to technique, or put-on displays of sympathy. Findings similar to those reviewed by Truax and Mitchell (1971) have been reported with regard to the premature dropping out of therapy as well. Therapists who have been judged to be personally warm, objective, and understanding have relatively low drop-out rates among a broad range of clients (Hiler, 1958; Carson and Heine, 1962; Baum, Felzer, D'Zmura, and Shumaker, 1966).

A more recent review of this area (Parloff, Waskow, and Wolfe, 1978) points to a growing literature that suggests that the therapist's general mental health also affects the success of treatment. These reviewers cite at least nine studies that indicate that the more evidence of psychological disturbance in the therapist (e.g., anxiety, defensiveness) the poorer the treatment results. In a related series of studies it has been found that special training procedures with therapists who may be anxious or in conflict about working with clients with a different socioeconomic background than their own can produce increased success rates (Bernard, 1965; Jacobs, Charles, Jacobs, Weinstein, and Mann, 1972). In these studies the training consisted of a variety of procedures to make therapists more sensitive to the expectations, special needs, and life-styles of these clients. Therapists were provided with direct information, attitudinal problems were openly discussed in staff conferences, and individual supervision focused on resolving deeper therapist fears and hostility. Such efforts appeared to be effective in producing important changes in therapists' behavior during treatment. Relative to "unprepared" therapists, they were generally more flexible in their approach, exercised care in using communications that were meaningful to clients, and they devoted increased efforts to reinforcing clients' motivations to remain in therapy.

In summary, we have seen in this section several areas of research that point to the importance of therapist personality factors. The evidence seems to be generally in keeping with widely held beliefs among therapists about such positive attributes as personal warmth, empathy, nondefensiveness, and objectivity. The reader should recognize, however, that these findings represent only the beginnings of an enormously complex area. As pointed out in the review by Parloff, Waskow, and Wolfe (1978) a great deal of further work is required. They suggest that the whole question of discovering how to *match* therapist and client characteristics to produce maximal treatment success may be a critical area for future research. For example, preliminary evidence indicates that similarities of economic and ethnic background (Siegal, 1974) and shared values and expectations about therapy (Beutler, Pollack, and Jobe, 1977; Warren and Rice, 1972) increase the chances for successful treatment. These findings illustrate some of the directions this topic is likely to take in the future as the profession attempts to investigate the subtle issue of the personal chemistry that takes place between clients and therapists.

CONCLUSION

After reading this chapter it is probably apparent that workers in the mental health field face many and varied pressures in their professional lives. After lengthy periods of formal training they must continue to vigorously keep up with new developments in the field. Constant attention to legal and ethical considerations is required. Awareness of one's own personality problems or areas of insensitivity is essential. Added burdens arise from the occasional interprofessional conflicts that occur. Finally, the therapist's role carries with it a responsibility to meet the needs of one's community and to continually improve services. In all, these represent a stringent set of requirements that makes the profession both challenging and fascinating.

PART TWO

THE INTAKE PROCESS
AND CLINICAL DECISIONS

CHAPTER THREE

THE INTAKE PHASE: FIRST CONTACT AND ASSESSMENT

Having considered some general conceptual, professional, and ethical issues in the first two chapters, we can now review more detailed aspects of the initial phases of the therapeutic process—managing the client's first contact with the agency or therapist and assessment of the client's problems. The general principles to be described are pertinent to a wide variety of therapy settings, be they, for example, a community outpatient clinic, a paraprofessional mental health specialist associated with a medical facility, or a junior high school counseling office. The specific techniques involved in these *intake procedures* will, of course, vary somewhat from setting to setting; however, issues common to most situations will be the focus of discussion.

In order to deal with the intake process in a step-by-step fashion, this chapter will be divided into two sections: a brief one dealing with the management of the client's initial contact with the therapist or agency and a longer section reviewing the principles and techniques of assessing the client's problems.

FIRST CONTACT WITH THE CLIENT

A number of important tasks must be accomplished in the opening stages of contact with the client. These include (1) a proper introduction to the therapeutic agency and a description of the general services available, (2) a review of the problems for which the client is seeking help, (3) an explanation to the client of the procedures involved in the intake process, (4) discussion of any pertinent professional or ethical issues, and (5) development of a preliminary agreement to proceed with the intake process. Each of these steps is designed to produce a clear, structured, and professional relationship with the client, and they give both the agency and client an opportunity to initially evaluate whether the available services fit the particular needs of the client. In the following sections each of these steps will be generally described, along with examples from a variety of settings.

Introduction and Description of Services

Most potential clients are unfamiliar with the workings of agencies that provide psychological services, while others may have formed romanticized or unrealistic impressions from popular literature or movies. Therefore it is necessary to present a concise and understandable description of the therapist's or agency's functions at the outset. This may prompt further discussion of any of the client's misapprehensions, which can then be clarified. In the following examples several different situations will illustrate the importance of such introductions in initiating a therapeutic process on an appropriate footing.

Example A A thirty-six-year-old woman comes to a community mental health clinic, on the advice of a friend, to discuss her fourteen-year-old daughter's underachievement at school.

> **Therapist:** Hello, Mrs. Smith, I'm Miss Dawkins. I'm a social worker here at the clinic.
>
> **Client:** Hello. [*Pause*] I'm sure glad that I finally got up enough nerve to come here. I'm really upset and worried, and I need advice. Are you a child psychiatrist?
>
> **Therapist:** No, a social worker is not the same as a psychiatrist. Although both professions work with psychological and social difficulties that people may be experiencing, social workers don't have a medical background. Our clinic staff has psychiatrists, psychologists, and social workers, however, and we work as a team. In this way, the clinic is able to be of service for lots of different problems. Once we get an idea of what the difficulties are, we can assign the most qualified person. You mentioned an interest in a child psychiatrist.
>
> **Client:** Yes, you see my daughter is having really bad school problems. She . . .

Example B A fifty-five-year-old man is a patient in the rehabilitation ward of a large medical hospital. He suffered a stroke six months earlier, which partially paralyzed his right side, and he has been undergoing the arduous work of physical rehabilitation for several months (exercise, retraining, etc.). The physical therapy staff have noticed his progressive sense of discouragement and lack of cooperation over the past several weeks, and they have requested that one of the paraprofessional psychology aides consult with the patient. The psychology aide comes to see the client in his hospital room.

> **Therapist:** Good morning, Mr. Jones. My name is Jim Brooks, and I am a member of the psychology staff here at the hospital. I . . .
>
> **Client:** Jeez. They really think I'm crazy, don't they? [*Indignant*] Can't you all just leave me alone?

Therapist: I know how you feel, Mr. Jones. Many people get the wrong idea when I come to see them. No one thinks you're crazy, but the people over in the rehab section are worried because you seem to have been pretty discouraged for a while.

Client [*Angry*]: You know what you can do with that whole bunch in rehab. There's this one therapist who thinks he's running the Green Bay Packer training camp. Thinks he's hot stuff. Five years ago I could have run circles around him.

Therapist: Yes, I know sometimes they come on pretty strong and get people upset with them. Part of my job as a psychology aide is to get in the middle of these kinds of situations and try to work things out. Lots of times a third person is in a position to notice how people might get on each other's nerves and maybe to make some helpful suggestions.

Client: Yeah, maybe. Let me tell you what he did yesterday. . . .

Example C A twelve-year-old boy is sent to see the school counselor because of his aggressive, rebellious behavior in class. Teachers have tried various forms of classroom discipline with him and have had several conferences with his parents, all to no avail. His earlier school records revealed no apparent problems, and his present teachers are at a loss as to how to manage him.

Therapist: Come on in, Frank, and have a seat. You've probably seen me around school. I'm Mr. Gonzalez.

Client: Yeah, I see you around. Don't you coach the basketball team?

Therapist: That's right, I'm an assistant coach. But my main job here at school is a counselor. If any of the students need advice about school-work, or if they've got things on their mind, they come to talk them over with me. I guess you know that your teachers are worried about the way it's been going with you this year, and that's why they asked you to see me.

Client: Who are you trying to snow man? Those _____ don't give a _____ about me. Nobody does, not even . . .

Note that in each of these illustrations, the therapists attempt with varying degrees of success to provide a concise and understandable statement of their role and function in the particular setting in which they work. The directness and candor of these introductions seem to elicit equally frank reactions on the part of the clients—responses that are not necessarily pleasant or acquiescent, but which at least initiate the relationship on an open and problem-oriented level. Note also that the introductions help to focus discussion on immediate topics of concern and therefore serve as an entrée into the next phase of establishing contact with the client.

Initial Review of the Client's Problems

A major issue during the first contact is whether or not the therapist or agency provides services that are appropriate to the client's problems. Thus a preliminary review of these problems is necessary. If it appears that there is a potential fit of problems and services, then this initial discussion serves as the beginning of the intake-assessment procedure. However, if it is apparent that the client's problems can be better treated by another agency, then this discussion should lead to a referral to a more appropriate setting or therapist. Regardless of the outcome, however, the therapist must listen to the client's description of problems with care and sensitivity.

To illustrate, let us continue with the examples from the previous section.

Example A (mother of underachieving fourteen-year-old)

Client: Yes, you see my daughter is having really bad school problems. She just isn't working very hard. I don't know what's gotten into her. She's always been at the top, but now she doesn't . . . Oh, I've tried everything . . . [*Starts to cry*].

Therapist: She really concerns you very much.

Client: And it's not only school. We used to be so close. Now she hardly talks to me. You know it hasn't been easy since her father left. . . . I thought I knew how to handle her, but now I'm so confused [*Crying*]. She gets so angry with me sometimes.

Therapist: Why is that?

Client: I don't know. Maybe I'm too strict, or not giving her enough guidance. Oh, I don't know, those sound like just words . . . I'm scared because she's all I've got. Can you tell me what to do?

Therapist: I know it's not easy raising a child by yourself. There are quite a few parents who come to the clinic to work on improving relations with their families, and it sounds like we may be of help to you. Let me tell you what would be involved. . . .

Example B (fifty-five-year-old stroke victim)

Client: Yeah, maybe. Let me tell you what he did yesterday. I was working out on the pulleys, and he came over and said I should have more weights on—and he marked that down on the chart.

Therapist: Yes?

Client: Well, don't you see? He's keeping a record of the evidence against me. He's not even trying to hide it anymore. But I had him spotted anyway. He's not so tricky.

Therapist: I don't think I understand. Can you explain some more?

Client: Listen, I want you to take a note to the FBI. They'll get it straightened out [*Very agitated and nervous*]. I'm not going to fight them, and their shrewd little plans, all alone.

Therapist: Yes, it sounds as if you need somebody on your side. And it also sounds kind of frightening and confusing. You know, sometimes after a person has had a stroke, and has been pretty much alone in the hospital for awhile, it's understandable that he'd get upset once in a while and maybe even misunderstand what others are doing.

Client: Yes, maybe. Are you talking about me?

Therapist: Yes, I am. I'm going to ask Dr. O'Hagan to come to see you this afternoon. He's a psychiatrist who has had a lot of experience in understanding these sorts of things. He'll be helpful and he's an easy guy to talk to. Is that okay?

Client: You do think I'm crazy, don't you? . . . Aw hell, I don't know, maybe I have been kind of screwy lately, just looking at these walls. Yeah, what the hell, send him up.

Example C (twelve-year-old boy)

Client: Who are you trying to snow, man? Those _____ don't give a _____ about me. Nobody does, not even my folks. They're so hung up with their fights, they don't know _____.

Therapist: You've got troubles at home and at school. . . . I'd like to help, if I can.

Client [*Exasperated*]: I don't want to talk about it.

Therapist: That's okay.

Client [*Pause*]: Hey, why didn't you call a time out at the end of the Central game?

Therapist: Yeah, we really goofed on that one. You interested in basketball?

Client: Well, I was thinking of trying out for the JV next year, but I don't know if I'm tall enough.

Therapist: You never know. Guys at your age grow a lot. Why don't you come to the gym after school today. It's a regular practice, but maybe you can get an idea of how it works.

Client: Yeah. Maybe I can make it.

Therapist: There will probably be time for us to get a Coke after the practice and get to know each other a little better.

Client: Okay. See you around. [*Begins to leave*] What could you do, anyway?

Therapist: Let's talk about it some more this afternoon when we've got more time.

As these examples try to demonstrate, each case takes its own direction early in the intake process. After the initial introduction and structuring, the therapists tried to have the clients describe what was troubling them. In the case of the distraught mother, this resulted in an emotional outpouring of problems concerning her daughter and a direct plea for help. The communication suggested to the therapist that the nature of the difficulties *may* be such that the agency could be of service, and she began to outline what is involved in the intake process (next section). In contrast, the paraprofessional psychology aide was rather surprised when the hospitalized stroke victim began talking about the bizarre-sounding material of hospital staff collecting evidence against him and his desire to contact the FBI. Recognizing the likelihood that this may reflect a disturbance beyond his therapeutic competencies, the paraprofessional initiated a referral process for a psychiatric consultation.

The case of the twelve-year-old boy illustrates a more subtle and cautious opening to the therapeutic process. Wary of the counselor and evidently unready to talk about troublesome material, he expresses considerable conflict with regard to entering a therapeutic relationship. Rather than pushing the process, the therapist expresses a willingness to maintain contact at a level acceptable and tolerable to the client. Underlying this approach is the assumption that as a trusting rapport develops, the twelve-year-old will feel secure enough to disclose personal problems and will perhaps enter into a working relationship with the counselor.

Review of Intake Procedures for Client

Following the client's description of problems and a preliminary decision to proceed, the next logical step is to provide a review of the intake procedures that are to follow. This review is important in that it is designed to accomplish several aims. First, it provides some structure and direction for the client's efforts in the early parts of therapy. Second, it communicates that the treatment processes will be systematic and understandable. Third, it frequently indicates that considerable effort, candor, and self-analysis will be required of the client right from the start of therapy.

Naturally, the specific procedures that are reviewed will vary from client to client, but in general this structuring should cover what will be involved in the *intake interview*, the possibility of *psychological testing*, and the likelihood that *other sources of information* will be tapped (e.g., interviews with family members, a medical examination, etc.). In addition, the client is informed that following the therapist's (or agency's) evaluation of this intake information, further discussion with the client will take place regarding mutually acceptable treatment goals and therapy procedures.

Let us continue with two of the case illustrations (omitting the stroke victim who was referred to the psychiatrist) in order to exemplify some variations of the structuring process.

Example A (distraught mother in community mental health clinic)

Therapist: . . . It sounds as if we may be of help to you. Let me tell you what would be involved. First, I would like to set up an appointment for you for what we call an intake interview, sometime in the next few days. You'll meet with Dr. Burgess, a clinical psychologist on our staff who specializes in parent-child difficulties, and the interview will probably last an hour or so. During that time you'll have an opportunity to go into the problems in more detail and go over some of the background—when things started going poorly, and so on. Dr. Burgess may also feel it important to talk to your daughter later on, but that's something the two of you can discuss more fully when you meet.

Client: Oh my! This really sounds complicated.

Therapist: Yes, I know it sounds that way, Mrs. Smith, but it's really not too bad. You see, it's important that we get as full a picture as possible in the beginning so we can then discuss with you the best plan of action.

Client: Well, I guess that makes sense. After this next interview, will they tell me what to do?

Therapist: I'm not sure. Quite frequently, the clinic also finds that taking some psychological tests or consulting with your daughter's school is helpful. As I said, generally, the more information that can be assembled, the better able we'll be to . . .

Client: You know, she doesn't know I've come here. I don't know how she'll be when she finds out [*Pause*]. And if my exhusband ever found out that I was coming here, he'd hit the ceiling—tell me all over again what a bad mother I am. He'd probably storm over here, all huffy and everything, and want to get to the bottom of it all.

Therapist: Yes, there is a lot to consider, and opening the subject with your daughter will be an important step. As far as your exhusband is concerned, let me tell you about our clinic rules about our records and protecting your privacy. . . .

Example C Frank has maintained contact with the school counselor for two weeks, principally by hanging around the gym during team practices. He has steadfastly avoided discussion of personal problems, but has become generally less defensive. One afternoon, while leaving the gym, the following conversation occurs.

Therapist: What's up, Frank? You're pretty quiet today.

Client: Nothing.

Therapist: Hey, c'mon. You say, "nothing." But it's written all over your face. Give a little.

Client: Aw, I don't know. . . . I screwed up today. . . . Aw, forget it.

Therapist: C'mon, Frank. We're friends.

Client [*Looks at therapist tearfully*]: Uh, uh. You know Jimmy, uh, the little guy you got playing guard, uh . . .

Therapist: Yes. Good ball player.

Client: Uh, well . . . you seem to like him a lot . . . I mean, you're always horsing around and kidding each other . . . I mean . . . I'll bet he doesn't mess things up.

Therapist [*Stops walking, and turns to confront client*]: Frank, I like you a lot, too. Whether you screw up or not, we're close friends, and nothing is going to change that.

Client [*Bursts into tears*]: I, I, uh, I'm so _____ up, Mr. Gonzalez. Uh, I don't know, anymore. I mean, I, I, what do I have to do to get straight?

Therapist: Let's keep talking, and keep being friends. . . C'mon, let's walk around, and you can fill me in on what's been happening. . . .

These cases involve different settings and markedly different schedules for the processes of initial contact, but they nevertheless illustrate the common necessity for providing structure and guideposts for the client. In the first example, the review of intake procedures that is provided represents a rather traditional outpatient clinic approach. A formal intake interview is scheduled, along with an alerting to the possibility of psychological testing and other consultations. A logical and appropriate rationale is given for these procedures, along with reassurance that the information will be discussed with the client with regard to the development of treatment goals and plans.

In the second example, formal scheduling of interviews and information gathering give way to the more fundamental issue of establishing a meaningful working relationship with a hesitant and resistant client. Although structuring of the procedures is limited to the brief "Let's keep talking," a tacit agreement to be friends also provides an emotional structure that permits the therapeutic process to continue.

Professional and Ethical Issues

As outlined at the beginning of this chapter, professional and ethical questions frequently arise during the client's first contact with therapist or agency. These may well be issues that require resolution before the client can feel ready to proceed with the intake procedures. Matters concerning fees, confidentiality, legal complications, involvement of family members, and so forth, all fall within this area.

On most occasions these questions are spontaneously raised by the client, but at times the therapist must anticipate some of them and introduce them for discussion. In either case, the same general principles espoused earlier of therapists' frankness and sensitivity are required in the management of these issues.

Proceeding with the two case illustrations, let us see how such issues are handled in these rather different situations.

Example A (distraught mother)

Therapist: . . . let me tell you about our clinic rules about our records and protecting your privacy. Things that you talk about with the staff of the clinic are confidential, and so are any records that the clinic may keep. Any of that information can be released only with your written permission—and there is a law in this state that actually protects this confidentiality. Just for completeness, I guess I should add that the only exception to these rules might occur if a crime is involved—and I'm only mentioning that to give you the full picture.

Client: Oh my! No! No crimes. But I'm really worried about my exhusband. He's so hotheaded. I don't want any more trouble from him. . . . It's going to be difficult enough with my daughter.

Therapist: I can appreciate that. Teenagers sometimes need a delicate touch. I might mention also that, with the kinds of problems you've mentioned, our clinic usually feels it important to get the teenager involved in any treatment, but that's something that you'll have an opportunity to go over with Dr. Burgess.

Client: Yes, well, I guess so. . . . You know, I came in here hoping to get some expert advice right away, but I guess it's more complicated than that. . . . But I've got to get this straightened out for my own peace of mind. . . .

Example C (twelve-year-old boy)

Therapist: . . . and you can fill me in on what's been happening.

Client [*Long pause*]: Jeez, I don't know how . . . I, I, . . . Do you, er, do you have to have parent conferences? I mean, er . . . [*Pause*].

Therapist: Frank, it sounds as if you've got a lot on your mind, and if it's stuff you want to keep just between us, that's okay. Later on, if there are things that involve your folks, we can talk about it, but I won't do anything without checking with you first.

Client: Yeah, okay [*Pause*]. I wish I could talk to my old man the way I do to you. . . .

Agreement to Proceed

Usually the "first contact" culminates in an explicit decision on the part of the client of whether or not to go ahead with the intake process. Issues pertaining to the services provided, the nature of the problem, ethical and professional concerns, and what will be involved in the intake procedures have been reviewed, and now the client is in a position to make a reasonably informed decision. As could be noted in the case examples, these "first contact" procedures have to be handled in a flexible and sometimes gentle fashion. However, the general principles of providing understandable information and establishing workable professional guidelines are the same for each case.

To complete this section, the two cases will be concluded with a review of how these "agreements to proceed" were managed.

Example A (distraught mother)

Client: . . . but I've got to get this straightened out for my own peace of mind.

Therapist: I can appreciate your concerns about getting to work on these problems. I think that once you get started with your intake procedures you'll feel better, because you'll be coming to grips with them.

Client: I feel a little better already, just having broken the ice.

Therapist: Do you have any questions about the intake interview with Dr. Burgess, or anything else?

Client: Should I bring my daughter?

Therapist: No. This first time, he will just want to talk with you, find out more about the problem, and make arrangements with you for any other information that may be important. Is that all right?

Client: Yes. When can we get started?

Therapist: How about Tuesday at two? I see that he has an opening then.

Example C

Client: . . . I wish I could talk to my old man the way I do to you. Sometimes he gets me so mad. I go crazy. I don't know what to do.

Therapist: We do feel pretty good about each other, don't we? Let's take some time, so you can tell me more about the problems. It might not be so easy, but if we can get things out in the open, maybe we can both figure out the best way to handle things.

Client: Yeah. The only problem is that I'm not sure if there's anything that can be done.

Therapist: I'm sure willing to give it a try, if you are.

Client: Yeah. I'd like to. Can we talk some now?

Each of these cases has now been brought to the point where the client and therapist are ready to embark on the next stage of the intake process. General information has been provided regarding what is involved in the gathering of intake information, and each therapist has also communicated that the client will be a part of the decision-making process as to any subsequent treatment. Finally, the cases also illustrate that each client came to a point of *commitment* to begin the therapy process — an important event in terms of the client's motivation and taking responsibility for treatment.

Having completed the initial contact, the client is now ready for the important and demanding work of the *assessment stage* of the intake procedure. This will typically involve the intake interview, psychological testing, self-observation techniques, and information gathering from other sources. The aim of the assessment process, of course, is to permit a detailed evaluation of the client's problems, which will then form the basis for the development of treatment goals and plans.

INFORMATION AND ASSESSMENT

The remainder of this chapter will be devoted to a description of the principal methods by which to assess the client's problems. These will include the intake interview, psychological tests, self-observation techniques, and information from others (family members, friends, teachers, etc.). The reader should recognize that the following material serves as a general orientation to these methods, but that a good deal more detailed background and supervised practice is required in order to acquire proficiency in these skills.

In the larger perspective of the overall therapy process, information gathered during this assessment stage forms the basis for the development of treatment goals and ultimately for the choice of treatment procedures with which to begin. It should be noted, however, that oftentimes this opening stage represents just the beginnings of a long process of identifying a client's problems. In some cases, where the issues are complex and subtle or where the client is especially defensive, the important areas of distress may not become apparent until well into therapy. Thus, as described in this section, the assessment stage represents an initial attempt to get enough relevant information with which to begin treatment on a reasonable footing. However, as therapy proceeds, both therapist and client should remain open to emerging problem areas and refinements of those already identified.

It can be noted that information from a variety of sources is utilized in the initial assessment (interview, tests, family information, etc.). Thus the practitioner must not only acquire competence in the specific technical skills involved in gathering data but also be able to organize the information into a meaningful and integrated description of the client. To accomplish such an integration, conceptualizations of personality dynamics and psychological maladjustment inevitably become involved. Thus, after having reviewed the assessment procedures individually in this chapter, a conceptual framework for organizing the information will be presented in Chapter 4.

The Intake Interview

After the "first contact" procedures have been accomplished and have resulted in an agreement to proceed with intake, the next usual step is the intake interview. Because of the rigors of scheduling, this is usually a one-hour session; however, individual circumstances may dictate a longer period of time or even several interviews. The intake interviewer is usually one of the more experienced practitioners at an agency, since in many settings this will be the individual who "presents" the case at the intake staff meeting. Such a presentation requires that the practitioner assemble all the data that is pertinent to the client, a process calling for sophisticated clinical judgments and abilities to conceptually integrate considerable amounts of information. In many clinic and hospital settings the intake interviewer will not be the person who eventually is the client's therapist, although this general rule will, of course, vary with the size of the staff and particulars of the agency.

An outline of a standard intake interview, which is applicable to a wide variety of settings and clients, is as follows:

I. Introductions, statement of purpose, and brief review of what is to be accomplished during the interview

II. Client description of problems
   A. Free running, uninterrupted account by the client
   B. Specific probes by interviewer, if not covered spontaneously by client
      1. When problems started
      2. Life circumstances at onset
      3. Suddenness or gradualness of onset
      4. Methods of coping with problems
      5. Client's perception of causes
      6. Prior professional treatment

III. Interviewer probes concerning effects of problems on current adjustment
   A. Interpersonal
   B, Work or school
   C. Community (legal, economic, social effects)
   D. Intrapersonal
      1. Physical (unusual eating, sleep, sexual patterns; psychosomatics; fatigue, etc.)
      2. Emotional (anxiety, depression, anger, etc.)
      3. Intellectual (inability to concentrate, poor judgment, misperceptions, etc.)

      4. Behavioral (impulsiveness, compulsions, inappropriate response patterns, etc.)

      5. Self-appraisals (low self-esteem, helplessness, self-blame, etc.)

IV. Brief review of client's social history

    A. Family

    B. Significant relationships

    C. Subculture

    D. Educational-vocational

    E. Significant events

V. Interviewer probes concerning client's readiness for therapy

    A. Commitment to change

    B. Level of insight

    C. Attitudes toward therapy

VI. Making arrangements for further information (where necessary)

    A. Psychological testing

    B. Medical consultations

    C. School or work records

    D. Interviews with family

    E. Self-observation procedures

VII. Closing summary and review of future procedures

Each of these steps will be discussed and illustrated in the following sections. Although space does not permit an example of an entire intake interview, it is hoped that the partial script will convey the essentials of the procedure.

Introductions and structuring As with the procedures involved in the first contact with the client, it is again necessary for the intake interviewer to identify himself or herself. In addition, a brief review of what is to be expected during the interview, and where it fits into the overall intake process, helps to define the situation for the client. Thus, although this opening phase of the interview need not be lengthy or detailed, sufficient information should be communicated to provide reasonable structure and direction for the client.

The following case illustration, involving a thirty-two-year-old man with problems of depression and suicide, takes place in a community outpatient clinic. Naturally, details of the interview might be different depending on setting and circumstance; however, the overall outline is probably applicable to a wide variety of situations.

Interviewer: Come in, Mr. Brown. It's good to see you. I'm Dr. Zackheim. Have a seat.

Client: Okay, thanks. I'm a little early. I hope that's all right.

Interviewer: Yes, that's fine. This will probably be a busy session, so we can use the time. I guess they told you the other day that this interview is to find out, in some detail, what brings you to the clinic, to get information about your background, and so on.

Client: Yes. I got that. I can fill you in on some of it, but there's a lot you'll probably have to ask me.

Interviewer: Sure. You also understand that, right now, we need to get as much information as possible? And that that might involve some psychological tests and maybe meeting with your family?

Client: Yeah, they told me when I was here last week, but I'm still not sure why you need to do all that.

Interviewer: In general, the reason is to get as full a picture as possible. After that, we'll have another meeting, where we can discuss what the best course of action seems to be.

Client: Yeah, that makes sense. That's the way I try to run my business, too. Get all the facts first.

Interviewer: Well, why don't we start, then? Tell me what brings you here.

Client description of problems It is quite likely that most clients have rehearsed this opening part of the interview. Therefore, in many ways, this initial description of problems represents the *client's formulation* of the difficulties and their causes — an analysis that can be of considerable importance in terms of later therapeutic decisions. Also, since this material has been rehearsed, one can assume that it has been, to some degree, censored and arranged so as to present an acceptable image of the client. This defensiveness is certainly understandable; however, in later parts of the session, the interviewer will likely attempt to go beyond this initial material in order to gain a more complete picture of the client's situation. In addition, the interviewer may find it important to note the degree of defensiveness displayed and the readiness of the client to work in an open fashion.

As suggested in the outline of the initial interview, the client's spontaneous account of problems is followed by probes into a number of specific areas: problem onset, life circumstances at onset, suddenness of onset, coping style, perception of causes, and prior treatment. Many of these areas may be sufficiently covered in the client's initial description, and therefore require no further investigation. However, where omitted or insufficiently described, the interviewer is usually quite direct in trying to elicit this information.

Interviewer: Tell me what brings you here.

Client: Well, doctor, it's this way. Two weeks ago, I tried to kill myself. Just turned on the gas, and wanted it to be all over. I was at my sister's house, and she got to me in time. Lucky, I guess. Really got her upset, and she said that I had to get some professional help. She's right. I'm really happy to have this opportunity to get things straightened out.

Interviewer: Yes. Fill me in some more on what happened.

Client: Well, there's not that much to tell. My girlfriend had just broken up with me, and I got real depressed and started drinking. Things just got worse and worse. Finally I just didn't care anymore, and that's when I did it. I can see now how dumb it was. I guess booze and depression just don't mix.

Interviewer: And it happened because of the breakup?

Client: Yeah, it really knocked me over. Here we had been going together real good—real close and everything. And then without any warning she told me it was all over. Didn't want to marry me. Didn't even want to see me anymore. I gave that girl everything. All my feelings. I always tried to do everything her way. And after all that she just dumps me. I can't figure it out. How could she do that?

Interviewer: It sound like it really came as a surprise to you. No hints that anything was wrong?

Client: No, nothing. It came out of the blue. That's what's so confusing. I had even asked her to marry me that evening, and you know, I was absolutely convinced that she'd say yes [*Pause*]. I was so stunned when she closed me out, I couldn't believe it [*Pause*]. I guess she finally realized how much I cared when I told her I was going to do myself in [*Pause*]. But even that confused me, because she still wouldn't see me. I'm still mixed up about it. I guess that's where you come in, doc; I need my head fixed up [*Laughs*].

Interviewer: Has anything like this happened to you in the past?

Client: No [*Pause*]. Well, yes, in a way, but it was different before. You see, I was divorced about a year ago. Had been married for twelve years, and one day my wife just packs up and leaves. Took our son with her. Said she never wanted to see me again, and left. No explanations. No nothing. Everything just came apart for me.

Interviewer: What happened?

Client: I tried to kill myself and ended up in the hospital. Cut my wrists, but I didn't do such a good job. They kept me in the hospital for a few months, but I never got to see the psychiatrist very much. After I got out, I was really living like a bum—drinking, not taking care of myself. Slipping fast. That's why I had such high hopes when I met _____. I thought we could really make it together [*Pause*]. You know, it really helps to talk to you about this. I need to get myself straightened out.

Interviewer: It sounds like things go all right for you while you're in these relationships, but then when they break up, you really go to pieces. Is that the way it is?

Client: Yeah, that's it. I'll be riding high, and then, crash. Depressed, drinking, and I don't care what happens.

Interviewer: What do you think goes wrong?

Client: I don't know. That's what's got me so confused. Things seemed to be perfect between _____ and me. We hadn't known each other more than a month, but it was right, I know that [*Pause*]. With my wife it was more complicated. She always seemed tense and dissatisfied. God knows, I tried. I'd do everything her way. I was the one who was always giving, but she just got worse and worse. I still don't know how she could blame me, after all I gave her. I don't know [*Laughs*]. There must be something wrong with me.

Effects on current adjustment Following the initial review of problems and symptoms, the focus of the interview shifts to an analysis of the quality of the client's adjustment. What areas of the client's life are adversely affected by these problems? How serious are the disabilities? Are the psychological and environmental conditions such as to bring about further difficulties or an impending crisis?

Also of importance here is information regarding the client's strengths and existing supports in the client's life. Evaluating the strengths, weaknesses, and areas of vulnerability in current adjustment patterns will be critically important in subsequent judgments regarding the goals of treatment and the most appropriate therapy.

Since these areas of concern are natural outgrowths of the client's initial description of problems, the topical transition in the interview need not be dramatic or forced. In continuing with a partial transcript of our illustrative case, note that the therapist manages this shift by responding to the client's statement of internal problems.

Client: . . . There must be something wrong with me.

Interviewer: Tell me about that. How do you see what's wrong?

Client: I'm not sure. I don't really know. I just have this feeling. I don't know if I can explain it.

Interviewer: Give it a try. It's important to explore as much as we can.

Client [*Pause*]: Well, it's like I was saying. I was really living like a bum. Just drinking, hardly going to work, taking money from my sister. I really hated that. I don't want to be that way, but, I don't know, I just kind of gave up. Almost got fired, but I guess I had worked there so long, they gave me a break. My sister's been okay about it, but her husband is putting pressure on her. He really thinks I'm a loser. Maybe I am. But she's all I've got. If she gives up on me, I don't know what I'll do.

Interviewer: If that should happen, what would become of you?

Client [*Nervous laugh*]: Oh, boy. I don't know. She's been kind of my backup, all my life. Even when we were kids she'd look out for me. . . . Wow, I can't even think about that . . . I don't know . . . I guess I would do an awful lot of drinking again. It would really be bad. . . . I guess the only thing that might save it, is to have someone like you to talk to.

Interviewer: If she gave up on you, that would be close to the end of the string?

Client: Yeah, I guess so [*Pause*]. You know, it's funny. I was just sitting here asking myself why. And it came to me. All my life I've needed affection from people. And more than ordinary affection. I really need it. It's always been that way. When I'm getting it, I feel great. But when it stops, like with my wife, I really come apart. . . .

This section of the interview continues with a further description of the client's affectional needs and how drinking and depression occur when these needs are not fulfilled by others. He also describes more fully the consequences of the depression-drinking pattern—irregular eating and sleeping, deterioration of personal hygiene, sporadic work schedule—all resulting in further despondency and loss of self-esteem.

Review of client's history   The transition from issues of current adjustment to a review of the client's background can frequently be a smooth and appropriate one. Having described present problems and their effects on life processes, a natural question that seems to arise concerns the historical roots of these difficulties. Thus, although a relatively brief period in the interview may be devoted to this review, it can provide valuable information regarding long-term patterns and trends in the client's life.

Interviewer: You mentioned before that it's always been this way for you. Tell me how it's been throughout your life.

Client: Oh, wow! I don't know. That would be hard to pick out. I don't know where to start. My wife, my folks? I meant before that I've had this need for affection as long as I can remember, even as a kid.

Interviewer: Tell me about that.

Client: Okay, well, let's see. I never got along with my father. I hate to say it, but I really think he was a nasty guy. Always drinking, always picking a fight with Mom, or one of us kids. I just stayed away from him as much as I could [*Pause*]. Now with Mom it was different [*Pause*]. I guess she was what you'd call a domineering mother. She really made me toe the mark—good grades, always be polite, don't dress sloppy. She really had me under her thumb.

Interviewer: What effects did all that have on you?

Client: Well, I was a real goody. I did what she wanted me to [*Pause*]. And now that I think about it, I stayed that way for a long time. Even in high school, jeez, I must have been sixteen or seventeen, I can remember always trying to please her—that was the big thing [*Pause*]. Oh, wow!

Interviewer: Judging from the expression on your face just now, something important just came to you.

Client: Yeah. It's been that way all my life. Trying to please everybody— my mother, my wife. You know, that's the way I've always tried to get affection. But, I don't know, somehow I got lost in it all. I don't know, it's all confusing.

The client proceeds to describe his unhappy marriage, mentioning his wife's progressive emotional withdrawal from him and his inability to understand why the relationship had deteriorated. He also mentions that during these years of the declining marriage, bouts of depression and drinking increased, which culminated in the suicide attempt when his wife divorced him.

Probes concerning readiness for therapy At this stage of the intake interview, the therapist has obtained at least an outline of the principal symptoms, their effects on current adjustment, and some information regarding long-range patterns in the client's life. Now, efforts are required to assess whether or not the client seems ready to engage in productive efforts to work on these problems in psychotherapy. Such issues as the client's apparent motivation to explore his life, willingness to change, and attitudes towards therapy come under consideration. Naturally, the therapist has been forming impressions on these questions throughout the interview; and this section can be a relatively brief one bringing together these issues.

Interviewer: Well, we've covered quite a bit, and I was wondering how you see the clinic being of help to you.

Client: Jeez, I'm not sure. I mean, I thought you would tell me [*Pause*]. I don't know, I look at it this way. Right now my life is a mess, and I kind of look at my coming here as my last chance. I mean, I've really screwed things up, especially this last year, with all the drinking and everything. God knows, I've tried, though. I really worked hard in my marriage—I gave and gave and gave—but it went sour anyway. I don't know if it was her or me, but it really tore me apart [*Pause*]. I guess I'm confused. Right now, I'm kind of lost, except that I know I can't go back to living the way I did this last year. What do you think I should do?

This material, coupled with the client's handling of earlier parts of the interview, suggests to the therapist a readiness to engage in psychotherapy. Dissatisfaction and expressions of distress over his current life, along with a felt need for professional help, indicate that he will be a motivated client. In addition, he seemed to approach much of the earlier probing in an open and nondefensive manner, again revealing at least an initial ability to take part in a frank and serious review of his problems.

Arrangements for further information At this stage of the interview, with most clients, the therapist is considering questions that are still unresolved. These pertain to issues that will have a bearing on the imminent decisions regarding therapeutic goals and the most effective treatment approach. These are also questions that cannot be easily answered during the intake interview, but rather require consultation with other professionals or information from other people. Hence, at this point in the interview, arrangements can be made for such outside contacts as a medical or neurological examination, psychological testing, meetings with family members, social service assistance, and so forth, as the therapist deems necessary.

As with earlier aspects of the intake process, the need for such additional information should be frankly explained to the client. This explanation can also include a review of the broader aim of gathering together as much data as possible with which to make effective decisions regarding therapeutic goals and procedures.

With the particular client used in the illustrative interview, two major questions confront the therapist. These pertain to the depression-suicide pattern in the client's life and to the possible physical effects of the apparent chronic drinking problem.

With regard to suicide, a very real risk is involved, since the client has related at least two such episodes in his life. What is the possibility, under the stresses of certain kinds of treatment, that another such episode may be triggered by therapy itself? How readily will this client react with depression-drinking-suicide if he undergoes another rejection (for example, from his sister)? While the therapist may have already formulated some impressions on these questions, a decision is made to arrange for psychological testing in order to gain additional information on these critical questions.

Regarding the chronic drinking problem and the associated self-care deficits described by the client, the possibility of undetected physical problems exists, and hence arrangements are also initiated for a thorough medical examination. Should physical disabilities be discovered, then a coordination of medical treatments with the planned psychotherapy would be necessary.

Interviewer: I need to bring up two things that are of concern, and tell you what I'd like to suggest. The first is this business of drinking and of not having taken care of yourself. I don't know if you've had a recent medical exam, but I think it's important that you get one. Sometimes people who have been drinking a lot develop physical problems, and we need to check that out.

Client: Yeah, okay. But I think I'm all right physically, it's my emotions that are all messed up.

Interviewer: Well, that brings me to the second concern. You've told me about twice in your recent life when you tried to kill yourself, and to tell the truth, I'm not clear in my own mind how prone you are to take that route to solve your problems.

Client: Wow, you don't pull any punches, do you?

Interviewer: You wouldn't want me to, would you?

Client: No, you're right, but I don't think I can answer that question.

Interviewer: I know. It's a tough one. And that's why I'd like you to take some psychological tests. They are not foolproof, but if you approach them in the same open way that you've talked to me today, we can probably get some more information that would be helpful.

Arrangements are made for the medical and psychological exams, with an agreement that information derived from these consultations may be made available to the clinic.

Summary and review of future procedures   The therapist is now ready to close the intake interview. In most instances this terminal stage involves a brief overview of what the client has talked about and an explanation of the next phases of the intake process. This explanation indicates to the client that information from the interview and other sources (psychological tests, medical exam, and so forth) will be assembled and reviewed by clinic staff and, further, that consideration will be given by the staff as to recommended goals and treatment (or referral to a more appropriate agency, in some cases). Finally, arrangements are also made for a future appointment during which the recommendations will be reviewed and discussed with the client.

Interviewer: Well, we've covered a lot today, and I think I've got a pretty good idea of the problems—the drinking, the times you got to the point of suicide, and how badly your life has generally been going lately. I should be getting the medical and testing reports by the beginning of next week, and then the clinic staff will go over it all at our intake meeting next Wednesday. I'd like to have a meeting with you after that to go over the staff recommendations, and see what you think of them. How about next Thursday at two o'clock?

Client: Fine.

Psychological Tests

The use of standardized psychological tests for the assessment of personality functions has a long and rich tradition in the areas of mental health, education, vocational counseling, and personnel selection. Such widespread usage has led to a proliferation of specific tests, and it is beyond the scope of this book to even attempt a review of these many instruments. Also, as suggested earlier, the administration and interpretation of most personality tests involve considerable technical skill that requires special training and supervised practice. For these reasons, this section will be limited to a general discussion of tests as they apply to overall therapy issues, with particular emphasis on the use of test information as an aid to decision making in the initial stages of therapy.

General issues in testing   One of the principal aspects of personality tests is that they present to the subject a *standardized* set of stimuli to which he or she is to respond. Ideally, administered under standardized conditions as well, the subject is thereby presumably minimally affected by extraneous or situation-specific influences. Responses elicited under these relatively constant conditions thus permit a comparison of an individual's performance with (1) that of other individuals or (2) with expected patterns of responding derived from theories of personality or psychopathology.

Many of the current-day personality tests use the first comparison process, that is, studying a subject's responses on the standardized test in relation to those of other groups of individuals—groups with certain characteristics of relevance to understanding the subject. Such tests, of course, require the compilation of *norms* that accurately reflect the performance of these comparison groups on the test, and the subject's responses are compared to these group norms in a careful, statistical fashion. For this reason, personality instruments that use this approach are frequently referred to as *objective tests*. One of the most widely used and carefully researched objective personality tests is the Minnesota Multiphasic Personality Inventory (MMPI), an instrument that compares a subject's responses on over five hundred items with those of patients from a wide variety of diagnostic categories (e.g., depressive, psychopathic, schizophrenic patients, etc.).

Standardized tests that evaluate an individual's performance primarily in relation to theoretically expected patterns of response place a greater burden of interpretation and judgment on the examiner. Most such tests present the subject with a relatively ambiguous set of stimuli (e.g., ink blots, pictures of unstructured social situations) and require that the subject impose a structure on the stimulus materials ("Tell me what you see in the ink blot" or "Make up a story to this picture"). The underlying assumption of such tests is that subjects will project or reveal their unique personality style and inner personality dynamics in responding to such unstructured materials. As such, these types of instruments are usually termed *projective tests*.

Of concern in the administration and interpretation of tests are the subject's attitudes and openness in taking the test. Naturally, attempts are made to engage the subject's cooperation, but nevertheless, either purposeful or subtle processes may occur that result in a lack of candor in responding. Such "faking" can be in the direction of masking or minimizing psychological problems (answering in a socially desirable fashion) or, under some circumstances (e.g., trying to gain insurance compensation), portraying oneself as more debilitated than is actually the case.

Various means have been utilized to minimize such effects and thereby to produce more meaningful data. For example, on some tests the specific personality functions being evaluated are disguised or hard to discern (as on the projectives), and hence subjects have a difficult time in knowing how to "fake good" or "bad." On some self-report inventories, the response choices available to subjects are limited, thereby in effect forcing answers into one of only several defined categories. In this way subjects are afforded little opportunity to minimize or hedge on responses. Perhaps the most systematic procedure to control for such "response sets" involves tests that independently evaluate test-taking style and then statistically correct the personality scores in terms of these test-taking factors. Such corrections are an integral part of the MMPI.

Objective and projective personality tests differ on a number of dimensions—notably, the type of information they provide, the way in which they are scored and interpreted, and in general, the scientific basis for the tests themselves. Thus in clinical settings the choice of which tests to use depends on the specific questions and circumstances that arise with each client.

Objective tests Objective tests typically use a self-report format, such that subjects indicate whether each item on the test is true or false about themselves. To illustrate, the following are several items from the MMPI: "It is safer to trust nobody." "I have very few fears compared to my friends." "I brood a great deal." An inventory of this sort has the advantages of being easily administered and scored. The results are most often interpreted according to reasonably precise statistical criteria and ostensibly indicate the extent to which the subject displays a particular trait or the similarity of his or her responses to those of a known diagnostic group.

Considerable research has been devoted to these types of instruments (particularly the MMPI), and these extensive data highlight both their strengths and shortcomings as clinical tools (Gynther and Gynther, 1976). On the positive side, they may serve with reasonable adequacy as screening devices for identifying broad symptom complexes or in making predictions about future behaviors (e.g., proneness to delinquency, likelihood of a psychotic episode, probable response to therapy). However, their usefulness in helping a clinician to understand the subtle personality dynamics or the specific emotional conflicts of an individual client is questionable (Kleinmuntz, 1967). It appears that, at best, the scores (or patterns of scores) on these tests may serve as a source of hypotheses about a client's areas of stress or vulnerability.

Projective tests Projective tests utilize relatively ambiguous stimuli to which subjects may respond in a free, interpretive manner. They presumably reveal deep and enduring aspects of personality organization and unique modes of perception. A variety of projective methods have been developed, including such techniques as indicating one's perceptions of ink blots (Rorschach Test), drawing a picture of a person, composing stories around pictures of unstructured social situations (Thematic Apperception Test), and creating endings for incomplete sentences. As can be noted, the tasks faced by subjects on such tests are quite a bit different than those encountered when simply responding true or false to items on the typical objective test.

This freedom of response on projective tests is a two-edged sword. On the negative side, these devices are notoriously difficult to score and interpret in a standardized fashion. Multiple dimensions of personality may be reflected, as well as a variety of environmental factors that are affecting the subject. Because so much of the interpretation depends on the skill of the examiner, it is virtually impossible to evaluate the adequacy of the tests themselves apart from that of the clinician who is using them (Exner, 1976). The assumption that projective instruments are tapping basic and enduring aspects of personality has also been questioned (Phares, 1979). The very ambiguity of the tests seems to make them susceptible to transient situational factors in the testing situation itself, or to guarded and superficial responding by some subjects. For these reasons the formal research that has been done on projective tests (literally thousands of studies) has been generally disappointing (see Sundberg, 1977).

Proponents of projective tests seem to acknowledge the poor research showing, but they maintain that the very nature of projective methods makes them difficult to assess (Exner, 1976). Rather, they emphasize that the free and multidetermined responses of subjects on these tests provide a rich source of personal information in the hands of a skilled clinician. Adherents of these methods contend that inferences may be made about subjects' needs, conflicts, areas of anxiety, psychological defenses, perceptual style, and the interplay between personality dynamics and environmental pressures. Such an array of information about a client in the early stages of therapy would, of course, be invaluable.

Clinical Utility of Tests

The use of personality tests can be a time-consuming and relatively expensive endeavor. Therefore most agree that they should be used judiciously and under circumstances where there is reasonable assurance that they will add useful information about a client to that already gathered from interview and biographical data (Sechrest, 1963). In general, research results have not provided a clear picture of which assessment procedures are most informative, and therefore clinicians are advised to exercise careful judgment in tailoring their selection of tests so as to focus on pertinent issues for each client (Sundberg, 1977). There does not appear to be a generally agreed-upon method for making such selections of tests. It may be useful, however, to outline some of the major types of questions that arise during the intake phase and to consider these questions in relation to objective and projective tests.

Diagnostic category Decisions concerning goals and treatment strategies in many instances may be dependent on the complex of symptoms and traits exhibited by clients, or the diagnostic category which they seem to fit. Thus, for example, a client who displays some unusual or eccentric conversational patterns in the intake interview may elicit concerns about a possible psychosis. On the other hand, these observed behaviors may reflect some more specific (and less serious) difficulties in social skills, or even a transient flippancy or defensiveness prompted by the interview itself. Resolving such ambiguities will likely play an important role in decisions regarding the initial therapeutic strategy to be used with such a client. Since some of the objective tests (particularly the MMPI) were designed to compare subjects' responses to those of various diagnostic groups, such an instrument might well be selected in the present example. Although research has indicated that such usage of objective tests is far from foolproof (Zelin, 1971), this test data may add a significant increment to information gathered from other sources.

Predictions of future behavior Is client A likely to attempt suicide? What are the chances that client B may develop delinquent patterns of behavior? How will client C probably adjust to incarceration? These and similar types of predictions about a client's reaction patterns in the future have an important bearing on treatment decisions. In many instances the answers to such questions may be reasonably apparent from biographical and interview data (Sechrest, 1963). However, where additional information may be needed, considerable research indicates that objective tests may enhance the clinician's predictive abilities and are the likely choice when faced with such tasks (Gynther and Gynther, 1976).

Degree of distress Treatment decisions oftentimes take into consideration the intensity of anxiety, depression, or similar emotions being experienced by a client. On occasion it is difficult to gauge the degree to which such distress is present from interview data. Clients may be overly guarded in revealing themselves, or they may feel that they are supposed to appear strong when discussing their problems, and so forth. Since treatment strategies themselves may differ considerably in the degree of stress they impose on a client, it is important not to overly tax an already severely distressed client. Thus psychological tests are occasionally called upon to help in making this assessment. On this issue it appears that both objective and projective tests may be of utility. Such self-report instruments as the State-Trait Anxiety Inventory (Spielberger, Gorsuch, and Lushene, 1970) and the Beck Depression Inventory (Beck, 1967) were specifically designed to make these sorts of evaluations, and they have received considerable research validation. On the other hand, clinicians are also likely to use projective tests for these questions. While the projective tests usually do not provide a standardized score pertaining to distress, they may provide clues as to the sources of anxiety and the mechanisms by which a client attempts to manage stress.

Psychodynamic hypotheses The planning of treatment strategies could be enhanced in many instances with knowledge about such issues as a client's defensive style, areas of conflict, characteristic ways of relating to people, inner needs, environmental stressors, and so forth. These are facets of personality functioning that are not likely to be revealed to any great degree in the course of an intake interview. The development of hypotheses regarding these issues could be useful in helping to focus therapeutic efforts into productive areas and in identifying special vulnerabilities of the client. For these kinds of questions the projective tests seem to fare better than objective instruments. Recall, however, the relatively poor research support for projective devices cited earlier and the necessary reliance placed on clinicians' individual interpretive skills when using these techniques.

Specialized issues This brief survey of questions that arise concerning treatment decisions is inevitably incomplete and oversimplified. It should be recognized that many specialized issues may arise in clinical work that require specific tests and assessment procedures. Problems related to mental retardation, poor school achievement, learning disabilities, and brain damage, to name but a few, may call for specially designed tests in order to identify particular cognitive and behavioral deficits and to help plan specific rehabilitation efforts.

The Use of Test Data with the Case Example

In the first half of this chapter the initial interview of a man with a history of two suicide attempts was presented. Let us briefly return to this case to note how psychological tests were used in gaining a clearer understanding of his problems. Of immediate concern were the following questions: What is the likelihood of another suicide attempt? How depressed is the client? How much personally stressful material can he confront in therapy without precipitating a crisis? These are questions to which the therapist has perhaps already formulated some tentative answers; however, because of the critical nature of the issues, the results of psychological testing can serve as important additional information.

Two objective tests were administered, along with one projective test. The Beck Depression Inventory was utilized to assess the severity of the client's negative, pessimistic mood and to identify specific symptoms associated with depression (sleep disturbances, loss of appetite, suicidal preoccupations, etc.). The MMPI was administered with two purposes: (1) as a screening device to obtain a general picture of the diagnostic classification that may be applicable and (2) using research based norms from an MMPI handbook (Dahlstrom, Welsh, and Dahlstrom, 1975) to assess this client's suicide potential. A projective instrument, the Thematic Apperception Test, was used in an attempt to identify inner need states and environmental stressors that may be related to the client's depressive-suicidal pattern.

The summary section of the psychometrist's (or tester's) report may serve to illustrate the utility of the test information:

Psychometric examination reveals a moderate to severe depression, which is characterized by deficits in self-care, regular work habits, and general activity level. A gloomy, pessimistic view of the future is coupled with clinical levels of anxiety, which together are producing a highly unstable emotional state at present. The strong anxiety did not become apparent during a routine interview, but the test data suggested intense preoccupations and fears about interpersonal rejection. This patient seems to be at a low ebb with regard to defenses and coping skills (other than the temporary relief afforded by alcohol) and is currently highly dependent on others for support and protection. Should these supports be withdrawn the test signs indicate the strong possibility of another suicide attempt.

Behavioral Observation Techniques

Recent years have seen a rise in techniques of systematic behavioral observations in the assessment of clients (see Ciminero, Calhoun, and Adams, 1977). An outgrowth of the expansion of behavioral therapies over the last twenty years, such observational techniques have as their hallmark the recording of discrete, well-defined units of behavior. This provides reasonably rigorous data as to the frequency of the behaviors or symptoms under study, as well as some hypotheses concerning the conditions under which they occur.

Several areas of difficulty are encountered with these techniques. Naturally, not all symptoms or problem behaviors are amenable to recording by outside observers. Such "private" symptoms as feelings of anger or depression cannot be directly measured. Similarly, it may not be feasible to have observers present under some circumstances. If such "private" processes are to be recorded, the subjects themselves have to be "observers" of their own behaviors and reactions, a procedure that necessarily raises questions about how reliably and accurately the data are gathered.

Other problems encountered in behavioral observation techniques are related to possible bias and irregularity by the observers. Since observers may employ different definitions regarding the occurrence of a behavior or may impose biased interpretations, it is important that clear and specific behavioral units be utilized. The degree to which observers agree is usually assessed prior to the actual observations, and data collection does not begin until the definitions of the units to be recorded are refined to the point where inter-observer agreement is high. Further difficulties arise in that the presence of an observer may alter the "natural" occurrence of the behaviors under study. For example, having a "stranger" in a classroom of children with behavior problems will probably prompt cautious, "company is here" reactions among the children and thereby mask their usual behavior patterns. This problem is usually dealt with in two ways: having the observer as a regular part of the environment so that initial inhibitions are dispelled, or recording the data unobtrusively (e.g., from behind a one-way mirror). This latter alternative, however, is frequently not feasible, either practically or ethically.

Two principal methods are employed in gathering behavioral information: time sampling techniques and continuous recording. In the former, selected time periods serve as the observation intervals. For example, on a busy ward in a psychiatric hospital a trained aide may randomly set aside five minutes every two hours to engage in careful recording of the behavior of a particular patient, and thereby accumulate data on a cross-section of behavior throughout the day. With continuous recording, a procedure is set up such that every occurrence of a particular behavior is noted, as for example with a client in a weight control program who keeps a record of how much and what type of food is ingested throughout the entire treatment period.

The advantage, of course, of direct observational techniques is that systematic data is collected on symptomatic behaviors over a period of time. Interpretive judgments and inferences are minimized (in contrast to those frequently required in psychological testing), and the increases and declines in the rate of problem behaviors can be studied in relation to changing life circumstances. In addition, these kinds of data also provide an opportunity to evaluate the behavioral or symptomatic changes that may result from treatment.

Behavior observations with the case example To continue with the client used to illustrate procedures in this chapter, the following observational techniques were instituted by the psychometrist who did the psychological testing. The client was instructed on how to keep an accurate log on the following occurrences: (1) when and how much alcohol he drank; (2) when and how intensively he felt depressed; and (3) the circumstances and who was involved whenever he felt rejected or "put down" by another person. His sister, with whom he was living at the time, was instructed in a time-sampling procedure of recording his mood at several intervals every day, noting episodes of drinking, and monitoring job attendance.

To illustrate the value of such material, the following partial data from the client's log for the two-day period following the psychological testing sessions are presented:

Thursday

7:30 a.m.: Woke up feeling kind of down. Needed a drink, but said no to myself. Fran [his sister] was grumpy at breakfast. Figured she was just tired. Mike [brother-in-law] said he couldn't pick me up after work because he has a meeting. Irritated and pretty depressed.

About 10:00 a.m.: Work was a bummer. Felt bored and depressed. Supervisor looked at me like I was not working fast enough. Needed a break then.

12:30 p.m.: Had two beers and a shot of whisky. Had lunch with Jimmy at Ryan's bar, and had some laughs.

4:00 p.m.: Feeling okay until now. Supervisor said he was putting me on another machine tomorrow. Said because Tom was sick. Asked him, why me, since I'd not been feeling well. He said you'll do it. Mad, depressed a lot.

4:30 p.m.: Back at Ryan's, can't remember how much drinking. Eight or nine boilermakers. Having a good time. The guys were really loose and kidding a lot.

11:00 p.m.: Needed a ride home. Called Fran. She sounded mad. Blew my lid and told her off. Drank some more. Really down. Got a ride home with somebody.

Friday

7:30 a.m.: Too sick to work, asked Fran to call in. She was cool, gave me the silent treatment. Took a long pull on the bottle, and settled down.

11:00 a.m.: Depressed and sick all morning. Watching TV. Fran made some eggs and said something nice. Trying to make it up to me for last night. Couldn't control it. I started bawling like a baby.

5:00 p.m.: Had good day. Opened up to Fran and told her how unhappy I was. Seemed to be getting through.

7:00 p.m.: Mike arrived, and gave me some crap about missing work. Doesn't understand how hard I'm trying. I just kept quiet. Fran took my side and Mike left, real upset.

11:30 p.m.: Watched TV with Fran, and went to bed. Feeling okay.

In studying this log, it is possible to arrive at some reasonably precise measures of the amount of alcohol intake and to make some judgments about fluctuations in mood. In a rough fashion, estimates can also be made of the degree of interpersonal rejection or acceptance he perceives in each of the reported incidents. In quantifying these data, the degree of depression, for example, was placed on a 0 to 5 scale, with the higher numbers representing more severe despondency. Similarly, the acceptance-rejection dimension was represented by a scale from +2 (strong acceptance) to −2 (strong rejection). To illustrate the interplay between mood and interpersonal process with this client, the depression and interpersonal data are plotted on the same coordinates in Fig. 3.1. As can be seen in this figure, a strong relationship is apparent between these two processes, suggesting (as did our earlier data on this client) that his episodes of depression may be triggered by interpersonal rejection and removal of emotional supports.

Not only does this type of analysis provide additional information for the pretherapy assessment of the client, it also establishes a multiple set of *baseline* measures pertaining to three major problem areas of his life. As such these measures, if continued during and after the treatment period, can represent a standard against which to evaluate therapeutic progress and success.

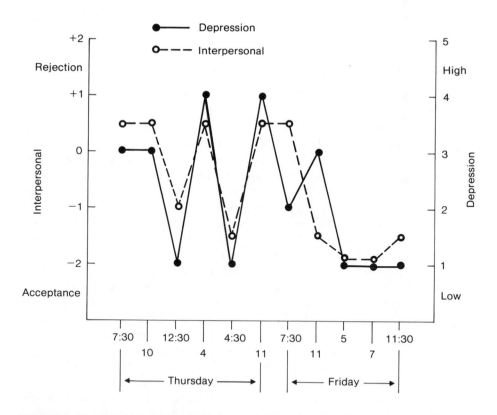

Figure 3.1 Graph of depressed client's moods and feelings of interpersonal acceptance and rejection. Data gathered from personal log of client over a two-day period.

Assessment and the Intake Process

This chapter has reviewed some of the principal methods by which to initiate a therapeutic contact and also to gather systematic information about a client's problems and current psychological status. Careful attention to these procedures, as well as analysis of the varied sources of information, provides the groundwork for some critically important decisions regarding therapeutic goals and procedures. Recall that in Chapter 1 a framework was suggested for organizing one's thinking about treatment goals: crisis management, behavioral change, corrective emotional experiences, and self-exploration. Preliminary decisions regarding which of these goals is most appropriate for a client are based on the intake information. As was also discussed in Chapter 1, the goals that are formulated dictate, to a large extent, the actual treatment approach with which to begin therapy with the client.

Prior to making these decisions, the therapist must be able to assess and organize the intake information into a formulation of the client's psychological-behavioral problems—a process that requires a conceptual framework of personality functioning and maladjustment. In the next chapter such a conceptualization will be presented.

UNRESOLVED ISSUES AND FUTURE DIRECTIONS

The entire field of personality assessment seems to be at a crossroads in current-day practice. There is still a strong, ongoing tradition to utilize a combination of interview data and psychological tests to evaluate clients. However, as noted in this chapter, each of these methods has its shortcomings and limitations. The increasing popularity of behavioral observation procedures seems to reflect attempts to overcome these deficiencies—too heavy a reliance on clinicians' inferences, assessments that are too vague and global, and questionable validity of test interpretations.

Some of the underlying assumptions of personality tests have been questioned, and it is these conceptual issues that probably will receive a great deal of attention in the future. The main area of contention has to do with the concept of *personality traits*. The critics' arguments proceed as follows: Many of the interpretations that are made from test scores refer to enduring personality traits of clients (e.g., client X is a habitually aggressive person). A growing number of theorists (e.g., Mischel, 1976; Endler and Magnusson, 1976) argue that the concept of long-term traits is not supported by research data. Rather, they argue that people's behaviors vary considerably depending on the situation they are in; thus personality assessment should focus on the likelihood of specific behaviors occurring under specific circumstances.

This "interactional approach" basically suggests that it is difficult to study personality variables alone. They can be assessed only in relation to specified circumstances and situations. Trait theorists counter this argument by maintaining that certain behavioral patterns do indeed recur over and over again in the lives of individuals—perhaps because certain situations also recur (or are perceived to recur) frequently in the person's life.

Whatever the eventual resolution of this debate, many contemporary therapists are becoming more cautious in their approach to personality assessment. Diagnostic test reports today are likely to focus on maladaptive behaviors that occur under specified circumstances, rather than as global traits. This trend towards specificity suggests that assessment involves increasing reliance on behavioral observations and careful analysis of the client's social ecology.

CHAPTER FOUR

THE INTAKE PHASE: EVALUATING INTAKE INFORMATION AND DECISION MAKING

INTRODUCTION

At this point in the therapy process we have reviewed procedures involved in the opening contact with the client, the initial interview, psychological testing, observational techniques, and the gathering of adjunct information from such sources as the family, medical exams, and so forth. This opening phase has two primary functions: establishing a professional working relationship with the client and accumulating sufficient information with which to understand the client's problems and make treatment decisions. Arriving at a formulation of the problems is a joint task faced by both the client and the therapist. The client supplies not only information and test data, but in many instances also takes an active role in interpreting the sources of stress and the long-term life patterns that are involved.

Evaluating and organizing the intake information into a meaningful picture is not an easy task. It requires skills in integrating data from a variety of sources, and additionally, it involves interpreting the information within a conceptual framework. This latter theoretical component of the process presents particular problems because of the many and varied conceptual approaches to understanding personality that exist in the field today. Rather than focusing on any one of these theories, the present chapter will suggest a general and eclectic framework that emphasizes an analysis of the client's *current adjustment patterns*. Such an approach should provide a basic orientation to client assessment that can later be refined and elaborated by the advanced student.

Four basic decisions are required at this intake stage of therapy: (1) Should the agency or therapist accept the client for treatment, or will the client be better served by a referral to another treatment source? (2) If accepted, what are the appropriate goals of therapy? (3) What will be the most effective treatment methods by which to meet these goals? and (4) Who will be the most effective therapist? Evaluation of the intake information is basically oriented toward answering these four questions.

In the following sections we will review the organization and assessment of the intake data, decision processes regarding the four questions cited above, and the providing of feedback and explanation to the client.

ORGANIZATION AND ASSESSMENT OF THE INTAKE INFORMATION

Data collected during the intake procedures, gathered from a variety of sources, provides a view of the client from several perspectives. Naturally, none of these sources has perfect validity. The client may be defensive in the interview, the psychological tests contain sources of error, and family reports may be self-serving. Hence a degree of caution is needed in evaluating this material. Perhaps the best rule of thumb is to look for consistencies across the various sources of information. For example, if in the interview the client speaks of high levels of debilitating anxiety, if this is also cited by family members, and if such indications are reflected in the test data, then we have converging evidence in support of this symptom. Conversely, when the data on a particular issue are conflicting or only partially consistent, the evaluation can be made only in a tentative fashion until further information is collected. Naturally, experienced clinicians also rely on speculation and hunches based on partial evidence; however, when these are included in an evaluation report, they should be recognized and labeled as such.

A convenient method by which to organize and interpret the intake data involves three interrelated areas of analysis. This is an approach used by many therapists to formulate an assessment of the client and is applicable to organizing a verbal presentation of the case to an intake staff or supervisor, as well as serving as an outline for written reports. The three areas are: (1) an *objective description* of the client's symptoms or behavioral-emotional problems, (2) an *evaluation* of the areas of living that are debilitated by these problems and an assessment of the degree of debilitation, and (3) an *analysis* of the factors that are producing and maintaining the problems and symptoms. Recommendations regarding treatment goals, type of therapy, therapist, or referral to alternate sources of help are outgrowths of this three-stage assessment process.

Objective Description of Problems

The objective description of the client's problems is the one relying most heavily on direct information and objective test data gathered during the intake procedures. The aim here is to describe as accurately as possible the symptoms, behavioral patterns, emotional reactions, conflicts, environmental stresses, and interpersonal-social factors that seem to form the basis of the client's distress and problems. Naturally, the particular focus will vary depending on the nature of the difficulties, but to some extent all of these areas are considered with each client.

Such descriptive material usually deals with "factual" components of the client's problems, such as readily observable reaction patterns, first-hand reports of emotions and attitudes, objective reports of the client's environment, and direct assessments from psychological test data. Relatively little inference or interpretation of underlying motivations or causal factors is called for in this section of the evaluation. Rather, careful attention must be paid to the frequency of occurrence and intensity of symptoms, as well as to the circumstances under which they occur.

Several other issues of concern should be covered in this descriptive material. One pertains to the length of time that the client has manifested these problems. In making therapy decisions later in this process, for example, it may make a difference whether the client has undergone a gradual onset of symptoms over a period of months or years, as contrasted with a sudden eruption of problems within the past few days or weeks. A second dimension that requires consideration concerns the primary locus of the difficulties—pressures and stresses from the environment that are producing problems or behavioral-emotional patterns that are characteristic of the client and probably would be manifested regardless of environmental factors. Again, such general considerations may well have a bearing on later decisions regarding appropriate areas of therapeutic intervention.

Naturally, the range of psychological difficulties with which therapists deal is extremely broad. In addition, each client presents a unique constellation of behaviors, emotions, and environmental factors, making it virtually impossible to offer a complete listing of the possible syndromes to be assessed. However, a compilation of the major classes of problems may be of assistance in orienting the student to the kinds of disturbances that are encountered.

The following outline is drawn from the American Psychiatric Association's *Diagnostic and Statistical Manual of Mental Disorders* (DSM III) (1980) which is the standard system for classification and diagnosis in the United States. The latest revision of the diagnostic manual contains some important improvements over earlier versions: (1) the symptoms associated with the various disorders are spelled out in greater detail; (2) an attempt is made to relate specific symptoms with more enduring personality patterns in the client; (3) the system requires a judgment about the severity of psychosocial stress in the client's life; and (4) judgments are required about a client's level of functioning in terms of the highest level of adaptation displayed during the past year. The following outline will not reflect these features of the system, nor will this section review some of the controversial aspects of the DSM III. For now, attention is drawn only to the vast array of problems that are covered. These problem areas are outlined as follows:

1. *Disorders usually first evident in infancy, childhood, or adolescence:* Includes problems of mental retardation, attentional deficits, various conduct problems (as for example, undersocialized aggressiveness), anxiety reactions, eating problems, disorders involving physical symptoms (e.g., stuttering, bed-wetting, sleepwalking), and such pervasive developmental disorders as autism.

2. *Organic mental disorders:* Involves impairment of brain functions that may result in deficits in orientation, memory, general intellectual functions, or changes in personality and emotional functioning. Includes symptoms associated with senility, substance-induced organic changes, and traumatic brain damage.

3. *Substance use disorders:* Deficits associated with either abuse of or outright dependence on such substances as alcohol, barbiturates, opiates, cocaine, amphetamines, and so on.

4. *Schizophrenic disorders:* Major behavioral and thinking disorders where the impairment is to a degree that ordinary life demands cannot be met.

5. *Paranoid disorders:* Includes serious problems involving delusions of persecution or delusional jealousy in which emotions and behavior are consistent with the content of the delusional system.

6. *Affective disorders:* Problems involving serious disorder of mood and related behaviors, which include mania, depression, and mixed (manic-depressive) symptoms.

7. *Anxiety disorders:* Involves generally neurotic disorders in which fear and panic are the major symptoms. Includes the various phobias, general anxiety states, obsessive-compulsive disorders, an posttraumatic-stress reactions.

8. *Somatoform disorders:* Problems involving physical symptoms for which there is no evidence of medical disorder, physical injury, or side effects of medication, drugs, or alcohol. Includes such neurotic categories as conversion reactions (e.g., a paralyzed arm) and hypochondria.

9. *Dissociative disorders:* Involves problems of memory about important personal information that go beyond mere forgetfulness. Includes such disorders as amnesia, multiple personality, and depersonalization.

10. *Psychosexual disorders:* Difficulties in sexual identity, unusual sexual attachments, child molesting, exhibitionism, sadistic or masochistic sexual patterns, or various problems in carrying out normal sexual functions.

11. *Disorders of impulse control:* Specific problems not covered in other categories, such as pathological gambling, kleptomania (compulsive stealing), and so forth.

12. *Adjustment disorders:* Varied maladaptive reactions to identifiable stresses that typically involve overreactions or prolonged symptoms to the stress. Includes such difficulties as depressive or anxious mood, work inhibitions, and social withdrawal.

13. *Personality disorders:* Generally maladaptive behavioral and interpersonal patterns of long standing that typically result in social or occupational problems and disruption. Included are habitual patterns of suspiciousness, social withdrawal, antisocial activity, dependency, narcissism, passive-aggressiveness, and so on.

14. *Conditions not attributable to mental disorders:* Problem areas that are treatable but that represent specific environmental adjustment problems rather than a mental disorder. Includes such difficulties as occupational, academic, or marital problems, bereavement, change in phase of life, and so forth.

It should be kept in mind that this outline was presented not as a vehicle for diagnostic labeling (although it is frequently used that way) but rather to introduce the reader to the possible range of syndromes that may be encountered. The difficult job of actually describing the behavioral, emotional, and situational aspects of each unique client's problems represents the major task facing the therapist.

Evaluation of Debilitation

The second step in client assessment involves an analysis of the areas of living that are adversely affected by the client characteristics described above. This analysis is still closely tied to the objective data, but obviously some degree of clinical judgment is also called for when evaluating the degree of debilitation. Three broad areas are usually considered in this evaluation: debilitated adjustment to the environment, impairment of mental and physical functions, and intrapsychic distress.

Adjustment to the environment obviously covers a broad spectrum of issues. An important concern here is the question of how the client's problems are affecting interpersonal relations. Are family and friends a part of the client's life? What is the quality of these relationships? Are others remaining steadfast and supportive? Are they frightened, angry, withdrawn, exploitive? Or are they behaving in ways that subtly foster even more severe debilitation of the client? Second, an evaluation of the ways in which the client's problems are affecting work/school performance, relations with coworkers, classmates, and supervisors, rate of absenteeism, and overall job security is another major area of concern. Third, an estimate of what might be called relations with the community is of importance. Included here would be such considerations as police-legal problems, financial complications (e.g., possible foreclosure, bankruptcy, need for emergency social assistance), difficulties with neighbors, and so forth.

It is almost a truism to say that many psychological problems stem from disturbed relationships with one's environment. Once symptoms or maladaptive behavior patterns are set in motion by this disturbed person-environmental interaction, the environment (family, boss, legal agencies, etc.) in turn reacts to the symptoms. These reactions can be benign, supportive, and constructive, or they can be rejecting, punitive, and destructive; in effect compounding the problems and perpetuating a process of continued or even worsening maladjustment. With this in mind, the evaluation of the client's psychological status involves not only how he or she is *currently* adjusting to the environment, but also where the processes seem to be going. If left untended, are there self-correcting factors occurring in the client-environmental interaction, or is the process destined for increased distress and more serious symptoms?

The second major area of evaluation pertains to mental and physical functions. Regarding mental processes, information gathered from psychological tests, work/school records, and reports from teachers, supervisors, and so on, are particularly helpful in assessing any intellectual performance deficits or any recent changes in these functions. Of special interest in these areas are data pertaining to unusual or illogical thought patterns, inabilities to concentrate or carry out sustained mental activities, memory or perceptual difficulties, or unusual problems of motivation.

Because of the seriousness of these types of problems, it is important that a careful assessment be made of the degree and generality of these deficits.

With respect to physical problems that may be related to the client's psychological condition, it is obvious that physicians' reports and prior medical records are of critical importance. Clearly, a wide variety of psychological symptoms have a physiological cause (e.g., certain nutritional diseases, biochemical imbalance, toxic disorders, brain damage), and these possibilities require careful medical diagnosis. In addition, even when physical symptoms are likely just side effects of psychological-emotional problems, an assessment of the physical disabilities necessitates medical consultation. At the symptomatic level, clinicians usually are attuned to such problems as sleep disturbances, changes in sexual function, unusual dietary patterns, obvious physical symptoms (e.g., paralyses, perceptual loss), possible drug and alcohol related symptoms, unusual states of consciousness, and, of course, reports indicating potential psychophysiological disorders (high blood pressure, skin disturbances, gastrointestinal symptoms, and so forth). In evaluating the severity of these types of problems and their likely future course, a carefully integrated assessment of psychological and medical reports is necessary.

The third area of evaluation pertains to the client's level of internal distress. Information on this issue comes largely from the client's self-report, from the psychological test data, and from observations made by the client's family and others. The principal emotions and drives to be assessed in this realm are anxiety, depression, low self-esteem, guilt, unusual sexual impulses, anger, loneliness, and the general meaning and direction attributed to one's life. As part of this analysis, naturally the quality and strength of these internal processes are estimated. In addition, how the client controls or expresses them, how they may conflict with each other, and how they interfere with daily functioning is also evaluated.

With some clients these assessments are of critical importance in that unusually strong distress may signal a high-risk situation. If, for example, anxiety is approaching intolerable, paniclike levels, the client may be prone to react in an impulsive, uncontrolled fashion in an attempt to gain relief, or may be driven into a psychotic episode involving disturbed thought processes, bizarre behavior, and withdrawal from reality. Similarly, depression raises the spector of suicide, while rage and poorly controlled sexual impulses obviously constitute potential risks for others. Thus, in addition to an analysis of how much a client is psychologically "hurting," this section of the evaluation frequently indicates the "danger signals" regarding high-risk problems.

To sum up, we are now partway through the suggested outline for the organization and conceptualization of intake information. The client's problems have been described in some detail, and the areas of debilitation have been assessed. The quality of current adjustment has been evaluated and the analysis has included attempts to estimate the likely course of adjustment in the future. The formulation is now at a point where the therapist takes what information is available on causal factors that underlie the current problems and makes some educated speculations about these roots. In this next section we frequently see the therapist's theoretical biases emerging, a process that can be helpful in gaining a deeper understanding of the client, but also risks imposing a point of view that is not completely consonant with the realities of the client's psychological state.

Causal and Maintaining Factors

Let us begin this section with a brief example that highlights the importance of this level of analysis. Each night, when put to bed, a three-year-old cries violently and shows signs of strong distress. Because of this, his parents sit with him for prolonged periods of time, until he finally drops off to sleep. Should they leave prematurely, the screaming returns with great intensity and continues until they reappear in his room. This pattern, having gone on for months, is obviously very disturbing to the parents and also totally disrupts their evening activities.

One day a well-meaning relative, who has had several courses in child psychology, casually remarks that the child's problem is obvious. The parents, by being attentive each time the child cries, have been inadvertently reinforcing this behavior; hence, over a period of months, the child's tantrumlike reactions have become progressively worse. The relative recommends that the parents put the child to bed, taking only a normal amount of time to get him settled. After that the parents should let the three-year-old cry and scream without reentering his room. The relative explains that by not rewarding such behaviors the crying should extinguish over a period of time and the family schedule can return to normal.

Three important issues can be raised with regard to this example. First is the general point that treatment recommendations are a frequent outgrowth of the analysis of causal and maintaining factors. In this case, viewing the child's symptoms as resulting from a simple reinforcement mechanism dictates a treatment based on extinction procedures. A second point pertains to the fact that the causal analysis, to a considerable extent, is colored by the particular theoretical point of view of the observer—in the present example, a behavioral orientation. The interpretation given by the relative seems to be consistent with the facts of the case, as far as they are known; however, one is left with the uneasy feeling that the analysis was presented too casually and easily, without sufficient efforts to obtain all the possible information regarding the child's problem. The danger in following a particular theoretical orientation too rigidly, of course, is that the therapist may selectively seek out only certain kinds of diagnostic information and thereby overlook important aspects of the case. This danger leads to the third point: the need for caution in avoiding premature conceptualizations, attending to all the relevant data, and considering the case from a variety of orientations before arriving at the one that fits the information most appropriately. In the present example, consider the potentially tragic consequences if the child's crying was not based on the reinforcement mechanism proposed by the relative. If, in fact, the child's distress was due to an anxiety-related issue (e.g., night terrors), how frightful it would be to simply leave him alone night after night to face the terror "cold turkey," under the mistaken assumption that all he was seeking was parental attention.

With this cautionary preface, a framework for analyzing the factors that underlie and maintain symptoms will be proposed. The five categories that compose this system are not meant to be mutually exclusive or all-encompassing; however, they may serve the student as a convenient set of guidelines for understanding the roots of a client's problems.

The first possibility to consider is that symptoms may stem from *biological-organic causes*, including brain damage, biochemical disorders, intake of toxic substances, nutritional deficiencies, or other physiological dysfunctions. Where correctable or controllable, such biological factors obviously dictate medical intervention. In addition, however, analysis of psychological-behavioral contributors to such problems (e.g., failure to follow a proper diet, alcoholism, resistance to a prescribed medical regimen, stressful life-style) serves to provide a more complete and potentially helpful picture of the underlying physical disorder.

Second, one may entertain the hypothesis that a client's problems are due to *behavioral or emotional learning deficits*, that is, lack of appropriate learning experiences that normally occur in the lives of individuals. Included in this general category would be deficiencies in the acquisition of various social or intellectual skills, failure to acquire appropriate controls and restraints on behaviors, or gaps in emotional development (e.g., absence of significant parental models or early emotional deprivation experiences).

A third category that may offer a means of understanding the processes that underlie symptoms is *inappropriate social learning*. In contrast to the previous category, which focused on the absence of certain learning experiences, this set of factors deals with clients who have learned deviant or ineffective behavioral-emotional patterns. An example of this level of analysis might be the client who has grown up in a family where the parents, because of their own problems, encouraged and rewarded an aggressive, domineering, and egocentric pattern of relating to siblings and playmates—a learned way of dealing with others that is producing considerable strife for the client as a young adult.

The fourth category of analysis pertains to *ineffective methods of coping with stress*. Throughout life people are faced with various forms or degrees of stress, both external (e.g., aggression from others, unexpected tragedies, possibility of failure, poverty) and internal (strong anxiety, guilt, insoluble conflict, etc.). Individuals usually evolve characteristic ways of coping with stressors, thereby overcoming or meeting environmental pressures and also maintaining a degree of internal equilibrium. Furthermore, most psychologically robust individuals have acquired effective and multiple coping strategies, such that in circumstances where one particular strategy does not appear to be working, another means of adjustment can be invoked. On the other hand, people prone to psychological difficulties may have developed insufficient depth of coping techniques (defenses) and hence become debilitated under stress, or they utilize defenses that themselves produce psychological or interpersonal problems.

Finally, the therapist may look for deviant *attitudes, morality,* or *philosophical orientations* as explanatory concepts. Factors such as these can obviously exert a major influence on the entire life-style of an individual, affecting relations with others, community, religion, and ultimately, the very direction and meaning given to one's existence.

It is recognized that the foregoing material is detailed and complex. Therapists have to take information from a wide variety of sources and arrive at an integrated description of the client. Hopefully, this suggested method of organizing and reporting the information, also outlined in Table 4.1, will serve as a helpful guide.

Table 4.1
The organization of intake information

Information gathered during intake: interview, tests, observations by others, consultants' reports, client's self-observations →

1. Objective description of symptoms and problems
   a) Frequency and intensity
   b) Onset and duration
   c) Circumstances under which symptoms occur
   d) Environmental factors and stresses

2. Estimated degree and focus of debilitation
   a) Adjustment to environment
   b) Mental and physical functions
   c) Intrapsychic distress
   d) Risk factors
   e) Strengths and environmental supports
   f) Likely future course

3. Analysis of causal and maintaining factors
   a) Biological-organic factors
   b) Learning deficits
   c) Inappropriate social learning
   d) Ineffective coping with stress
   e) Deviant attitudes, morality, philosophy

→ Treatment decisions

TREATMENT DECISIONS

The three-stage process of organizing and evaluating the data on the client is now complete. The individual therapist (or the intake staff at a clinic or hospital) has obtained (1) a reasonably objective description of the client's symptoms, behavioral problems, and/or internal areas of distress; (2) an evaluation of the areas of living that are debilitated by these problems, as well as estimates of the degree of debilitation; and (3) an analysis of the factors in the client's history that brought about the problems, as well as processes in the client's current life that are maintaining them.

The intake process has progressed to the point of decision making regarding treatment or referral. Should the client be accepted for treatment? If so, what should be the goals and most effective therapy approach? Who would be the most appropriate therapist? As will be seen in the next sections, there is at least partial research evidence that can serve as an aid in making some of these decisions, but with others, therapists still have to use clinical judgment, theory-based assumptions, and plain common sense in answering these questions.

Acceptance for Treatment

The decision to accept a client for treatment or to refer the client to another agency is based on numerous factors. Foremost, of course, is the question of whether or not the therapist (or agency staff) has the competencies and experience to work with a particular problem. A second issue pertains to the availability of alternate sources of treatment in the community that may be more appropriate for the client. And third, also obvious, is the current treatment load of the therapist; that is, does acceptance mean a long waiting period before treatment can actually begin?

Also involved in this decision are more complex issues concerning the likelihood that the client will remain in treatment and will profit from it. Such questions are particularly relevant when the work load of the therapist (or agency) is approaching its maximum. Under these circumstances, the concern becomes the difficult one of providing services for the most likely beneficiaries, while referring or delaying treatment for others. Difficult as such decisions may be, the limited and overcrowded mental health facilities in many communities unfortunately force this issue upon us.

Considerable research evidence is available pertaining to clients who have relatively poor prospects of profiting from treatment or who are likely to drop out prematurely. As might be expected, those who are unmotivated for therapy or who have been coerced into seeking help are relatively poor risks. Additionally, clients who view their problems as caused by physical or environmental factors rather than personal psychological processes, or who do not have a reasonable understanding of treatment also have a reduced likelihood of success (see Garfield, 1978).

Numerous studies have also shown that, generally, the more disturbed a client is, the less likely he or she is to seek out therapy, be accepted, stay in treatment once it is started, or profit from treatment (Garfield, 1971, 1978). This suggests the paradoxical situation that those who ultimately receive complete treatment are the clients who are least likely to need it. As we saw in a previous chapter, evidence also indicates that individuals from poor socio-economic and educational segments of the population are less likely to be accepted for treatment (Garfield, 1978; Korchin, 1980). Recognition of these shortcomings in mental health services has led to many contemporary efforts to expand treatment facilities and to develop more effective approaches with underserved clients (e.g., Goldstein, 1973).

A number of well-designed investigations have studied ways of improving low-income clients' attitudes and expectations about therapy. The usual procedure is to meet with a client prior to treatment, and during this session to accomplish several aims: (1) explain the overall process of psychotherapy; (2) describe and explain the specific procedures that will be involved; (3) provide a description of the roles to be played by both therapist and client; and (4) forewarn the client about possible problems with motivation and resistance to treatment. In general, the studies in this area report positive results in terms of lowered drop-out rates, more positive treatment outcomes, and generally high client satisfaction with treatment (Heitler, 1976; Lorion, 1978). These benefits are also seen during actual treatment sessions themselves in that "prepared" clients are more communicative, exploratory and show more initiative than do "unprepared" clients (Heitler, 1973).

An interesting sidelight in these studies is the finding that "prepared" clients are seen as more attractive and less threatening by their therapists. This result seems to highlight the importance of doing preliminary work on attitudes with both clients and therapists—in effect, to lower the barriers on both sides of the fence. Although not definitive, the research suggests that such double preparation may indeed maximize the attractiveness of treatment for low-income clients.

Needless to say the decision to accept a client for treatment is a complex one, involving consideration of client variables, available resources, and therapist qualifications. Fundamental to weighing all these factors, however, are therapists' ethical responsibilities to provide appropriate services to those in need and to work in one's community to continually improve mental health resources.

Goals of Treatment

The decision to accept a client is followed by consideration of the goals of treatment. Again, multiple issues operate in this determination, including, of course, the nature and severity of the client's problems, causal and maintaining factors, and the client's capabilities and motivation for treatment.

As indicated in Chapters 1 and 2, specific goals are usually developed in consultation with the client. Understandably, these should be tailored to the client's needs and particular life circumstances. In addition, the treatment objectives should be well defined and, where possible, have criteria of success specified for each. In this fashion the stage is set for focused and cost-effective treatment.

Unfortunately, this ideal approach to goal setting is frequently not possible at the intake stage of therapy. Not enough relevant information may have been gathered, or some clients may be too distressed or confused to formulate long-range goals. Indeed, with some complex cases, the relevant problems may not yet have come to light. Thus in many instances the early stages of therapy itself may be used to "home in on" and refine the goals of treatment.

In Chapter 1 a framework of four broad classes of treatment goals was proposed. These classes may be viewed as first approximations to the specific sets of objectives that are gradually developed with each client. The four classifications should thus be viewed as a tentative set of guidelines to aid students in conceptualizing the various directions that therapy can take. These broad classes of goals are: (1) crisis management, (2) behavioral change, (3) corrective emotional experience, and (4) self-exploration and change. Now that we have had an opportunity to review intake and assessment procedures, we can examine these goals more closely. As will be seen in future sections, decisions regarding the aims of treatment dictate to a large degree the initial therapy strategies to be used.

Goals of crisis management Most therapistss or agencies get their share of psychological emergencies—clients who for one reason or another require immediate help to forestall impending disaster. In many such instances the crisis aspects of the situation are apparent, and the information gathered during intake serves only to provide specific details of the high-risk condition.

The term *crisis*, of course, is subject to varying interpretations; however, most clinicians generally agree upon several broad categories that are so designated. The first pertains to clients who have had a "normal" history but who have recently undergone an overwhelming traumatic experience with which they are unable to cope. The precipitant may be an unexpected death of a loved one, severe battlefield conditions, the breakup of a relationship, loss of job, victimization as in rape or physical assault, and so forth. The feature of all such events, however, that defines them as a crisis is the client's marked debilitation of even routine functions, or the risk of some impulsive, destructive reaction (to self or others) that only would compound the tragedy.

A second category pertains to clients who are undergoing what may be termed, "runaway emotions"—negative affective states of such extremity that abilities to concentrate, pursue logical thought processes, exercise adequate judgment, or maintain appropriate controls on behavior are impaired. High states of anxiety, depression, and anger seem to be the principal offenders here, and as discussed above, these highly charged emotional states increase the vulnerability of the client to even more serious consequences. These risks of impulsive "acting out," suicide, or a psychotic adjustment are of principal concern and thus require immediate management.

There is obviously overlap of these clients with those in the first category (normals under severe situational stress); however, in this second group, we frequently encounter individuals who have had a history of psychological maladjustment. Representative of this type of client is one who for a long period of time has displayed the neurotic symptoms of avoiding even routine problem situations in their lives, rigidly not thinking about disturbing emotions, impulses, or fantasies and continually focusing only on trivial pleasantries. This incomplete sketch of a hysterical neurosis is thus characterized by the long-term use of repression and avoidance as mechanisms for coping with internal and external difficulties. Occasionally in the lives of such clients, these repressive defenses are not adequate in dealing with particularly strong emotions or an unusually provocative situation, and the client is dramatically confronted with intensely disturbing feelings, thoughts, or impulses. Perhaps it is the client's lack of practice in managing such personal confrontations or the sudden shock of a wrenching change in one's self-perception, but a frequent outcome is debilitating levels of fright, guilt, or anger. The accompanying sense of becoming overwhelmed and being unable to manage or understand these reactions is what makes this a crisis situation, in what in this example can be termed a "decompensating" neurotic client.

A third category of clients for whom crisis management is the appropriate treatment goal, are those with acute psychotic reactions. Psychoses generally refer to conditions in which an individual is seriously distorting or is withdrawn from reality, engaging in illogical thought processes, displaying markedly inappropriate emotions, or is apparently undergoing bizarre or grotesque experiences. Many therapists distinguish between acute and chronic phases of psychosis (particularly in schizophrenic syndromes), with the latter pertaining to withdrawn, underresponsive, largely unemotional vegetative states as might be seen in many long-term residents of state mental hospitals. In contrast, "acute" phases of psychosis usually refer to highly emotional, bizarre, and active episodes of psychotic symptoms that frequently occur in the early stages of the disorder. Because these acute episodes often involve intense emotions, unpredictable behavioral outbursts, and primitive forms of thought, they can be considered as threats to the safety of the client and others, and thus they constitute crisis situations. (Clients displaying the chronic syndrome, being relatively inactive and unresponsive, do not seem to represent crises in the same immediate sense and therefore call for other treatment goals; see below).

The last category of clients requiring crisis management are those with acute psychoticlike reactions resulting from specific physiological insult. "Bad trips" from drugs, alcoholic delerium tremors, reactions to toxic substances, or highly disturbed states related to brain damage fall into this group. Again, overwhelming emotions, uncontrolled and unpredictable behaviors, or illogical thought process may combine to produce a temporary but highly volatile situation of considerable risk to the client and others.

Having reviewed these various client categories, we can now step back and gain some perspective on the commonalities and risk factors involved and thereby consider some of the specific goals of crisis management. First, note that the categories typically involve strong negative emotional states with which the client cannot cope. Second, each category implies a relatively high risk of impulsive and ill-considered behavioral acting out. And third, in varying degrees, the categories describe debilitation of logical thought processes. These areas of deficit dictate, then, the three principal goals of crisis management: (1) reducing emotional levels to a point where the client does not feel overwhelmed by them; (2) enhancing controls on behavior by strengthening the client's self-monitoring and self-restraining capabilities, or where necessary, imposing external restrictions to aid in behavioral control; and (3) strengthening the client's rational problem-solving approach to both inner conflicts and environmental stressors.

A review of treatment techniques by which to accomplish these goals will be presented in Chapter 5. Suffice it to say for now that, although crisis management may represent relatively short-term, focused treatment in emergency situations, both the technical and emotional demands on the therapist are immense and require a unique kind of commitment.

Goals of behavioral change Many clients who enter treatment do so because they seek help with a specific, identifiable symptom or behavioral pattern that is producing difficulties in their lives. Such clients are frequently uninterested in or incapable of a wide-ranging uncovering and analysis of hidden fantasies, deep emotions, or childhood traumas. Rather, they are hopeful of receiving focused and direct help for a circumscribed problem.

The prospect of focusing treatment on symptom removal touches on an important conceptual controversy that has rippled through the field for several decades. Therapists who adhere to a psychodynamic view of therapy argue that merely treating symptoms or bringing about behavioral change is doing an incomplete job. Such therapists suggest that therapy should treat the underlying emotional conflicts that are causing the surface problems. This viewpoint has been called the "medical model" because of the analogous processes that occur in some physical illnesses: for example, a fever (symptom) that is caused by an underlying viral infection. The other half of the controversy is represented by behavior therapists, who argue that removing troublesome symptoms or changing inappropriate behaviors are valued goals of therapy in and of themselves. Underlying this point of view is an attempt to build a scientific basis for treatment that deals with observable (and measurable) behaviors rather than inferred constructs such as unconscious processes, id-superego conflicts, and so forth.

While this controversy is of general theoretical interest, it seems to recede into the background in the everyday, practical decisions that take place in a mental health facility. Consider the following two cases, which illustrate how practical, clinical judgment takes precedence over dogmatic allegiance to either the medical or behavioral models.

Mr. Smith is a twenty-five-year-old bachelor who comes to a clinic at the suggestion of friends. He is seeking therapy because he feels that he is too shy, socially inhibited, and emotionally restrained. He wants help in becoming outgoing, assertive, and more "loosened up" emotionally. On the basis of the intake interview, psychological tests, and family information it seems reasonably clear that he has been a quiet, retiring individual all of his life, such being the general climate and expectations within his family while growing up. Indeed, his parents also seemed to be introverted and unexpressive, thus providing consistent role models for his personality style. Given this background and the absence of other apparent problems in Smith's life, he appears to be a good candidate for a direct, behavioral approach to his difficulties—one that focuses on developing and practicing new social skills and encourages the lowering of inhibitions on emotional expression.

Now consider a second client, Mr. Brown, also a twenty-five-year-old bachelor, who comes to the clinic with exactly the same complaints (he is shy, socially inhibited, and emotionally restrained) and who, at the suggestion of friends, wants to become "loosened up." In Brown's case, however, as the intake information and test data are reviewed, a different set of background factors becomes apparent. Both of his parents were extremely abusive alcoholics, who frequently and unpredictably beat him throughout his upbringing. He reports being very disturbed by frequent nightmares involving uncontrolled, homicidal aggression in which he is sometimes the victim and sometimes the aggressor. Finally, the psychological tests also give strong indications of preoccupations with violence and grotesque forms of bodily injury.

Although Mr. Brown's characteristics are somewhat overdrawn, he is certainly not the type of client with whom a therapist would casually agree to his wishes to become more emotionally "loosened up" and unrestrained. A reasonable supposition in Brown's case is that his inhibited and constricted behavioral style serves the important function of controlling some awesome and potentially destructive emotional patterns in his personality.

The point being made here, then, is that merely attending to symptoms and directly observable behavioral patterns is insufficient in deciding on behavior change goals—even if the client specifically requests them. The therapist (or intake staff) must take the larger perspective of evaluating the observable behaviors and symptoms in terms of the apparent background factors and the current emotional status of the client. In Mr. Smith's case, the goal of helping him to change some maladroit social behaviors and methods of self-expression seems appropriate and in keeping with the evidence that he never had the opportunity to learn more satisfying interpersonal skills. Mr.

Brown's case, however, seems to call for a much more cautious approach and a more complex set of goals, which take into account the emotional vulnerabilities in his personality.

The foregoing material on choosing behavior change goals serves as a cautionary introduction. We can now review the types of problems for which these goals seem appropriate, keeping in mind the important assessment issues covered in the previous discussion.

Two broad classes of behavior problems/symptoms seem to be appropriate for behavior change goals: (1) difficulties stemming from behavioral deficits and (2) difficulties associated with the frequent use of inappropriate behaviors. In the first category there is a relative absence of certain adaptive response patterns, because the client never learned them, they were lost because of injury, or because the client is fearful of using them. Thus, with such "deficit" problems a substantial portion of therapy is devoted to teaching and practicing the desired response patterns, effecting a transfer of such learning to naturalistic settings, and reducing anxiety associated with these behaviors. The second group of problems are usually more complex in that the goals involve removing an undesirable behavior pattern and replacing it with a more appropriate one—a therapeutic endeavor that again most likely includes training, practice, transfer, and the management of anxiety, in addition to techniques to remove behaviors.

Within each of these general classes a wide range of problems are amenable to behavior change goals—some very specific and simple (e.g., a facial tic) and others more complicated, involving multiple behaviors, complex conditionings, and issues of self-regulation and cognitive control (e.g., alcoholism). It is impossible to list all the problems that fit these categories; however, perhaps mention of some representative instances will give the reader a sense of the wide range of applicability of behavioral goals. In the following material the two general classes will be distinguished, along with indication of the complexity of the processes involved (specific, intermediate, or complex).

Within the category of behavioral deficits, some examples of specific problems are the following: (1) a car accident victim, a year after a head injury, who continues to have some problems in perceptual-motor coordination that affect such skills as handwriting, using eating utensils, shaving, and so on; (2) a six-year-old child who has been a bed wetter all of his life; and (3) a middle-level business executive who has intellectual and verbal skills but feels unpracticed and unsure of himself when making a public address (e.g., a sales meeting or a speech at his club).

At the level of intermediate complexity, behavioral deficit problems can be illustrated by such clients as the following: (1) a shy, recently divorced middle-aged man who is unsure about how to form new relationships, go about dating, and generally manage heterosexual affairs; (2) a nineteen-year-old college sophomore who has been moderately depressed because she feels unable to organize her study habits and get the most out of her course work;

and (3) the parents of an unruly and rebellious eight-year-old, who sense that they have been inconsistent in methods of discipline.

Clients who represent complex behavior deficit problems are exemplified by the following: (1) a forty-year-old recent discharge from a mental hospital, currently living in a community half-way house. Having been in the hospital for fifteen years, this client has literally forgotten even such basic skills as dealing with a clerk at the grocery, maintaining an apartment, adhering to a work schedule, and so forth; and (2) a six-year-old autistic child who has never developed language, is completely incontinent, and exhibits virtually no controls on behavior.

In the general category of changing inappropriate behavior patterns we can again roughly arrange the problems on a complexity dimension. Specific difficulties can be represented by the following: (1) a chronic cigarette smoker seeking help in overcoming this unhealthy habit, and (2) a client suffering from muscle-tension headaches whose physician recommended biofeedback techniques. Problems in intermediate complexity include: (1) an otherwise adjusted client who has a phobia of riding in elevators; (2) a middle-aged father of three who frequently struggles with strong erotic impulses pertaining to women's shoes; and (3) a person with a recently diagnosed case of diabetes who is resisting appropriate self-care routines (dietary restrictions, administration of insulin, etc.). Problems at a complex level can be exemplified by: (1) a long-term alcohol abuser who is seeking to not only change his drinking patterns but also to develop new ways to cope with anxiety and frustration and restore a satisfying interpersonal climate in his family, and (2) a highly driven, competitive, and anxiety-ridden businessman whose heart condition requires that he change his life-style to a slower, more relaxed pace.

As can be noted from the foregoing, the goals of behavior change apply to a wide range of problems. In some instances a single and specific behavioral pattern is treated, while in others a wide range of interrelated problems are dealt with. Regardless of the complexity, however, a careful assessment of background factors, emotional correlates, and the general psychological status of the client is required in arriving at a determination of behavioral goals of treatment. The therapy techniques that have been found to be most helpful in achieving these goals will be reviewed in Chapter 6.

Goals related to corrective emotional experience The set of goals related to corrective emotional experience applies to a relatively small number of clients when one considers the broad range of problems that are covered in the mental health area. Nevertheless, individuals who come under this treatment goal frequently have highly visible and dramatic symptoms and often display equally dramatic positive responses to treatment.

A central feature of clients for whom corrective emotional experiences are an appropriate goal is a history of abuse, exploitation, or rejection by others. Such negative interpersonal experiences have in turn led to generalized attitudes of cynicism and mistrust of people and expectations that future interpersonal encounters will have similar outcomes. In addition, these attitudes and expectations prompt a variety of "protective" social behaviors, which are designed to ensure against further hurt or exploitation but paradoxically frequently result in increased interpersonal strife. The net result of such syndromes is that having been interpersonally dealt a bad hand to begin with, the client sets in motion processes that tend to perpetuate negative experiences and an even more cynical view of people.

The principal treatment goal with such clients is to utilize the *therapeutic relationship* itself to teach the client that (1) not all people are exploitive and rejecting; (2) the client's generalized protective behaviors tend to make the situation worse; and (3) under appropriate circumstances it can be safe to trust others and to enter into mutually respecting and affectionate relationships.

A variety of life circumstances can lead to this general syndrome, and as in earlier sections, several examples of commonly occurring patterns will hopefully provide some of the specific characteristics. Perhaps the most dramatic of such cases are young people (from eleven to sixteen years of age) for whom virtually all previous contacts with adults have led to their being rejected, punished, or ignored. Thus future encounters with adults most likely involve a combination of resentment, fear, and expectations of more harm. Furthermore, if such encounters cannot be avoided (e.g., teachers at school), a variety of protective behaviors can be observed, including: (1) being openly provocative and challenging (in effect, directly testing the strength of one's opponent); (2) being exploitive (beating the other to the punch); or (3) remaining surly, withdrawn, and passively aggressive ("I won't play your game"). As can be imagined, such behaviors have a high likelihood of provoking counteraggression or rejection by others, thereby fulfilling the client's expectations about the nature of the adult world. Were such patterns to extend into adulthood, the basis for an alienated, socially withdrawn life-style would likely be established.

A second group of clients who fit this general picture are young or middle-aged adults who have undergone one or more intimate relationships in which they ultimately felt psychologically abused and abandoned. With some individuals such experiences may result in a cynical, mistrustful set of expectations about people in general. The behavioral consequences of such patterns, while not as visible as those of the adolescents described earlier, may be equally maladaptive. Subtle characteristics involving emotional reserve, sensitivity to trivial slights or oversights, frequent prompts for reassurance, interpersonal tactics that test others' sincerity, and so forth, tend to produce added burdens to future relationships.

A last example of clients who come under corrective emotional experience goals are the elderly and isolated. As will tragically happen with some individuals of advancing age, the death of a spouse and only periodic contact with grown children leaves them alone, inactive, and directionless. Among persons who have few friends or little contact with group activities, such circumstances are frequently associated with depression, hopelessness, and feelings of abandonment—reactions that work against seeking new social contacts and productive activity. Treatment goals with these clients thus involve reversing the view that the social world is closed to them and prompting interests and motivations towards engaging activities.

As can be noted from these examples, treatment goals that involve corrective emotional experiences apply across virtually the entire age range. However, actual treatment procedures (to be covered in Chapters 7 and 8) are frequently a demanding emotional-interpersonal experience for the therapists, regardless of the client's age, since most such individuals enter therapy mistrustful of others, including the therapist.

Self-exploration and change goals Self-exploration and change goals are somewhat more complex than those described earlier. As will be seen, they also involve some of the other goals—particularly those involving behavioral change.

By way of introduction, let us begin with the fact that many clients seek treatment for a variety of psychological problems that, from their point of view, are ill-defined. The client frequently cannot specify any particular set of behaviors or identifiable emotional patterns that need to be changed. These clients do not seem to be in a crisis situation, nor do they communicate unusual attitudes and expectations about people. Despite the absence of such specifics, these clients exhibit signs of psychological distress—anxiety, depression, loneliness, a sense of being unfulfilled, and so forth—that are every bit as real as the problems described in previous sections. Such conditions may be particularly disturbing to clients because they cannot readily identify the reasons for their distress.

As a first approximation to understanding these clients, let us theorize about some of the underlying processes that may be involved. Some individuals lead exceptionally hectic, demanding lives and literally devote all of their attention to responding to the immediate pressures of the job, school, or household. Their daily schedules are so filled with reacting to momentary external demands that they rarely have the opportunity to introspect, to appreciate the subtleties and nuances of interpersonal relations, or to stand back and evaluate their lives in broad perspective. With such individuals, relationships with other people and reactions to one's own inner, emotional stimuli tend to become routinized, automatic, and uninspected. Under these conditions, then, when interpersonal affairs are going badly or when internal processes come into conflict or turmoil, the person is literally unpracticed in analyzing and understanding what is going wrong.

Now let us extend this line of reasoning one step further. Consider individuals who have many of these same characteristics, but in addition have had life experiences that prompted severely painful emotions—so agonizing that it became safer to avoid thinking about them. Such individuals develop styles of thinking (defense mechanisms) that, in effect, keep them from attending to these threatening emotions. Quite likely, these clients also have become adept at avoiding provocative situations or at manipulating relationships in such a way as to keep these emotions from being aroused. The unfortunate consequences of these various avoidance maneuvers is that they exact a heavy toll in terms of deficits in personal problem-solving abilities, restrictions regarding engaging in stimulating activities, and limitations in the quality and depth of interpersonal affairs.

We are talking here, then, about clients who have deficits in awareness about the behavioral and emotional patterns in their lives; and especially those patterns that are related to negative emotions and psychological pain. As can be imagined, when these patterns lead to intra- or interpersonal problems, the client has difficulty in recognizing the offending behaviors and emotions and feels helpless in being able to solve the problems.

The first general goal with such individuals, therefore, is to have the client (and therapist) identify and analyze the maladaptive behavioral-emotional patterns, followed by the second goal of bringing about appropriate changes in these patterns.

The term *insight* has traditionally been attached to the first goal; however, this general label is just a convenience for a rather complex and multifaceted concept. We can ask the question, "Insight into what?" and come up with several different answers depending on the nature of the client's problems. At the risk of oversimplification there are at least three overlapping types of problems that can be delineated, each of which answers this question from a somewhat different perspective.

The first category pertains to the clients whose principal difficulties seem to lie in the interpersonal realm. Their initial reasons for seeking help are usually some vague realization of failure in relating to others, along with considerable confusion as to why this should be so. They ask such questions as: "I seem to get along with people all right, but why can't I keep any deep and lasting friendships?" or, "Our marriage seemed to be progressively coming apart, and I have this feeling that somehow it was my fault, but I'll be darned if I can figure out why"; or "I'm forever freezing up when I meet new people, and then inside, I get frightfully angry at them. Isn't that crazy?" Exploration and insight with such individuals most likely would focus on uncovering: (1) the specific modes of behavior the client uses in relating to others, (2) the subtle, and perhaps conflicted, communication patterns that develop in relationships, and (3) the likely impact such patterns have on others. After these patterns are elucidated and analyzed, the client and therapist can negotiate which of them should be changed, and thereafter pursue the second set of goals—that is, actively working toward establishing new and more satisfying modes of relating.

A second category of client involves those whose propblems seem to be largely internal. These are usually related to vague but strong emotional conflicts or fear and guilt associated with certain emotions and impulses. Typical statements in describing their plight are: "Most of the time I'm at war with myself. I can feel tremendous forces pushing and pulling me emotionally, and they leave me totally exhausted"; or "Even looking at a stupid television program that involves violence drives me up the wall. I become paralyzed by fear"; or "I'm completely locked up and frozen over. I know that I'm capable of feeling, but for the last year or two I've been nothing but a robot." Insight with such individuals will focus on specifying and elaborating the emotions involved, identifying the cues and situations which trigger the turmoil or fear, gaining an understanding of the origins of the conflicts, and analyzing the defense mechanisms by which the client has thus far dealt with them.

Achieving insight into these areas is again followed by the second set of goals, that is, bringing about changes in emotional reaction patterns and habitual ways of coping with them. Such changes may involve becoming desensitized to the anxiety associated with certain emotions; learning to face and deal with emotional issues directly, rather than avoiding them; recognizing the defenses that may have been appropriate in an earlier traumatic period of one's life but are no longer necessary; and developing new and appropriate ways of expressing emotions and impulses.

A third perspective on insight applies to clients who fit into what might be termed the "every person" category. These are individuals who at some point come to the realization that their lives are routine and boring, that satisfactions and accomplishments that once were important have lost their impact, and that life is passing by without much direction or meaning. Such clients may be functioning without apparent disabilities, and yet they are searching for untapped potentials within their personalities and a redefinition of their existence. In contrast to the previous clients there may not be any *specific* interpersonal or emotional patterns that require elucidation; rather, what appears to be called for here is a broad-based self-exploration and analysis of personal philosophy, sources of emotional responsivity, and aspirations for the future. Following these kinds of "insight," the prospects for change are many and varied (and difficult to summarize). Clients may, for example, elect to develop new ways of relating to people, or reconsider vocational and educational aspirations, become involved in long-dormant creative activities, or simply work toward a more profound appreciation of their present lives.

Conclusion As described in this section, the process of helping a client achieve insight sounds mechanical and straightforward. Nothing could be further from the truth. When one considers that it frequently involves the first deep, honest, and realistic self-inspection that occurs in a person's life, some of the drama can be appreciated. The fact that very intense areas of anxiety are often exposed indicates a process of considerable delicacy and risk. Working with a client through such a potentially tortuous time in his or her life requires a full measure of professional skill. The principal therapy techniques that are applicable to self-exploration and change goals will be reviewed in Chapters 9 and 10.

Type of Therapy and Therapist

Having reviewed the major treatment goals and the types of problems for which they apply, a discussion of therapy decisions can now take place. Just as each of the goals needs to be tailored to the specific characteristics of the client, the particular therapeutic strategies that are adopted likewise require adjustment to individual needs. However, as implied in the previous section, major classes of treatment can be identified as appropriate to each of the therapy goals. These will be briefly mentioned here, with more ample description of the specific techniques involved reserved for the remaining chapters.

In the last several decades an unusually large and varied number of treatment modes have been developed, making it difficult to classify them in an integrated system. It seems possible, however, to conceptualize four broad strategies of therapy that parallel the four general treatment goals described earlier. These categories can be termed supportive therapy, behavior modification, relationship therapy, and insight therapy. As we go into these strategies in succeeding chapters, it will be noted that considerable overlap exists among them. They all have a common core of the therapist establishing positive rapport with the client. Many specific therapeutic techniques are shared. Depending on their particular needs, some clients may require a combination of these treatment strategies. Despite these overlaps, the four-way system being proposed appears to be justified on several grounds: (1) each therapy mode is organized to meet somewhat different sets of client needs; (2) individual treatment techniques, even though they may be utilized in several of the therapy strategies, are sequenced and emphasized in different ways; and (3) such a proposed system, which incorporates a wide spectrum of theory and specific therapeutic techniques, may have instructional value in aiding students to develop an organizational framework for understanding this very complex field.

Each of these broad strategies will be briefly summarized on the following pages, with more detailed descriptions provided in subsequent chapters.

Therapy emphasizing supportive techniques This general approach refers to a coordinated set of procedures for the achievement of crisis management goals—reduction of high levels of negative emotions, control of impulsive behaviors, and mobilization of a rational, problem-solving approach to difficulties. Treatment procedures principally involve such techniques as active and directive guidance, environmental manipulation to reduce external stress, relaxation procedures, arranging for medication, imposing controls on behavior, fostering self-monitoring and self-control techniques, focusing on reality issues, and rehearsal of instrumental coping behaviors.

Clients in a crisis condition usually feel overwhelmed by frightening emotions, fantasies, and impulses—to the detriment of a systematic and thoughtful approach to problems. Supportive techniques involve an overall strategy of helping the client to "put a lid" on feelings, while at the same time enhancing reality-oriented, problem-solving behaviors.

In general terms, clients in crisis seem to require what might be termed a strong, active, "take charge" therapist who they feel can temporarily assume responsibility for helping them through an overwhelming situation. Therapeutic contact thus may not be on a regularly scheduled basis; rather, the therapist remains available until the crisis subsides. Such an approach may possibly foster dependency on the therapist, which if prolonged could prompt other complications; however, in the short run such issues take a second priority to dealing with the immediate crisis.

Therapy emphasizing behavior modification techniques Behavior modification techniques comprise a wide array of procedures that are generally based on learning principles. To a large extent, analogues of these procedures have been experimentally examined in the laboratory, and a substantial proportion of them have also received research attention in clinical settings. Thus, as a group, these techniques are among the most validated of all the procedures in psychotherapy. As the title suggests, these procedures are primarily appropriate to behavior change goals, but we see them represented to some extent in other therapy strategies as well.

The hallmark of behavior modification treatments is their attempt to scientifically understand the factors that govern undesirable behaviors and troublesome reactions in the individual client. Systematic and rigorous analyses of the stimuli and environmental conditions that affect maladaptive behaviors are an integral part of the approach. Similarly, therapeutic procedures with each client are carefully evaluated in order to assess their affects on problem behaviors. If, for example, such "functional analyses" indicate that a particular procedure is not having a measurable effect on a targeted behavior, the therapist will most likely reassess the situation and try another treatment procedure—which in turn will be evaluated. Thus, in essence, a data-based treatment program is evolved for each client. Specific treatments are generally based on principles drawn from classical and operant conditioning, observational learning, and the allied areas of self-monitoring and self-control. These latter topics are defined by their emphasis on clients' abilities to regulate and change their problem behaviors.

During the last decade, several important trends have occurred in the behavioral area. Recognition of the importance of verbal mediation in the control of many behaviors has resulted in efforts to extend learning-based treatments into the less accessible realms of language and thought patterns. Related to this is a parallel development of capitalizing on the client's abilities to fantasize or imagine certain stimuli or situations—mental events that can then be utilized to promote behavioral change. A third development that also reflects the growing sophistication of behavioral approaches is the attempt to treat highly complex, multidetermined disorders (e.g., alcoholism). Such endeavors involve the appropriate use of a variety of behavioral techniques, timed and sequenced in a proper manner (see Goldfried and Davison, 1976).

Therapy emphasizing relationship issues Therapy emphasizing relationship issues is suggested for clients with corrective emotional experience goals. It is probably the least defined of the therapy emphases, and few specific techniques can be uniquely identified with it. This is so because the central purpose of this type of therapy is the development and fostering of a deep and healthy relationship with the client — a process that normally must be adapted to the special characteristics of each client.

Because of this focus on the relationship itself, there may be no special agenda of personal issues, symptoms, or behavior problems that is set. Similarly, therapy meetings with many clients may not be scheduled on a regular weekly basis; rather, they may be arranged in a more spontaneous fashion, depending on the special requirements of the developing relationship. Finally, in keeping with this spontaneity, therapy meetings may not take place within the formal confines of an office. Instead, contact is made within any setting that will promote the relationship — for example, a ball game, shopping trip, or the neighborhood hangout.

The development of a positive relationship with clients needing corrective emotional experiences is frequently a difficult and stormy process. Recall that such clients have typically undergone prior relationships in which they have been rejected and exploited; hence they bring into therapy expectations of further hurt, as well as protective social behaviors designed to keep others at a distance. The therapist is therefore quite likely to be a recipient of these protective behaviors, and further, will undoubtedly have to go through a series of "tests" — some blatant, some subtle — designed by the client to evaluate the therapist's genuineness and caring.

The choice of therapist in this kind of treatment seems to require special care. An individual who tends to be inflexible, technique-oriented, or overly concerned with changing specific symptoms will probably have difficulty. In contrast, a therapist who is attuned to interpersonal processes, who can be honest and nondefensive, and who is capable of genuine rapport with clients will probably have reasonable prospects of making progress. This interweaving of therapist personality and treatment procedures is a particularly fascinating aspect of relationship therapy.

Therapy emphasizing insight Therapy emphasizing insight is applicable to self-exploration and change goals as described in the previous section. As suggested earlier, it is probably the most complex of the therapies in that it involves two broad stages — the first aimed at discovery of relevant problem behaviors and emotional patterns and the second aimed at bringing about modification of these patterns. In general terms this set of procedures is an outgrowth of what have been termed "dynamic" schools of therapy (Freudian, neo-Freudian, Rogerian, gestalt, existential approaches) and are so designated because of their emphasis on studying the relationship between observable symptoms and underlying emotional-motivational forces.

The insight stage basically involves the question, "How do you get persons to take a deep, honest look at themselves, without rationalization, distortion, or getting overly frightened?" This can be a particularly difficult process when one considers that many clients have established long-term patterns of nonexploration, or have developed well-ingrained images of themselves (however unrealistic), which they rigidly try to preserve. Complicating the process further is the likelihood that areas of living involving strong anxiety are being investigated, thus prompting clients' resistance to the entire process.

Three classes of procedures can be identified as the therapeutic tools for promoting insight. The first pertains to a variety of *verbal techniques* that are used to help clients attend to and rationally analyze their behaviors, emotions, and fantasies. These techniques can range from relatively nondirective reflection of feelings to active confrontation and interpretation by the therapist. A second class of procedures pertain to an analysis of the *unique relationship* that the client establishes with the therapist. Based on the assumption that people tend to repeat their habitual behaviors, emotions, expectations, and defenses in each new social encounter, the therapeutic relationship itself thereby becomes a vehicle for self-exploration. Such insight techniques have developed out of the psychoanalytic concept of transference, and more recently from the interpersonal mechanisms studied in transactional analysis. A third class of insight techniques encompasses a range of procedures designed to have clients *directly experience* emotions and impulses of the moment. Colloquially called "getting in touch with feelings," such immediate experiences help reduce inhibitions and defenses and basically enhance the client's appreciation and understanding of the emotional roots of symptoms and conflicts. Techniques here include such procedures as the psychoanalytic process of free association, various gestalt exercises of fantasy production, and introspective, meditational experiences.

Underlying the use of the various insights techniques are several less tangible but important issues. Considerable clinical judgment and sensitivity are required in tailoring these procedures to each client. Some individuals enter insight therapy with high motivation, a willingness to take emotional risks, and a reasonable understanding of what is involved in the process. Such clients may thrive with relatively mild, largely nondirective efforts. On the other hand, some clients may enter the process with considerable skepticism, resistance, or anxiety and thus may require more active and confrontive procedures. In any case, most insight therapists seem to agree that the therapist's humanity and trustworthiness as perceived by the client are important factors in treatment. Considering that the insight process is essentially an unsettling and sometimes frightening entry into one's personal unknown, often involving intimate areas of living, we can appreciate the client's need to be assured that the therapist is not an insensitive clod, or worse, a person who may take advantage when one is exposed and vulnerable.

Toward the close of the self-exploration stage of this therapy, successful clients achieve a high level of self-analysis in which they can identify the patterns of behavior and emotional reaction that are creating difficulties in their lives. They most likely also have an understanding of some of the historical roots of these patterns and an appreciation of how destructive they are for contemporary adjustment. With this knowledge they are now in a position to make realistic judgments as to which of these patterns should be changed, and in what direction such changes should take place.

A number of current-day theorists seem to agree on an important short-coming of traditional insight therapy. This concerns the largely unsubstantiated assumption that once insight is achieved by a client, adjustive and appropriate behavioral patterns will somehow emerge (e.g., Wolberg, 1967; Martin, 1977; Phares, 1979). This unresolved issue has led to suggestions that active attempts to have clients develop more effective behavior patterns be an integral part of insight therapy. Phares (1979, p. 353), for example, cites his observation that more and more therapists seem to be combining insight and behavior change methods with many of their clients. In this light, then, we can consider a somewhat broadened view of self-exploration therapy; that is, after maladaptive behaviors and reaction patterns have been identified during the insight phase of treatment, a second phase involving systematic attempts to modify these inappropriate patterns may be reasonably included with many clients.

EXPLANATION TO THE CLIENT

We are now approaching the close of the intake process, having taken the client through the initial contact with the therapist, the gathering of information via the intake interview and other means, organizing and evaluating the information, and preliminary decision making regarding therapeutic goals and overall treatment strategy.

The process most likely will end with a meeting between intake worker and client. At this session the intake worker is usually prepared to provide a summary of the evaluation and to indicate to the client recommendations for treatment goals and type of therapy. Ample explanation, in keeping with the client's ability to understand, is given for these recommendations, along with a general outline of what may be expected in therapy. In keeping with the principle of informed consent, the client should therefore be apprised of the treatment procedures that would likely be involved, possible alternative therapies, any risks involved, probable length of treatment, and the costs involved.

SUMMARY

After reading this chapter, the student may be left with the impression that deciding upon goals and treatment approach is a straightforward and inflexible

Table 4.2
A proposed system for conceptualizing treatment goals and strategies

Client	Goals	Treatment emphasis
Severe situational stress; decompensation; prepsychotic; acute psychosis; psychoticlike toxic reactions	Crisis management (reduce affect, control of impulsive behaviors, foster rational problem solving)	Supportive therapy (active, directive guidance, relaxation techniques, environmental manipulation, self-control procedures, reality oriented problem solving)
Specific, identifiable behavioral disorders	Change behavior (correct behavioral deficiencies, replace inappropriate patterns)	Behavior modification (classical conditioning and operant techniques, modeling, self-regulation procedures)
Reactions to rejection and exploitation; elderly isolates	Corrective emotional experiences (change interpersonal expectancies, reduce debilitating social behaviors, foster affectionate, trusting relations)	Relationship therapy (therapist uses interpersonal skills to develop relationship with client)
Distress or symptoms with no debilitating behavioral or emotional patterns apparent to client (subtle interpersonal deficits, defensive avoidance of threatening emotions, dissatisfaction with life-style)	Self-exploration and change	Insight therapy (verbal insight-promoting techniques, analyses of therapeutic relationship, procedures to enhance direct emotional experience); behavioral-emotional change

matter. It is considerably more complex than this. First, the system of goals and treatments that is presented here reflects the "state of the art" as interpreted by this author rather than a scientifically developed framework. Second, often clients do not fit cleanly into one or another of these categories, thus posing an added challenge to therapists' judgments and decisions. Third, the treatment approaches that are outlined represent relatively ill-defined and sometimes overlapping territories. In sum, the reader should recognize, as stated in Chapter 1, that the proposed system of client problems-goals-treatments is only a "first approximation" to developing specific aims and specific therapy programs for each client. In this sense, the content of this chapter may be used as a rough set of guidelines that help practitioners to develop an initial orientation to client problems during the intake phase. The difficult work of developing specific aims and treatments for each client should evolve from this framework as more detailed information is gathered during the early phases of therapy. Table 4.2 summarizes the main essentials of the proposed system.

PART THREE

FOUR TREATMENT STRATEGIES: SUPPORTIVE, BEHAVIORAL, RELATIONSHIP, AND INSIGHT TECHNIQUES

CHAPTER FIVE

TREATMENT ORIENTED TOWARD CRISIS MANAGEMENT: SUPPORTIVE THERAPY

INTRODUCTION

Put yourself in the following situation. You are out for a pleasant day at an amusement park, and you are looking forward to an exciting trip on the roller coaster. It is billed as the "World's Scariest Ride," and it really is an immense and dramatic superstructure. But you have been on it before and found the experience exhilarating. Coming out of the first big dip, you are indeed high. Suddenly, the car starts making a strange noise, one that you had not heard on previous trips. The car is not braking the way it should as it approaches the big turn. You can feel the entire superstructure vibrating in an ominous fashion. You are eleven stories above the ground in a runaway vehicle, and in a flash you just know that the whole thing is coming apart.

Helplessness. Impending crash. Panic! Amid the screams and crying, thoughts are racing too fast to think clearly. Senseless impulses jump into being. "Should I leap out of the car?" "If I stay frozen, I'll be all right." "A dark pit is forming underneath my body." "Save me!"

A trivial little fantasy perhaps, but it seems to capture some of the emotional qualities of a person in crisis. A sense of impending disaster, along with a feeling that one is helpless to do anything about it, seems to be the central aspect of this psychological state. Added ingredients are unusually strong emotions, deficits in being able to think clearly, and the tendency to behave impulsively. Taken together, these characteristics define a condition of high vulnerability and risk.

Supportive therapy, the subject matter of this chapter, is a set of procedures that is designed to help people in crisis. This treatment approach is not necessarily one that will bring about a long-range "cure" of psychological difficulties. Rather, it may be viewed as relatively brief and focused emergency therapy aimed at assisting individuals through an especially difficult episode in their lives. Recall that in Chapter 4 the principal goals of crisis management were outlined as follows: (1) reducing emotional levels to a point where the individual does not feel overwhelmed; (2) strengthening controls on behavior to lessen the risk of impulsive and ill-advised actions; and (3) enhancing a rational, problem-solving approach to both inner and environmental stressors. From this perspective we can see that treatment may not even remove or reduce stressors. Instead, the focus is on restoring psychological equilibrium, fostering effective coping behaviors, and preventing desperate or tragic attempts to deal with the crisis.

Settings for Supportive Therapy

Many traditional mental health agencies are not organized to handle psychological emergencies very effectively. A facility that is open only from eight until five, that has a waiting list, and that is scheduled to see clients on a weekly basis is hardly capable of stepping in quickly and decisively during a crisis. In addition, many such traditional agencies are staffed by practitioners whose treatment orientation is one of relatively long-term personality and behavior change. In contrast, crisis work requires a setting in which a therapist is available on a twenty-four-hour basis, in which lengthy administrative procedures can be short-circuited in the interest of timely intervention, and in which contact with the client can be maintained on a flexible basis as needed. Caplan (1961) estimates that most crises resolve themselves within six weeks (sometimes disastrously); therefore treatment needs to be focused during this unstable period.

Butcher and Maudal (1976) present an interesting historical overview of the emergence of various crisis facilities over the last forty years. These include the development of short-term treatment approaches to quickly deal with battle-related stress during World War II; the rise of special facilities during the 1940s to deal with psychological problems of bereavement; the establishment of clinics and telephone "hot lines" related to suicide prevention during the 1950s; and, also during the 1950s, the development of general crisis clinics associated with large metropolitan hospitals and mental health agencies. Butcher and Maudal also point out that during the 1960s and 1970s there was a rapid expansion of the "free clinic" movement, so called, not because of economic issues, but because of the nontraditional focus of these agencies. Counseling related to drugs, gay rights, the draft, pregnancy, and so forth, were but a few of the specific types of agencies that were developed during these years. Many of these "free clinics" arose spontaneously to meet urgent community needs and frequently were staffed by concerned laypeople rather than professionals. The anti-establishment attitudes of many of the youthful clients of this era made these nontraditional facilities a particularly important source of help for troubled young people of that turbulent time.

Such are the diverse historical roots of crisis-oriented therapy. Many of the innovations of these earlier facilities have now become established as standard procedure in contemporary community agencies. Many neighborhood mental health clinics and community hospitals have a special section devoted to the management of short-term, emergency situations. Such crisis facilities usually have twenty-four-hour-a-day access, a schedule that permits "walk in" clients to receive immediate attention, therapy teams that can go into the community to render assistance on short notice, and a corps of specially trained para-professionals and informed laypersons, along with a professional staff, who can make rapid and supportive contact with distressed individuals.

CRISIS THEORY

Most people manage their daily lives in a reasonably efficient manner. Work and school tasks are accomplished through well-practiced routines, social obligations are met, biological and emotional needs are satisfied, and occasional stresses or obstacles are overcome with only moderate discomfort. In short, a kind of personal equilibrium is maintained as people cope with environmental and internal demands, pursue long-range goals, or simply indulge in the art of living.

At times, however, this equilibrium becomes severely disrupted. An individual is confronted with environmental or internal stresses for which no adequate coping behaviors are available. When such stresses are reacted to as major threats to the individual's psychological or physical safety, a crisis is internally experienced. The phenomenon really defies a simple description, since it is a complex mixture of inner feeling states and reactions. However, one of the leading theorists in this area (Caplan, 1964) suggests that four stages can be identified in the typical crisis situation: (1) at the onset of a crisis, the individual reacts with heightened emotionality and tension, and attempts are made to deal with the situation with habitual coping behaviors; (2) as the individual discovers that these usual ways of handling stress are not effective, further tension, confusion, and anxiety are generated; (3) intensified efforts to restore equilibrium, accompanied by even greater levels of emotionality and distress, may involve novel solutions, seeking help from others, or escaping the situation; and (4) the failure of these more extreme attempts to reduce stress results in disorganization and severe emotional disruption.

Caplan's overview can be elaborated by a consideration of the major factors that seem to contribute to crisis reactions, as shown in Fig. 5.1. Starting at the top of the figure, we can see that four interrelated sets of factors come into play: (1) the type and intensity of the stressors (environmental or internal); (2) the person's psychological and biological vulnerabilities to stress; (3) the types of coping mechanisms available to the individual; and (4) the effects that these coping strategies have on reducing or removing the stress.

Let us review each of these factors in turn and consider how they interact with each other. This kind of theorizing is of some importance for the student of psychotherapy. It may not only provide a conceptual framework for

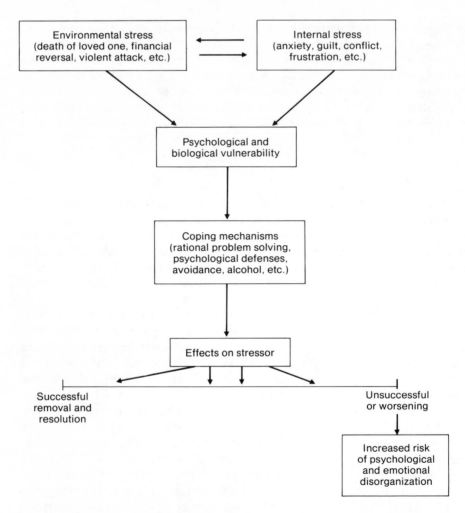

Figure 5.1 Factors in crisis development.

understanding crisis situations, but also help define some of the practical clinical issues that need to be evaluated with each client.

External Sources of Stress

To begin at the top of Fig. 5.1, environmental stressors of a magnitude to produce a crisis reaction are frequently identifiable without too much difficulty. Tragedies that can befall any one of us, such as death in the family, being the victim of violence, or failure at an especially important endeavor, are some typical examples. It is possible, however, to go beyond such obvious illustrations and do a more careful analysis of what it is about some stressors that make them high-risk triggers of a crisis reaction. Researchers in this area (Lazarus, 1966; Seligman, 1975), in studying the nature of stress, point out several common denominators that make certain situations particularly disastrous. These factors are: being helpless to do anything about the situation; being alone in facing the stress; the suddenness or unpredictable nature of the tragedy; and a sense that the stressor may unexpectedly reoccur. Thus, apart from the sheer magnitude or intensity of the stressful life events, these other factors seem to play an important, if not critical, role in producing the intense emotional disruption and disorganization of a person in crisis. These components of crisis situations are important considerations for a therapist engaged in supportive therapy. On occasion the environmental stressors in the life of a client may appear, to the outside observer, as minor or even trivial. However, if that stressor prompts reactions of uncontrollability, aloneness, and unpredictability, the central ingredients of a crisis situation may be present.

Internal Sources of Stress

It is probably true that we cannot separate environmental and internal sources of stress, since we each perceive and react to situations in our own unique ways. Note that at the top of Fig. 5.1 these sources of stress are connected by arrows, thereby indicating the interrelationship between the two. However, for purposes of analysis it may be profitable to discuss internal stressors as a distinct category. As one might expect, these precipitants of crisis, stemming from the more private world of emotions and personality dynamics, may not be easily identified. Nevertheless, they can be as awesome and overwhelming as some of the most severe external tragedies.

Having to rely on individuals' descriptions of inner experience, we can perhaps draw some examples from accounts of such crises that are portrayed in literature. In Arthur Miller's play *Death of a Salesman*, Biff, the young high school athlete, has a bright future in front of him. He is personable, gets on well with adults, and is a hero to his classmates. In his father's eye, Biff is the one son who will be the success that he never was. Biff idolizes his father, and he has grown up with the image that life is sweet and easy and that all one has to do to get ahead is to be "well liked." Catastrophe strikes. Biff accidentally walks into a seedy hotel room where he discovers his father's sexual affair. An overwhelming reaction of revulsion accompanies his sudden realization that all he has admired and worshipped in his father over the years has been a sham. Indeed, the very basis on which he built his own personality crumbles, and he is left empty and in despair. One leaves this play with the sense that this pivotal experience in his life is one from which Biff will never recover.

Camus describes a crisis with different characteristics in his short story *The Adulterous Woman*. In a remarkably subtle fashion Camus portrays a businessman's wife, whose existence is very conventional, circumscribed, and safe.

One day, almost by chance, it seems, she accepts his invitation to accompany him on a business trip to North Africa. During the ensuing travels strange and gradual transitions start to take place. She begins to experience the stirrings of vague but strong feelings that are buried deep within her. Her perceptions of the world around her seem to be somehow getting out of focus. Perhaps it is the change of scene, or the new people she encounters. She is not sure. It is uncanny and frightening, but the gradually emerging process is also fascinating to her. It reaches its climax late one night in the bedroom of a small desert hotel. Her husband sleeps quietly beside her and the light of the moon slips gently through the window. She recognizes all at once that up until this point her life has been without emotion or a sense of her own individuality. The tragedy of wasted years overwhelms her.

These two episodes from literature, so different in time course and outcome, share some important features regarding internal precipitants of crisis. In each instance the individual is faced with a dramatic and new confrontation of the self. Habitual ways of behaving, perceiving, and feeling are no longer viable. The person is now faced with either a void or a new conception of the self that may be too frightening or depressing to cope with.

Some differences between the two examples also have important implications for understanding internal crises. Note first that Biff's situation involved a single wrenching experience that reordered his perceptions of his father and himself. On the other hand, Camus's heroine seemed to approach a climactic moment in her life in gradual stages, with really no dramatic incident to serve as a precipitant. The point, of course, is that a therapist doing crisis work may not always be able to discern any clear-cut incident or trauma that has triggered the crisis. Rather, the crisis may occur as a result of a slow accumulation of changes taking place emotionally, or a gradual erosion in the effectiveness of a client's coping mechanisms. A second difference pertains to the aftermath of each crisis. In Miller's play, the tragic consequence is Biff's long-term reaction of cynicism and aimlessness in his own later life; whereas at the close of Camus's story we are left with the view that the heroine's life is just now beginning. The second point of emphasis, therefore, is the notion that internal crises are not inevitably tragic, but rather represent periods of upheaval and disruption in one's life that can have disastrous or beneficial outcomes. As stated earlier, the task of the supportive therapist is to assist the client in gaining positive resolutions to stress—an aim that can perhaps be seen more clearly by referring back to Caplan's four stages of crisis. Recall that in Caplan's third stage, the individual has found that the usual coping mechanisms are ineffective to reduce stress, and now (under heightened tension) seeks new solutions. Left to his or her own devices, a frightened or confused client may rely on inappropriate or destructive solutions, whereas under the supportive help of a therapist, some new and creative means of dealing with stress may be discovered.

Vulnerability to Stress

Research over the last thirty years has produced evidence indicating that individuals differ markedly in their susceptibility to stress. Further, this evidence suggests that heightened susceptibility may be caused by a variety of factors, both biological and psychological. Thus, in order to understand an individual's reaction to crisis, it is important not only to consider environmental and internal sources of stress, but also to assess the person's long-term vulnerabilities. For this reason, the overall model of crisis portrayed in Fig. 5.1 includes such a set of risk factors.

Physiological effects Vulnerability based on biological factors can be seen in a variety of forms. The classic work of Hans Selye (1956) on the General Adaptation Syndrome provides a basic perspective in this area. Selye outlines three stages of physiological reaction to stress: (1) an *alarm* reaction, occurring at the onset of stress, that involves the rapid mobilization of bodily energy systems (release of epinephrine, increases in blood pressure, heightened muscle tone, etc.); (2) a stage of *resistance*, during which biological systems function in a sustained "emergency" state so as to cope with the continuing stress; and (3) an *exhaustion* stage, in which actual tissue damage or physiological depletion occurs as a result of operating at chronic stress levels.

The exhaustion stage in Selye's model can be viewed as the biological counterpart of a psychological crisis. At the physiological level, bodily defenses and coping mechanisms are no longer operating in an adaptive fashion, and one is, so to speak, left at the mercy of the stressors. To more fully understand the relation of this dicussion to crisis theory, two physiological systems that appear to be especially vulnerable to this exhaustion syndrome need to be mentioned. First is the pituitary-adrenal system, so called because these two major endocrine glands are involved. Among many other functions related to maintaining physiological equilibrium, these structures coordinate the production and secretion of a variety of hormones (such as epinephrine and adrenal steroids) that affect most internal organs, including the heart, and also general activity level, muscle tone, and alertness. Disruption or damage of this sytem therefore has widespread effects on one's energy levels, physical robustness, psychological mood, and mental acuity.

The other physiological system of particular relevance here pertains to a large array of biochemical substances in the brain that are generally referred to as neurotransmitters. These biochemical agents (e.g., dopamine, serotonin, and norepinephrine) are essential to the efficient transmission of neural impulses in brain tissue; as such they are fundamental to virtually all mental functions—perception, memory, logical thought, emotional status, and so on. Disruption or depletion of these neurotransmitter systems can have profound effects on one's adjustive capacities, including such symptoms as deep depression, manic excitement, hallucinations, or disordered and illogical thought processes. To the extent that such disruption of brain functions occurs, we can perhaps see the biological foundations of a crisis state.

To return to our discussion of biological vulnerability, we can take a closer look at some of the factors that may make some individuals more susceptible to crisis reactions than others. Three general areas have been identified by researchers:

1. The first set of factors is a direct outgrowth of Selye's work, and perhaps is the most obvious. Individuals who have undergone long-term and severe stress by virtue of their life-style, occupation, or exposure to dire environmental circumstances may be physiologically on the verge of the exhaustion stage. Actual damage to the adrenal glands or the depletion of brain neurotransmitters, for example, may render the individual without the biological reserves to face even a moderately stressful situation. In effect this may be a kind of "last-straw" phenomenon in which these critical physiological functions can no longer support efforts to mobilize effective behaviors, causing the individual to succumb to psychological disorganization, depression, or panic.

2. Research over the last several decades also points toward genetic factors in this area For our purposes the findings of inherited predispositions for some types of schizophrenia, manic-depressive disorders, and certain forms of depression are especially pertinent (Gottesman and Shields, 1972). The personality disorganization, aberrant thought processes, and disruptive emotions of these disorders implicate the brain neurotransmitter systems. Experimental evidence (see Snyder, 1978) points to biochemical abnormalities in the brain as the specific physiological factors that are genetically transmitted in these disorders. It is reasonably clear, then, that persons with such genetic predispositions toward disorganization are especially vulnerable, and even a mild stressor may be sufficient to provoke a crisis reaction.

3. The area of substance abuse, particularly the use of hallucinogenic drugs or chronic alcoholism, has implications for the vulnerability issue. The hallucinogens and long-term alcohol consumption have effects on the brain neurotransmitter systems, with alterations in the normal functions of these systems being responsible for the disordered thoughts associated with being high or drunk. An unresolved question in these areas of research is whether or not these abnormal neurotransmitter processes are totally reversible, or whether repeated use of drugs or alcohol produces an increasing susceptibility to biochemical disruption in the brain. The weight of evidence in this rapidly expanding area of investigation suggests that some semipermanent effects may occur (Chafetz and Demone, 1974). Thus individuals with such histories of substance abuse may be unusually susceptible, on a biological basis, to the disorganization and disruption of crisis reactions.

Needless to say, the supportive therapist working with a client in crisis must be sensitive to these areas of physiological vulnerability. Careful assessment of such possible factors, gathered from the client's history and current mode of living, is essential in the development of an appropriate treatment plan. Specifics as to these assessment procedures will be discussed later in this chapter.

Psychological effects As stated earlier, it is difficult to realistically separate physiological from psychological processes when discussing vulnerability. However, for purposes of clarity, a separate discussion of psychological vulnerabilities may highlight some additional factors in this complex area. Our discussion can be conveniently organized around three general sets of processes that seem to produce heightened risks of crisis reactions: (1) the rearousal of early traumatic emotions, (2) the gradual development of a personal sense of helplessness in one's life, and (3) the erosion or loss of social support systems.

Psychoanalytic theory tells us that traumatic experiences that we have as children represent the kinds of ghosts that we carry within us into adulthood. As children we are, by definition, vulnerable; thus traumatic events in these tender years are frequently left unresolved and also have a particularly strong impact. In a sense these "ghosts" remain as specific pockets of fear and anguish in our emotional makeup, and we frequently go to great lengths to hide from them or disguise them in some fashion. This type of theorizing has received some research support, especially in the area of loss of parents in childhood and the consequent anxiety concerning separation and emotional attachment that are experienced in the later years of such children (Bowlby, 1973).

From this line of thinking, then, it is apparent that when stresses occur in a person's life that rearouse memories of an early trauma, a twofold emotional impact takes place: the emotional response to the realities of the present stress and the perhaps far more upsetting response to the earlier, unresolved tragedy. Consider the example of a twenty-three-year-old woman who is involved in a relatively minor car accident. Although not seriously injured, her reaction is a prolonged fit of uncontrollable hysterics followed by a severe bout of depression. This exaggerated reaction does not make sense until we discover that as a seven-year-old she witnessed the violent death of her father in an automobile accident—an event that she was able to describe as having had a profound effect on her life.

A second, more general set of processes that contribute to psychological vulnerability concerns the concept of a personal sense of helplessness. This notion has been around under a variety of labels for many years—feelings of inadequacy, absence of a sense of competency, and so forth—and in recent times it has been extensively investigated by several researchers (Abramson, Seligman, and Teasdale, 1978; Bandura, 1977). The research findings indicate that individuals who are exposed to stressful circumstances *over which they have no control* tend to display behavioral and motivational deficits. These deficits can perhaps be best summarized by the attitude, "What's the use of trying, I can see that my efforts will have no effect in overcoming this stress."

Applying these research results to natural life circumstances, we can envision some individuals who have undergone many such "helplessness-inducing" experiences and hence meet most new situations with a defeatist and pessimistic attitude. As might be expected, such an approach to life's demands almost ensures further failure experiences, and so the process feeds on itself. Little wonder, then, that when such persons encounter a major life stressor they are especially vulnerable to feelings of incompetence, anxiety, depression, and helplessness—that is, the essential components of a crisis reaction.

The third set of processes concerning psychological factors in vulnerability is the area of social support systems. Earlier in this section, in discussing factors that increase the likelihood of crisis reactions, the disruptive effect of feeling "alone" was mentioned. Let us take a closer look at this issue. Most individuals have relationships with family and friends that serve, in times of stress, as emotional supports. Others can serve as sources of guidance and as sounding boards with whom to discuss possible solutions to problems, or perhaps more basically, as providers of encouragement, empathy, and shared responsibility. In such supportive contexts, the individual facing stressful circumstances finds it easier to maintain psychological equilibrium and tolerable levels of tension—and hence can more effectively deal with the stressor. As with the other sets of factors mentioned above, considerable research supports these general assertions, with the majority of such studies finding that, in fear-provoking situations, individuals actively seek out other people. Even the mere presence of others, without them making any overt intervention, seems to reduce fear (Wrightsman, 1972).

Vulnerability to crisis reactions due to social isolation therefore is an important area of concern for the supportive therapist. Individuals who live alone, who are introverted, or who are alienated from friends and family seem to be particularly susceptible. Assessment of the degree of alienation and the possibility of quickly mobilizing others to provide support thus become important issues in developing a treatment plan for the distressed client.

Coping Mechanisms

We are now approaching the close of the theoretical description of crisis reactions. Having discussed the sources of stress and the factors that lead to heightened vulnerability, we can now discuss the actual coping behaviors that are used to deal with stress, and their effectiveness (bottom of Fig. 5.1).

Whether or not such behaviors are actually reducing stress is obviously an important issue in our understanding of crises.

The quality and effectiveness of coping behaviors are difficult to judge in any general fashion, because so much depends on the specific situation facing a client. Sometimes, for example, keeping quiet and doing nothing may be the most efficient way to handle a particular stressor; under other circumstances, such an approach proves to be disastrous. This problem of situational specificity thus requires that the therapist assess each client and stressor in an individual fashion, rather than attempting to make global judgments. For purposes of a theoretical discussion, however, perhaps a somewhat different mode of analysis and evaluation can be used. Two interrelated issues may be considered and assessed: (1) the process by which coping behaviors are decided upon and (2) the penalities one has to pay for using particular coping strategies.

With regard to the means by which an individual decides on how to manage a stressor, consider the following examples. Person A, overwrought and very tense, nevertheless attempts to make a rational and realistic evaluation of the stressful circumstances, thinks through the various options of how to deal with the situation, considers the possible outcomes of each choice, makes a decision based on these analyses, and then acts. Person B, equally tense and disturbed, becomes preoccupied with the feelings of tension themselves and can only seem to think about immediate ways to relieve this inner disturbance. Issues pertaining to the stressor and how to deal with it effectively are largely ignored. A temporary solution is arrived at (e.g., get drunk, leave the stressful situation) and the individual does experience some tension reduction — only to face it again as the short-lived escape comes to an end. Person C, faced with the same stressor, almost immediately gives way to feelings of being overwhelmed, cannot seem to think clearly, is convinced that disaster is looming, and behaves in an impulsive, unthinking way.

These examples are provided to illustrate variations in the degree to which a systematic and logical approach to stress management is utilized. Quite obviously, the more rational and planned the approach, the more likely will be an effective resolution of the stress; conversely, the more impulsive and irrational the approach, the greater the probability of a disastrous and tragic outcome.

The second, related issue to be considered here pertains to the penalties an individual pays for the use of various coping behaviors. The term *penalty* is used in a general sense to refer to negative "side effects" that occur as a result of an individual's attempts to deal with a crisis. Such negative effects can occur in various realms of living: (1) negative effects on the individual's own psychological state (e.g., feeling guilty over a course of action); (2) deleterious effects on other people (e.g., family or friends becoming angry and withdrawing support); and (3) effects which in the long run only make the stressor itself more severe (e.g., studying for a critical exam — the more delay, the less time to prepare).

Summary of Theory and Practical Implications

From the foregoing theoretical material, one gets an appreciation of the complex factors that may be operating in crisis situations. If a supportive therapist is to intervene effectively, an assessment of all these factors should be made in an attempt to fully understand the client's dilemma. This kind of evaluation is, under the best of circumstances, difficult. Under emerging crisis conditions, with time urgency, limited sources of information, and a client who may not communicate effectively, the task is particularly difficult. Nevertheless, the therapist attempts to make judgments in the following areas:

1. *Sources of stress.* External, internal, or a combination of both? Severity, predictability, and temporal factors (sudden, unexpected, gradual onset, etc.)? Degree of social support available? Client's immediate emotional reaction to stressor?

2. *Vulnerability to crisis reactions.* Past and present physiological reactions? Family history of crisis reactions? Similarity of current stressor to earlier traumas? General feelings of inadequacy or helplessness? Use of drugs or alcohol?

3. *Coping mechanisms.* Those being considered in current crisis? Processes by which they were arrived at? Are there penalties associated with each? Likelihood of success? What is likely to happen if coping strategy is unsuccessful? Tendencies toward disorganization and impulsivity?

Based on these considerations, the supportive therapist attempts to formulate a treatment plan that will best help the client negotiate the present crisis. After the next section, in which several typical clients in crisis are portrayed, the remainder of this chapter will discuss the processes and techniques involved in supportive therapy.

CLIENTS NEEDING SUPPORTIVE THERAPY

The theoretical material suggests that virtually anyone may experience crisis reactions in their lives, depending on the severity of stress, the coping behaviors available, and other factors in stressful situations. Thus therapists need to be generally sensitive to potential crises with all their clientele and avoid the pitfall of making prejudgments based on diagnostic labels or casually observed symptoms. Despite this overall caution, however, there appear to be several categories of clients who are especially susceptible to the disorganization and impulsivity of crisis reactions. These, of course, are individuals who display the types of vulnerabilities and ineffective coping behaviors that were described in the previous section. These high-risk clients were also briefly cited in Chapter 4 in our discussion of intake decisions, and they were described as falling into four general classes: (1) persons under severe situational stress; (2) persons undergoing acute disorganization and distress induced by physiological insult (e.g., brain damage or a "bad trip" from drugs); (3) decompensating neurotic persons who experience a panic reaction when their usual psychological defenses fail to function; and (4) individuals in an acute psychotic state who are undergoing intense fear, disordered thought processes, and bizarre inner experiences.

In the following paragraphs, a brief case illustration from each of these categories will be presented. These examples were chosen to provide naturalistic accounts of crisis reactions and also to highlight the interplay of the various theoretical factors discussed in the previous section.

Severe Situational Stress

Mrs. D is a thirty-six-year-old housewife who has devoted most of her married life to raising two sons, maintaining her home, and participating in modest social activities with a few other families with whom she and her husband have contact. Other people see Mrs. D and her family as living a stable, organized, and seemingly contented life.

However, as with most families, life is more complex than it appears on the surface. Although Mrs. D does not consider herself to have psychological problems and although others perceive her to be "normal," there have been times when she has felt very "moody and blue" and "down on herself." On most of these occasions her husband has been able to restore better feelings by being supportive and attentive, but it seems in the last few years that it has become progressively harder to snap out of these moods. Recently, she has even felt surges of a brooding anger toward her husband because he does not seem to try hard enough to help with her feelings.

If we make a deeper examination of Mrs. D and her marriage, some underlying destructive processes can be seen. The gradual and insidious nature of these problems make them difficult for Mrs. or Mr. D to fully understand, yet they are reacting emotionally to them in a progressively more negative manner.

Mrs. D began her relationship with her husband sixteen years ago. She had always been generally insecure within herself, unassertive, and emotionally dependent on other people. During their courtship and the first year of marriage, she was ecstatic over the fact that someone like her husband could actually feel affection and closeness for her. During those early years, however, at a time when Mr. D frequently had to work long hours in establishing his business, Mrs. D would occasionally experience some pangs of insecurity and neglect. When she communicated these feelings of neglect to her husband, his reaction was a sense of confusion and conflict that was rarely expressed openly. He wanted to be reassuring, but he also experienced a gnawing resentment that she was making him feel guilty. He could not quite understand the deeper needs and anxieties in his wife's personality. His usual behavior during these episodes was to openly express affection and support to her, but what was less apparent was that some of the resentment was also showing in his occasional sullen withdrawal.

An interpersonal pattern thus was established early in this marriage that slowly became magnified as the years passed. Mr. D seemed to say the right things to reassure his wife, but her insecurities and periods of depression were fed by the increasing alienation and withdrawal she sensed in her husband. As she communicated her feelings more openly (sometimes now in the form of tearful accusations of his lack of caring), he emotionally withdrew even further. The growing alienation in the later years has come to pervade all aspects of the relationship—from not being able to feel comfortable in routine conversations at dinner to a kind of mechanical, nonintimate approach to sex.

The whole process has now reached a point at which Mrs. D's daily existence is one of inner desperation. She fluctuates between fright, despondency, and anger. Her entire adult life has been focused on her marriage, and not much else has meaning for her. Her desperation reaches a peak when at the supermarket, she overhears a conversation between two of her neighbors in which they are gossiping about seeing her husband with another woman. The ultimate blow is struck, and the bottom drops out for her. Nothing is left but a long, agonizing descent into an exhausted and helpless depression.

When her sons come home from school that afternoon, they find her stuporous and unresponsive. With the help of neighbors, an ambulance is called to bring her to the emergency room.

Crisis via Physiological Insult

"Oh, did I ace that mother _____ exam. Everything he asked I went over ten times last week. I was loaded for bear—and, pow, I shot it all out on that little, old exam booklet! Hey, appreciate you guys inviting me over to your . . . er . . . seance. I've been studying so _____ hard these last few months, I don't know which way is up. . . . Don't laugh, but I never used any stuff like this in my life . . . you reckon it's all right? . . . Look at me, Mom, nineteen years old and I'm popping one for the first time. . . .

"_____, I'm not getting high. I can't let go. It's like I'm crazy, always been that way. No don't laugh, I'm serious. . . . I've been under the gun man, like in a way you wouldn't understand. Ever since grade primo, I've been the one. 'You'd better do good, you'd better not mess up, make your momma proud.' . . . No, damn it, it was different from you all. She *never* let up. . . . If only she wasn't so hard about it, like a damned vulture, just sitting there watching, waiting for you to _____ up. . . . Even in high school—listen to me, I can't stop talking—I'd hit the books all night, every night. I'd be so tired I'd crawl into bed . . . and then, oh _____, I couldn't even sleep good. I'd have these nightmares. . . . Huh? Yeah, give me another one, that first didn't do nothing. . . .

"I don't know. I'm all screwed up. You guys do okay, but _____, you're not screwed up like me. . . . Why do I have to push it so hard? The old vulture will get me if I let up. Hee, hee! Oh _____! That's it! The old vulture, she's not dead yet. . . . No, damn it! I won't take it easy. It's all there, in green and blue. What a waste! What a miserable, mother_____ waste! C'mon, gimme another. It's all coming clear. . . .

"Oh, jeez! Quick! Get it off me. They're all over me. Who are you? My head it's floating away. Oh, jeez, help me! I'm not a vulture! My head. Plutarch's coming. Oh God, save me!"

Decompensating Neurosis

The rules were very clear to Miss N when she was growing up. Her parents, especially her father, were the absolute authorities in her life. Her parents saw their mission as one of raising dignified and clean children, pure of body and mind. Emotions, physical needs, and even youthful exuberance were to be held carefully in check. Young minds were to be totally occupied with productive and saintly activities, and even the suspicion that one was engaging in frivolous or unwholesome thoughts was followed by a severe tongue-lashing, or worse, her father's strap. Miss N's upbringing was thus permeated with the idea that we must all guard against the evil side of our being, for without this constant restriction, terrible and hateful forces from within would be unleashed.

The physical beatings by her father occurred with some frequency during Miss N's preadolescent years. She was reduced to a whimpering, helpless state each time they happened, and she was completely confused because usually she had done nothing to deserve them. The painful welts on her legs and buttocks would be somewhat soothed, however, when later he would hold her closely on his lap and talk about purging the evil from their bodies.

Miss N entered her adolescent years an understandably tense and inhibited individual. She had developed an array of defenses to which she rigidly adhered in order to protect herself from a deep wellspring of anxiety associated with her parents and an even more ominous fear that something dirty and disgusting might reside within her personality. Thus she filled her waking hours with endless ritualized activities, thereby preventing opportunity for idle and possibly dangerous thoughts. She also avoided unnecessary contacts with other people of her age, feeling much safer when engaged in formal school activities or returning to her structured environment at home.

During her senior year in high school, a lonely and isolated Miss N begins to undergo a subtle transition. It starts with a vague recognition that her life is a somber and limited one. And further, she is becoming aware that her classmates, many of whom are spontaneous, outgoing, and emotional individuals, are not bad or evil. The contrast between their enthusiasm and joy of living and her own constricted way of life is becoming progressively more obvious. She feels a hungering for others and a desire to "come out" of herself.

In a sense, these inner stirrings are prompting her to let down her defenses somewhat.

As a first step, she is determined to go to the spring dance at school, the first such event she has ever considered attending. She is fearful and unsure of herself at the dance, but when one of her classmates asks her to dance, she is grateful for his attentions. As he holds her on the dance floor, however, she feels a sudden rush of emotion and then is totally overwhelmed by a combination of physical attraction, disgust, and sheer terror. The ghosts, the childhood fears, the long-standing yearnings, all so carefully hidden behind her defenses, have burst forth, and she is in panic and in a crisis.

Acute Psychotic States

Off and on for quite a few years, Mr. A has been wrestling with a peculiar problem. In his mind's eye, he pictures all objects in the world as being kept in their correct place, and in proper relationship with one another, by a vast complex of electrical forces. In some strange fashion he senses that his inner thoughts are kept in separate and orderly compartments by these same forces. They are so real to him that at times he can almost see the vast network of electrical conduits holding everything together. He is not sure how he arrived at this particular view of himself and the universe, but he remembers first starting to think about it when he was eleven years old—the time when his father had a "nervous breakdown."

Mr. A has not talked about these thoughts with others for fear that he could not explain them very well. Usually he just continues his solitary existence, merely trying to eke out enough money to live on from whatever job he happens to have at the time.

He is not sure why it happens, but there have been times in his life when the electrical forces seemed to lose their power—and the result was an awful mess. Objects blend together, events get out of order, and time seems to take on a cosmic quality. Even more peculiar to Mr. A on these occasions is his feeling that his thoughts actually "become" the blend of objects and events that he sees in the environment. Sometimes he wonders how others are reacting to these uncanny changes in the way things operate in the world.

In thinking about these occasional "power failures," Mr. A can remember some confusing incidents, such as the time he was being inducted into the army. He does not recall what actually happened, but he, along with thirty or so other men, was standing naked in a room. A loud voice had yelled, "Come this way, the doc is ready for you." The milling crowd started through the door. To Mr. A one door was the same as all others. So he proceeded to leave by another exit, followed by three other stragglers in the group. He and his little entourage created quite a stir as they wandered into the main lobby of the reception center.

Life has not been going well for Mr. A this last month. He has been struggling to keep his perceptions and thoughts in order, despite what seems to be constant pressure for his systems to deteriorate. For some reason it is more frightening this time, and he desperately wants someone to help him hold things together. His new job as a messenger is a challenge, but he is unsure of his capabilities. There are so many details to remember.

On his first trip today, he delivers the package to the wrong office. He is afraid to bring it back to the dispatcher. Everything is getting confused; the very air around him is highly charged. The electrical forces are not getting weaker this time but are instead becoming almost overwhelming. He feels caught in their web and is too frightened to move. Even a little twitch may destroy the world. He can see the people that are crowded around him. "Why are they moving and talking? Don't they realize that everything may explode? Oh good, here come the police; they'll get it straightened out."

Summary of Cases

The case sketches were presented to highlight, in a naturalistic way, the various factors discussed in the theoretical model of crisis. As can be seen in these illustrations, the factors do not operate in isolation but must be viewed in relation to one another and evaluated in the perspective of the client's overall life.

In the first example, that of the woman who becomes severely depressed, we can see the effects of a major trauma—her husband's infidelity. However, this severe external stress occurs in the context of considerable internal stress stemming from the mounting feelings of neglect and alienation that have developed in her marriage. On the vulnerability issue, we can discern some long-standing psychological processes (passivity, dependency, lack of interests outside the marriage) that increase her susceptibility. And finally, with respect to coping strategies, the slow erosion of her marital relationship over the years illustrates the deleterious consequences of her ineffective means of dealing with the stress of loneliness and her need for affection. These long-range processes have occurred so slowly and privately that friends were quite surprised at the "sudden" onset of depression. Indeed, the accumulation of problems was so subtle that even the client and her husband could not see them clearly. All they really knew was that they were becoming progressively less happy with each other.

The second case also illustrates the effects of a single traumatic incident (a bad trip from drugs) bringing on a crisis reaction. Again, as in the first illustration, we get a sense of some long-standing internal stresses in the life of the client. However, here the client seems to have coped with his mother's chronic pressures for school achievement in an adequate, albeit hard-pushing, fashion. Although distressed by his mother's attitudes, it is certainly possible that in future years this client would resolve or "grow out of" these problems. Unfortunately, a convergence of circumstances (just finishing a big exam, being exhausted, turning up at a drug party) bring about a highly dangerous, drug-induced psychotic episode.

In the example of decompensating neurosis, we see a somewhat different balance among the crisis-producing factors. The external event (dancing with a boy) hardly can be considered a major stress in and of itself. However, this minor incident triggers a devastating array of internal stressors with which this teenager cannot cope. Feelings and impulses that had been carefully buried behind a rigid set of psychological defenses suddenly confront the client, and she is emotionally overwhelmed. Because of the very severe family background we could also estimate that she was psychologically vulnerable to a crisis reaction, particularly so during her senior year, when she began to gradually "let down" her defenses.

The last case is presented to illustrate crisis in an individual who has been marginally adjusted throughout most of his life. Most likely the victim of physiological vulnerability (based on a genetic predisposition), Mr. A's thought patterns and mode of perceiving the world appear to be tenuous. Most of the time he has been able to keep his unusual thoughts to himself, and he has survived through a series of temporary and unskilled jobs. During times of increased stress, however (as when going for the Army medical exam), his borderline thinking processes deteriorate even further into a markedly illogical mode. The most recent incident, involving the anxiety and confusion of a new job, is too much for him, and a severe and risky psychotic state is precipitated.

OVERVIEW OF SUPPORTIVE THERAPY

The crises described in the previous section perhaps convey the highly volatile and dangerous situations into which the supportive therapist enters. Literally anything can happen, because people in crisis have been pushed to the extreme. The therapist has to be prepared for the worst and must institute measures to prevent disaster from occurring. Will the depressed housewife attempt suicide? Is it possible that the temporarily deranged college student will get a gun and start shooting at all the vultures that he "sees" around him? Perhaps the terrorized high school girl finds it safer to withdraw into a dreamlike fantasy world, where neither her emotions nor external reality can get to her. Will the catatonic man in the last example, trapped in his system of electrical forces, suddenly plunge through the office window seeking an escape?

In this brief section, we will consider two general aspects of supportive therapy: (1) the therapist's overall approach and responsibilities and (2) the usual sequence of therapeutic tasks encountered in this form of treatment.

The Therapist's Approach and Responsibilities

Needless to say, the therapist who assumes responsibility for a client in crisis faces what amounts to life and death issues. In this sense, although the period of treatment may be relatively short, a complete commitment to the safety and psychological survival of the client is required. Translating this principle into everyday practice thus can mean irregular work hours, lengthy phone conversations late at night, leaving the safety of one's office or home to meet emergencies as they are developing, and being able to maintain one's own equilibrium and good judgment in the face of deteriorating and sometimes terror-filled situations. Certainly many therapists are unable or unwilling to meet these basic tenets of supportive therapy.

Furthermore, the supportive therapist must be able to step into a crisis situation and "take charge." Psychological emergencies frequently call for direct and firm action and rapid mobilization of family, friends, or other agencies to assist in the crisis. A passive, overly cautious or nondirective therapist may only add to the confusion, or frighten a client even more. On the other hand, a "strong," calm, and directive therapist may be the only buoy that a client can hang on to in an otherwise turbulent and crumbling situation.

This necessity for rapid and decisive intervention places an added burden on the therapist: the necessity of making a fast and accurate evaluation of the client, the risk factors, and the overall crisis situation. One may not always be able to afford the luxury of lengthy psychological testing or extensive history gathering from family members. Assessing current mental status, suicide potential, sources of stress, and so forth, thus become important skills for the supportive therapist. Naturally, these assessments may not go into detail or detect many subtleties, but the principal components of the crisis situation need to be identified and evaluated rapidly and accurately.

Herein also lies one of the added risks facing the supportive therapist. Since the therapist does "take charge" and the client and others do, in large measure, follow the therapist's directives, mistakes tend to get magnified. Should the therapist make an inaccurate evaluation or exercise poor judgment in giving advice, the crisis may become even more severe—only increasing the risks involved for the client.

To summarize, then, the supportive therapist enters a crisis situation with the aims of restoring equilibrium, preventing a tragic outcome, and bringing the client to a point at which he or she does not feel overwhelmed by the current stress. An important aspect of these aims is also to help the client utilize effective coping strategies to deal with the current stress. Supportive therapy, on the other hand, is not usually oriented toward trying to resolve long-term psychological problems in a client's life. After the crisis subsides, the supportive therapist may encourage the client to seek assistance for these more chronic difficulties, but such treatment is generally of another sort (to be covered in other chapters).

Sequence of Therapeutic Tasks

Before proceeding to the specific techniques involved in supportive therapy, it is important that the reader gain a perspective on the overall process. When are the techniques to be applied? To what purpose? Is there a usual order of events that take place or a hierarchy of priorities that must concern the therapist? Although the answers to these questions may vary depending on the specifics of each crisis, there appears to be a general progression of phases in this therapeutic approach. These phases may merge into one another in a gradual fashion in actual practice, but they can be outlined as follows.

Phase 1: Evaluation of risk, stabilization, and mobilizing protective forces A crisis reaction, almost by definition, is an unstable condition. The extreme emotions, the sense of being overwhelmed, and the feeling of helplessness literally impel the client to get some sort of relief. All too often that relief is sought in tragic avenues—as we have already seen, in suicide, psychosis, or impulsive and destructive behaviors. Quite clearly, then, the first tasks facing the therapist are to evaluate the risks involved, protect the client from such tragic consequences, and to reduce the immediate distress to manageable levels.

Phase 2: Identification of sources of stress As the overwhelming emotions begin to subside somewhat, the client may be able to talk about (sometimes only partly coherently) the immediate precipitants of the crisis, and the client and therapist take the first step toward a logical analysis of the stressful situation. As indicated earlier, these sources of stress may be external situational factors or stressors coming from within the personality of the client. Quite frequently, the internal sources are the more difficult to identify. During this phase the client's emotional level may fluctuate dramatically—at times becoming calmer as he or she works toward a rational understanding of the crisis, and at times giving way to the extreme emotions of phase 1.

As part of the therapist's quest for as much information as possible in this phase of treatment, all other sources (family, friends, coworkers, participants in the immediate situation, etc.) are also tapped.

Phase 3: Consideration of coping strategies As the therapist and client gain an understanding of the factors that are contributing to the crisis, their analysis proceeds to an investigation of the methods by which the client has attempted to deal with the current stress. These methods of coping may be oriented toward dealing with the immediate external stressors or they may pertain to psychological defenses that attempt to protect the individual from current internal stressors. The effectiveness of these coping strategies are evaluated by both client and therapist, with the general orientation that perhaps there are more suitable methods of coping available.

A transition is thereby instituted in the emotional approach of the client, from one of helpless giving in to the stress to one of active problem solving. This transition is frequently difficult and gradual, since the client may still feel overwhelmed; however, as the possibilities for more effective control are considered, the client's high distress levels begin to subside.

During the latter part of this phase, the more effective coping behaviors are identified and decided upon. The relative contributions of client and therapist to these decisions vary considerably from case to case depending on the mental and emotional status of the client. If possible, having the client do much of the rational analysis and problem solving seems preferable, since this seems to foster a sense of control and mastery. However, in many instances clients may be in too great a turmoil for such systematic and thoughtful activity. In these instances, the therapist may be quite directive and specific in giving advice and in guiding the future course of action.

Phase 4: Implementing new coping behaviors and environmental manipulation: With the support and guidance of the therapist, the client now proceeds to put the new coping strategies into practice. In some situations this may be preceded by considerable discussion with the therapist as to how best to implement these new behaviors, the possible pitfalls, and the various environmental reactions that are possible. For some novel behaviors, it may be necessary to engage in practice and rehearsal with the therapist prior to their actual use in the environment.

Concurrent with these developments, the therapist may take active steps to "prepare" the client's environment for the new behaviors in order to maximize the likelihood of success. Thus, where appropriate, conferences with family, employers, or other relevant parties are utilized to arrange for supportive and understanding reactions.

Phase 5: Consideration of possible outcomes Of course, life is not as simple as is implied in the preceding paragraphs. Some clients may not be able to put new behaviors into practice. In some situations, the factors are such that there is nothing that one can do to reduce the stress. In other crises, the new behaviors that are attempted by the client turn out to be ineffective or even make the situation worse. Obviously there are no guarantees in life, especially in the tumultous atmosphere of crises.

For these reasons the client and therapist review the possible outcomes of the new course of action, including those that are negative. This phase of treatment is based on the assumption that it is better for the client to have anticipated and faced the most dire of the possible outcomes while still in the relative safety of therapy rather than be unexpectedly confronted by them later on. In a sense the client may thus become more emotionally prepared to face the continuation of stress and perhaps not be overwhelmed again should this happen.

Phase 6: Follow-up contact, arrangements for therapy on underlying problems, and termination This last phase of supportive therapy is important for several reasons. Once the client proceeds to use the new coping behaviors, the therapist has responsibilities to monitor their degree of success and to remain available for further supportive contact should it be needed. Clients may undergo a temporary easing of the crisis reaction once a new set of coping behaviors is instituted, only to revert to disorganization again should a setback occur. Thus the therapist may need to provide continued support and guidance until the new approach to the stressors is firmly established.

As part of this last phase, the client may begin to profitably consider the long-range factors that have contributed to the crisis and, where appropriate, make arrangements for therapy aimed at resolving such underlying problems.

Although supportive therapy is generally relatively brief, the client's contacts with the therapist can be very intense, and understandably, strong dependency may develop. After therapy ends, the client may become overly frightened at being alone or may lose hope that the stressors can be managed. New coping behaviors that appear to be working under the guidance and support of the therapist may suddenly seem to be flimsy once therapy ends. For these reasons, special care is exercised in the termination process, with the therapist helping the client to anticipate "going it alone," cultivating other sources of support, gradually reducing the frequency and intensity of therapeutic contact, and "leaving the door open" should future contact be needed.

AN ILLUSTRATIVE CASE

Having reviewed the various tasks and phases of supportive therapy, let us consider a case example that illustrates their application. The reader is urged to pay particular attention to the different therapeutic tasks that are accomplished in each phase. In addition, it would be instructive to note the specific treatment techniques that are used as the therapy progresses. These techniques will be more formally outlined in the concluding section of the chapter.

The crisis-oriented treatment administered to Miss N (labeled as the decompensating neurotic in a previous section) will be reviewed. This case was chosen because the sources of stress are, to a considerable extent, internal; that is, they come from her own emotional dynamics. The application of supportive techniques to such an internally based crisis is perhaps more elusive than when applied to crises brought about by situational stress. Hence it is hoped that a more subtle appreciation of supportive therapy will occur via this case illustration.

Recall that Miss N, a high school senior, had undergone a severely restrictive upbringing under an authoritarian and punitive father. She seemed to harbor intense anxieties connected with parental punishment and had even stronger fears that evil and despicable forces within her personality might be unleashed if she did not keep them under tight rein. Her crisis reaction occurred when, prompted by desires to "let down her defenses a little," she danced with a young man at a high school party. The sudden and overwhelming rush of intense inner emotions while on the dance floor was the beginning of Miss N's crisis.

No one noticed when Miss N quietly but hurriedly left the dance. Had they paid attention, they would have seen a face frozen in shock and fear and an uncontrollable shivering. Somehow she made it home, her mind and emotions racing. Met by her parents as she entered the house, the confrontation was too much. Her shrieking and wailing were uncontrollable. When she tried to explain, her words were unintelligible. The panic was real and all-pervasive. The family physician was called. She was given a sedative, and she slept. The next day she was withdrawn, almost stuporous, and unresponsive to her parents' questions and those of a doctor during a medical exam. In the afternoon, after a period of increasing agitation, another panic attack occurred, and the physician recommended that a therapist be brought in for an emergency consultation. The first meeting took place that evening in the therapist's office.

Therapist: Nancy, I know some things are upsetting you very much, and I'm here to help you. My name is Howes, Mary Howes. I'm a doctor, and I'm going to help. We'll work it out. Try to relax a little. I'll be with you. . . . Try to settle down some and tell me what happened.

Client [*Weeping and agitated*]: I, I, ugh, who, I, I . . . [*Long wail*]. . . . Daddy?

Therapist: Your father and mother are in the outside office. They'll be here. It's okay, we're all here. Try to relax. You're going to be okay. I know that you're frightened right now, but it'll get better. I'll help you calm down. . . . Listen to me. My name is Mary, and I'm a doctor. . . . Breathe deeply and let yourself relax a little. . . . That's it, deep regular breaths. Relax your arms. . . . Good, you're doing fine. Relax some more. That's fine. . . . Just listen to me, and keep relaxing. You're doing well. I'll be with you and help get it under control. . . . Tell me, Nancy, how old are you?

Client [*Still weeping and agitated*]: Seven, uh, uh, seventeen, I, I, uh, I, clean, uh, they, ugh, they . . . seventeen, I, scared! [*Shivers*]

Therapist: I know, Nancy, it is scary right now, but we'll work it out together. Here, put on this sweater. Keep breathing deeply. That's it. Relax. That's it. It's going to be all right. . . . And you're a senior in high school?

Client [*Slightly calmer*]: Yes.

Therapist: You're doing fine. Relax some more, and keep listening to me. That's good. Breathe deeply. It's settling down a little now. . . . Which school do you go to?

Client: Lincoln.

Therapist: Do you like it there?

Client [*Suddenly becoming very agitated again*]: Over, over, ugh, I, can't, I, I, . . .

Therapist: It's okay, Nancy. It's okay. Don't think about that now. Listen to me. Relax. Just like you were doing before. Yes. Fine. Get a grip on it. Breathe deeply and calmly. That's the way. . . .

The therapist's attempts at stabilization are proceeding very gradually, with some retreats, but as the session goes on, Miss N becomes somewhat less agitated and disorganized. Note that she seemed able to answer specific, factual questions. However, when the therapist makes the error of asking her if she likes her high school (a more vague and feeling-oriented question), Miss N seemed to become frightened and disorganized again.

After approximately an hour of primarily stabilization procedures, the therapist judges that Miss N may be able to tolerate talking about the crisis situation itself. Her intent here is to gain more information about Miss N's current emotional and intellectual status and the various risk factors that may require immediate attention.

Therapist: Nancy, I need to know some things about what happened the other night. Whatever it was seemed to shake you up pretty badly. And we both need to figure it out so we can decide how to handle it. Was that the first dance you'd been to?

Client: Yes. I don't go out very much [*Tearful and nervous*].

Therapist: What happened when you first got there?

Client: Not much. I don't know. . . . I was just standing around with some of the other kids. . . . Uh, you know [*Starts to cry*]. I'll never be able to go back. . . . I'm scared . . . dirty . . . Do I have to talk?

Therapist: I'll help you with it, Nancy. I know it's hard, but you'll feel better if we talk it out. You were standing with the other kids, and then what happened?

Client: Well, I don't know, I, you know, I was watching Karen dancing. She was having a good time, you know, just letting it go. I could see Mr. Baum watching her too. He made me nervous.

Therapist: Who is Mr. Baum?

Client: He's the assistant principal. Uh, ugh [*Agitated*]. He scares me. Uh, uh, but, you know, Karen didn't seem to care. I really, I don't know, I just started to feel funny. I, er, I don't know. . . .

Therapist: I know it's hard to put into words, but try.

Client [*Pause*]: Well, you know, I guess, er, I wanted to be like Karen, but, I don't now . . . it was like I couldn't stand for Mr. Baum, you know, to be staring at me that way. I was . . . I, I remember getting real scared. . . . Ah! Oh gee. I'm really feeling scared inside.

Therapist: It'll be okay. Do what I said before . . . try to relax, breathe deeply. . . . That's it. . . . Am I pushing too hard?

Client [*Laughs nervously*]: I don't know. I, er, well, I am feeling better, but, you know, I, I don't know what's happening to me.

Therapist: When you get those scared feelings, what kinds of things go through your mind? What do you feel like doing?

Client: I don't now. I just kind of, uh, you know, get lost. . . . Uh, I just want to hide; make them go away, I don't know. . . .

Therapist: What are your plans for when you go home this evening?

Client: Do I have to go now?

Therapist: No, not at all. We can stay together as long as you'd like . . . until you kind of get a grip on things. . . . I guess I was really asking if you're going to be okay when you go home.

Client: I think so. I'm really tired. I need to take a shower, er, wash my hair. Then I think I can sleep. . . . I, er, I, you know, I just don't think I can stand them asking questions. Don't get me wrong, I, er, . . .

Therapist: I understand. I'll talk to them, just kind of generally explain. I guess you kind of need your folks right now, but I guess they shouldn't rock the boat. . . . Is that okay?

Client: Oh thank you, yes. You just don't know my father. . . . I, er, I guess, I, I just get so mixed up, but, er, can I come back and see you?

Therapist: I want you to very much. We'll get it cleared up. Let's meet tomorrow, and I'll give you my number in case you need to call me before then. Call anytime you need to. . . .

This session lasted approximately fifteen more minutes, after which the therapist had a half-hour meeting with Nancy's parents. She explained to them the need for their supervision and support of Nancy and the importance that they not probe or place additional stress on their daughter. The therapist also learned from them that Nancy had no previous history of suicidal behavior or impulsivity that they were aware of.

This information, coupled with the fact that Nancy did not express ideas of suicide or destructive impulses, suggested that supervision at home was a feasible course of action. It was also recognized that the client was still subject to bouts of panic and disorganization but that in calmer moments she seemed to be oriented and capable of appropriate intellectual functions.

The therapist noted that Nancy was responsive to interpersonal support and indeed seemed eager to maintain therapeutic contact. At the same time, it was judged that an immediate return to school would probably place too much stress on her. The overall picture therefore indicated a continuation of brief but intensive supportive therapy until Nancy's emotional turmoil subsided and she could gain some rational control over the stress. An appointment was made for the next day.

Therapist: Good morning, Nancy. How did things go last night?

Client: Okay, I guess. I really slept. I couldn't believe, you know, my mom and dad. At breakfast they were really nervous, but they were, you know, trying to be so nice. I don't know, I just, I didn't know how to act with them . . . er, er, just kept quiet, mostly.

Therapist: You seem pretty talkative now. Is everything okay between you and me?

Client: Yeah, but, but, I don't know, if I know what, what happened. Something just came over me, you know, er [*Agitated*], like, uh, uh, like something outside of me. . . . uh, God maybe, you know, uh, uh, I was so scared. . . . I, I . . .

Therapist: Nancy, lots of times when we experience new feelings, er, or we see ourselves in a new light, it seems strange and unreal. And frightening. . . . Do you get what I'm saying?

Client: Yes, but, I don't know, uh, uh . . . I think so.

Therapist: I think that's what happened to you. . . . It won't be easy, but I think we can figure it out. Do you feel ready to try?

Client: Yes, but, I don't know where to start.

Therapist: Well, let's start with some of the things you mentioned last night. . . . You were at the dance. You kind of felt that you . . . you wished you could be like Karen. But you were afraid of what Mr. Baum would think.

Client: I can't remember it all. Uh, you know, uh, it's just that scared feeling that stays with me. . . . I don't know, I've always been shy and afraid. I, I, never even thought much, you know, about things except for school. . . . Ugh, I can't even think about school now, I can't, . . . I don't know . . . Ugh!

Therapist: Try to keep working at it.

Client: I was getting sick, you know, of myself. . . . Just letting life pass me by. . . . I, I, was trying, kind of, trying . . . trying to be like the other kids [*Starts weeping*]. But, I, I, uh, I'm different. I don't know, uh, uh. . . . And then Bucky asked me to dance. [*Crying*] I didn't want to. I was afraid . . . ugh [*Very agitated*]. I couldn't even say no.

Therapist: You're doing fine. It's difficult, I know.

Client [*Crying*]: And it was, you know, a slow dance. Oh! Oh!

Therapist: It's okay.

Client: I never touched a boy before. I don't know. . . . It's not right. . . . But there I was, I could feel him, ugh, you know, ugh, it wasn't right. . . . Everything started spinning. I just had to get away. . . . I couldn't think; I can't think now. . . . Ugh! . . . I, I, am I going crazy? I, I . . .

Therapist: No, you're not. What's more, it took a lot of courage to tell me. . . . You're going through what a lot of young people go through—

starting to come out of your shell, finding out about yourself. . . . Sometimes it's a hard and frightening thing to do, and . . .

Client: But, my father, . . . my mother . . . [*Crying*]. I don't know. . . . Uh, uh. They, he, uh, would, would, uh, call it ugly . . . bad . . . uh. . . . I'm feeling sick again.

Therapist: That's part of finding out about yourself. Kind of untangling who you are from what they want you to be. . . . You've got your own feelings and needs, and there's nothing wrong with them. . . . To tell the truth, it sounds like your folks have been pretty tough on you.

Client: I don't think it's right for me to talk about them, but . . .

The client goes on to talk about the restrictiveness and punitiveness of her parents and her consequent patterns of anxiety and guilt. She gradually begins to acknowledge that her recent feelings of panic have been due to a combination of factors: her "trying to come out of her shell," not knowing how to deal with newly emergent feelings, being terrified at her parents' reactions to these changes, and not knowing how to act at school. The morning therapy session ends with an agreement to discuss possible ways of dealing with these complex problems. Another meeting is scheduled for later in the afternoon. After a brief review of the main sources of stress in the afternoon session, the client continues to describe her feelings of helplessness to do anything about them.

Client: I'm not very good at this, Dr. Howes. Uh, uh, I keep coming back, you know, to the same thing. Everything, it all, uh, becomes confused. I, I, just want to run away; you know, it's too much . . . [*Nervous laugh*]. Why are you shaking your head?

Therapist: I was thinking just the opposite. Here you've just come through a kind of frightening and confusing experience, and you've really made tremendous progress. You've got a good idea about some of the stresses and strains behind it all, and you've got a good grip on your emotions. . . . Sure, it's confusing . . . there's still a lot to work on . . . but don't be so hard on yourself. . . . Let's take it a step at a time.

Client: Well, I guess, you know, I've always run away from things. Never, I, never, you know, faced up to things. I don't know, it was easier, uh, uh, easier to, you know, just get lost, lost in, like homework or, maybe reading. Uh! That wasn't so good, huh?

Therapist: You're right. There probably are some better ways . . . to face things, and handle them more directly. . . . Seems like you've already taken the first step . . . just like we were doing before . . . not letting your emotions run away with you, and kind of stopping to analyze all the parts of the problem . . . and now, figuring out the best ways, for you, to meet the problems.

Client: Uh, it sounds okay, but, I don't know . . .

Therapist: Okay. Look. Right now, you've got it kind of divided into three problems. How to handle your parents, uh, how to face things at school, and, uh, uh, how can I describe it, er, how to handle your own feelings, when you kind of open up to yourself. You know what I mean?

Client: Yes, I think I know; but it's so much, it's, it's . . . well like my dad . . . he'll never change . . . it's impossible. . . .

Therapist: Nancy, hold it a second. What you just said . . . it's impossible . . . that's part of the problem. That's the old thing about running away from things . . . just sort of giving up. Try to catch yourself when you do that. . . . Let's work at it, think about it. . . . There's got to be a better way.

Client: Okay, Dr. Howes. I'll try.

Therapist: Let's start with your parents. I guess they'll want some explanation. They really seem concerned. Let's talk about some ways that you can deal with them. . . .

The next two sessions were devoted to discussions of a variety of possible approaches that the client might take toward her parents and schoolmates. The emotions of helplessness and fright seem to subside considerably, and they are replaced by more routine feelings of hesitancy and nervousness at the prospect of taking some active steps at managing difficult situations.

In the interim, the therapist also had, with the client's knowledge, several consultations with her parents. These sessions proved to be difficult in view of their rigid, moralistic attitudes toward Nancy and their strong feelings that any compromise of their convictions might in some way cause their daughter to go astray. Despite such unbending attitudes, they did seem to display genuine affection for Nancy and a great deal of anxiety over what they described as Nancy's recent "attack of nerves." Under considerable pressure from the therapist, they tentatively agreed that, over the next period of time, they would try to simply be "good listeners" and "understanding parents" whenever Nancy tried to explain her plight. The therapist concluded, however, that any such lessening of parental pressures was likely to be short-lived in the absence of more extended consultations or therapy involving the whole family.

On succeeding days, two further sessions with Nancy involved rehearsal and role playing of some new behaviors.

Client: No, it just doesn't sound right. Er, you know. It's okay when we just talk about it . . . it seems okay . . . but I don't think I can, you know, talk that way.

Therapist: Nancy, you've been talking that way—very straight and direct—with me for three days now, and you've been doing it well. Now, come on, don't get all tightened up again. We're going to practice. You know it makes sense. . . . You'll get it in your own style. I know it's a change, but let's see how it goes. . . .

Client: Oh well [*Laughs*]. Okay, but it'll sound dumb. Okay . . . Mom, Dad [*Laughs*]. . . . This isn't going to work.

Therapist: Come on, come on [*Laughing also*], let's get serious. You won't win an Emmy this way. Let's get with it.

Client: Okay, okay. Boy, you're no fun. Let's see now. . . . Listen you creeps. . . . Oh, no [*Laughs*]. I didn't say that. . . . I really didn't mean that. . . . You won't tell them . . . [*Serious*]. Okay, I'll try. . . .

Therapist: Get in the mood. You're at home, and they want you to talk to them.

Client: Mom, Dad, er, er, it's hard to say, uh, but I've been thinking . . . [*Nervous laugh*]. There's been a lot on my mind, I don't know. It's just that I'm trying, you know, to grow up. Er, er [*Very serious*], and I've been, er, losing my way. I haven't, you know, done anything wrong, but I got so scared [*Weeping*]. . . . Part of it was, I, I, was, uh, uh, afraid of myself . . . I don't know why . . . and, part of it, oh, oh, part of it was you scared me [*Crying*]. . . . Dr. Howes says it's complicated, but that, uh, uh, I'm not sure, uh, I should keep working on it . . . we can all work on it. . . .

A total of three more sessions brought therapy with Nancy to an end. The first of these meetings took place two days later, after the client had returned to school and had initiated more open discussions with her parents. The remaining sessions were scheduled a week apart and were utilized to evaluate Nancy's overall adjustment and to review her degree of success with new coping behaviors. At these follow-up sessions Nancy had reestablished control over emotional and intellectual functions and had, to a large extent, returned to her rather restrictive and inhibited life-style. However, a window to the deeper aspects of her personality had been temporarily opened, and she was seriously considering longer-term therapy in the future.

SPECIFIC TECHNIQUES

In the sections to follow, the principal treatment techniques of crisis management will be presented. They will be discussed in relation to each phase of supportive therapy as outlined earlier. It is hoped that this approach, along with references to the illustrative case, will provide the reader with both a summary and an appreciation of the practical application of these techniques.

Techniques of Initial Evaluation, Stabilization, and Protection

Events are typically happening in a hectic and deteriorating manner when the supportive therapist first steps into the picture. Therefore several initial tasks must be accomplished concurrently: a rapid evaluation of the client and the overall situation, the initiation of procedures to restore psychological equilibrium in the client, and the institution of protective measures to prevent a tragic outcome of the crisis. Thus, in this risk-laden opening phase a variety of therapy techniques may be utilized.

Initial evaluation Korner (1973) suggests that six areas of client functioning should be immediately assessed. Information pertaining to this evaluation is gathered by directly interviewing the client, observing the client's behaviors and reactions, and questioning others regarding the client's current adjustment and previous history.

First, the therapist makes judgments regarding the client's present *intellectual resources*. Which functions are capable of adequate operation and which are in deficit? Is the client oriented as to time and place? Can the client describe the events surrounding his current situation? Is he capable of providing details? Are thought processes logical or do bizarre and unusual mental events seem to predominate? Does the client seem to display a potential for rational analysis and self-inspection?

Second, the therapist evaluates *interpersonal responsiveness*. Amid the emotional upheaval of the crisis, does the client react to the presence of the therapist or others? Is the presence of certain individuals sought or rejected by the client? Does interpersonal support seem to provide a measure of relief or reassurance? Are the principal figures in the client's life available and capable of offering support?

Third, the client's *emotional status and impulse control* are evaluated. Although the client is in a state of emotional upheaval during the crisis, a careful analysis may reveal particular areas of vulnerability or strength. Has the client totally given in to the severe emotions, or is she capable of at least temporarily gaining control over them? Does the client appear to be able to tolerate the disabling emotions, or does she seem to be on the verge of behaving impulsively in order to gain relief? Is the client communicating, even in a disorganized way, thoughts of suicide or other destructive acts? How has the client handled stressful situations in the past? Is there a history of self-harm, explosive aggressiveness, or psychosis in the client's life? Does the client display emotional qualities that can serve as positive resources in coping with the crisis, for example, affection for others, a sense of family responsibility, religious commitments, a potential for assertiveness and indignation, or a resilient sense of humor?

Fourth, Korner suggests an analysis of the client's *hope structure*. Does the client perceive the current crisis to be the "end of everything," or are there areas of living that hold promise for the future? If one set of important goals has been negated, are there others that can be substituted? Does the client's history reveal a pattern of long-term optimism or pessimism? Are there particular factors or individuals in the client's life that seem to prompt either of these attitudes? Does the client seem capable of using future hopes to sustain him through the current crisis?

A difficult area of evaluation involves assessment of the fifth area, the client's *motivation for self-help*. Can the client mobilize energy and personal resources to participate in treatment actively and to eventually function independently outside of therapy? Such judgments may be based largely on observations of the client's efforts to respond to the therapist. Despite the emotional turmoil, does the client attempt to answer even rudimentary questions? Does the client try to gain mastery over emotions or make efforts to analyze the situation? In other spheres of living, does the client try to maintain simple self-care behaviors, meet work or household responsibilities, and so forth? The fact that some clients in crisis may be motivated for self-help, but may be unable to display such desires because of their current condition, makes this an especially difficult area to evaluate.

Sixth, Korner suggests an assessment of the degree to which the client may be *overdramatizing the crisis*. As with the previous area, this represents an extremely difficult evaluation, one that may not be made with some surety until the crisis has actually subsided. Hence, cautious and conservative judgments that give the benefit of doubt to the client are called for here. Needless to say, however, supportive therapists may occasionally encounter clients who tend to exaggerate the stress that they are under or who engage in histrionic displays for ulterior motives (attention getting, as a weapon against family members, etc.). As suggested, the supportive therapist may entertain the hypothesis of such a pseudocrisis with certain clients; however, until clearly confirmed, risks should be minimized by adopting a supportive approach to the client.

After reviewing these six areas of evaluation, it is clear that the therapist must now integrate these assessments and arrive at some global and complex conclusions. What are the immediate risks of disastrous outcomes (suicide, psychosis, impulsive acting out)? How much supervision and protection does the client require? Is hospitalization necessary? How rapid and intensive does the supportive therapist's intervention need to be? How much of a supportive function can others in the client's life be expected to assume? What are the areas of strength in the client that can form the basis for effective treatment and self-help? As we saw in the case of Miss N, the therapist attempted to make many of these assessments during her first meeting with the client and her parents. On the basis of these evaluations it was judged that the client could return home under the supervision of her parents.

Stabilization Perhaps the most difficult part in all of supportive therapy is helping the client to reestablish psychological equilibrium and control over extreme emotions. This difficulty stems from a variety of sources. First, keep in mind that most clients in crisis have previously attempted to cope with a deteriorating situation, and have failed. Thus there are strong elements of helplessness that are an integral part of the client's reaction. Second, by definition, a crisis in essence represents a felt threat to one's physical or psychological survival, and hence the reaction is profound and all-encompassing. Finally, once a client gives up in attempting to cope with stress and succumbs to the emotional disorganization of crisis reaction, the rampant emotions seem to impede the ability to devise new and more effective coping behaviors.

As a preliminary to considering specific techniques in this area, recall from the theory section of this chapter some of the main factors that contribute to crisis reactions: a sense of being alone in facing the stress, a feeling of helplessness that the stress is insurmountable, and fears of the unpredictable future course of events. These factors, coupled with some general principles of establishing emotional control, form the basis for the techniques to be described.

Perhaps basic to most of the procedures to be described is the very *presence* of the therapist. Apart from expressions of concern, support, and encouragement, the physical and psychological proximity of another individual who is remaining steadfast provides a strong base of reassurance for the client. Of course, the type of presence and the nature of the therapist's communications play a major role in reestablishing equilibrium. In a general sense, however, the therapist's own calm and stable demeanor, soothing voice quality, and emotional closeness exert an ameliorating effect on the client.

In this interpersonal context, there are several specific procedures that may be employed. *Talking the client down* from a severe emotional state with a calm, reassuring, and sometimes repetitive train of talk seems to have a threefold effect: the direct induction of relaxation, diverting the client's attention away from distressing inner processes and onto the calming therapist's presence, and the introduction of more optimistic content into the client's stream of thought. In the case example, recall the therapist's repetitive and intrusive statements, such as, "It will be okay," "Try to relax," "We'll work it out," "Don't think about the bad things right now." These seemed to gradually induce a reduction in Miss N's extreme emotions to more manageable levels.

Other direct means of "taking the edge off" extreme emotions involve *muscular relaxation procedures* (wherein the therapist engages the client's attention on consciously relieving tensed muscle groups); *engaging in diverting activity* (taking a walk, jogging, some form of game or sport, and so forth, depending on its appropriateness for the client); and the use of various *physical* means of inducing a reduction in tension (a hot bath, a neck rub, etc.). Finally, within this category is the possible use of medications, requiring, of course, prescription and consultation by a qualified physician.

As the client steps back from the raw edge of panic or emerges from despair and becomes more able to communicate with the therapist, several additional stabilization techniques come to the fore. The therapist can guide, to some extent, the type of conversation that takes place. *Focusing on real events and concrete reality*, even in a trivial or minimal way, exerts pressure on the client to begin using rational thought processes. At the same time, *avoidance and discouragement of emotional expressions* and guiding the client's attention so as to *minimize preoccupation with fantasies* of a hopeless future should further reduce the immediate emotional upheaval. As communications are thus directed and gradually expanded into the realm of logical, cognitive processes (and away from emotions and fantasies), the client may acquire the beginnings of a sense of mastery over the inner turmoil of the crisis reaction. As part of this entire process, the therapist can encourage this emerging sense of mastery and hope by starting to orient the client toward the later phases of treatment—analyses of the sources of stress and the development of effective problem-solving strategies.

Protecting the client The last of the immediate tasks confronting the therapist is to relieve the stress and to arrange appropriate supervision and care. Naturally, the type and degree of such protection depends on the initial evaluation and the nature of the situation. In this context, then, the risk factors in the client's current situation (suicide potential, degree of emotional and intellectual disorganization, impulse control), as well as strengths and external resources, become the focus of attention.

A rather wide variety of protective measures are available, ranging from relatively mild to severely restrictive. Some general principles should be kept in mind regarding decisions on these measures. First and most obvious is the necessity to invoke sufficient supervision of the client to prevent harm to self and others. On the other hand, measures that are too restrictive and controlling may only contribute to the client's sense of helplessness and thereby impede the future phases of therapy.

Proceeding from the relatively mild to the more restrictive, the following protective measures may be considered. First is a *temporary removal from stressful circumstances* or the therapist's *manipulation of external stressors*. These procedures may involve such things as having the client take some days off from work or school, move in with a friend, or change his or her locale so as to reduce further stressful input. In addition, the therapist may actively intercede with sources of stress in an attempt to reduce the pressure or to have others temporarily assume responsibilities normally falling on the client.

The imposition of *behavioral prescriptions* and *scheduling* the client's activities can also be viewed as protective measures. Many individuals in crisis are disrupted from their usual routines, and in effect are aimlessly drifting in an unstructured and frightening void. By providing a clear and defined structure on activities (pleasant and tension reducing where possible), the therapist may help divert attention away from fruitless preoccupations and at the same time instill at least a rudimentary sense of control and predictability in the client's daily schedule.

Direct supervision by family or friends is an important measure in client protection. Naturally, such individuals will require some instruction regarding the risks involved and the client's vulnerabilities, as well as procedures to be utilized should the situation worsen. These instructions should include specification of the immediate aims of the protective supervision, the types of tension-reducing behaviors that may be used, and contingency plans for obtaining rapid assistance if needed. Included under this heading would also be the occasional need for hospitalization or referral to a detoxification center (for severe substance abuse) or other related facilities that can provide close supervision and medical consultation.

Analyzing Sources of Stress

Once the client's needs for stabilization and protection have been met, the emphasis of therapy shifts toward reestablishing inner controls on emotions and dangerous impulses. The aim here is to decrease the sense of disorganization and helplessness by helping the client mobilize logical and purposeful thinking patterns. As a first step in this direction, the client is actively encouraged to engage in a rational analysis of the stressors that precipitated the crisis. Such an analysis may involve consideration of environmental and interpersonal factors, as well as inner areas of distress. Since the client is typically emerging from the crisis reaction slowly and hesitatingly, the rational analysis proceeds in a gradual fashion.

First, the client is prompted to *identify the main components of the stressors*. In a sense, this task involves a general description of the current situation and attaching verbal labels to its major aspects. From the client's point of view, what had been a vague, amorphous mass of agony now begins to dissolve somewhat into more understandable terms. As the client engages in this analysis of the stressors, it is likely that feelings of panic and disorganization may be understandably rearoused; hence the therapist may have to periodically utilize some of the stabilization procedures described earlier. In the illustrative case, recall that under the therapist's guidance Miss N was able to identify three areas of stress: her parents, her school, and her own feelings.

Following the development of a logical overview of the stressors, *clarification of details* may proceed. The therapist, using direct questions, requests for elaboration, and prompts for deeper analysis, encourages further use of rational thinking processes and a growing feeling of control over the inner disruption. These procedures may then be extended into a mutual *analysis of the implica-*

tions of the current stressors in the client's life, along with a *focusing on the positive factors* that also exist. The development of this broader, more balanced perspective sets the stage for the next phase of treatment—that which addresses issues of how to best cope with the present crisis situation.

Analysis of Coping Behaviors

A natural follow-up to the analysis of current stressors is a consideration of how the client has handled this stress. This phase of treatment may involve several transitions, with the focus of discussion beginning with a review of the present ineffective coping behaviors and then proceeding to the task of developing more succesful strategies. The phase concludes with attempts to bring the client to a point of commitment to try the new behaviors in dealing with their present problems.

Continuing with the use of direct questions and requests for description of behavior, the therapist initiates this phase by focusing the client on a *self-evaluation of coping style*. What did the client hope to accomplish? How was a particular mode of response decided upon? Did any planning occur, or was the reaction an automatic, impulsive one? What were the factors that contributed to the failure of these behaviors, and what aspects of the approach represented strength and positive adjustment?

Coupled with this self-analysis is the *active teaching of a problem-solving approach* to life's stresses. Such general principles as restraining one's automatic impulses, systematically considering behavioral alternatives, and evaluating the possible outcomes are put forth by the therapist. When viewed by clients in the context of their present problems, these principles do not necessarily come across as abstractions but rather may be learned as specific steps in finding solutions to stress.

The stage is now set for *encouraging the discovery of more effective coping behaviors*. The client, having analyzed the current stressors and having acquired some general principles of problem solving is guided toward putting this knowledge to work. Here again, the actual implementation of this phase is far more difficult than is suggested in these paragraphs. The client may still be frightened or despondent and may continue to give way to disorganization. Regardless of this resistance, however, the therapist's firm guidance and continued insistence on rational analysis may gradually orient the client toward a systematic problem-solving approach.

The specific techniques utilized here may be varied, depending on the client's emotional status and motivation. Enlisting the client's efforts in a mutual search for effective behaviors seems to be most beneficial; however, the therapist may also use suggestion, direct advice, and teaching by example with clients unable to take the initiative in this process. An important side effect of these considerations of coping strategy is an increase in the client's optimism and hope for a restoration of equilibrium and personal mastery, along with a concomitant drop in feelings of helplessness and pessimism.

This phase concludes with attempts to bring the client to the point of commitment to try the new coping behaviors. Such an endeavor requires the mobilization of the client's energy and motivation through encouragement and emotional support as well as helping the client to overcome anxieties related to directly confronting the stressors.

Implementation of New Coping Behaviors

Even under calm and benign circumstances, putting newly developed behaviors into practice is not an easy task. During periods of high distress this becomes an especially difficult matter, and therefore a gradual and supportive approach is taken in this phase. The therapist and client may have come to an agreement on what is likely to be an effective course of action, and now efforts are devoted to preparing the client for the successful execution of this strategy.

Approaching this task in a stepwise fashion, the technique of *verbal rehearsal* is an appropriate beginning. Here, therapist and client "talk through" the behaviors to be undertaken, anticipating possible reactions from others, how these reactions will be handled, points of vulnerability, and so on. Following such planning, a period of *behavioral rehearsal* might ensue, in which the client actually practices the new behaviors in the therapy setting. Here the therapist may play the roles of significant others in the client's environment to more closely simulate real-life conditions. With the case of Miss N we saw the therapist encouraging the client to practice a new style of conversation with her parents.

Prior to actually testing new behaviors outside the safety of therapy, where appropriate, the therapist may *prepare the environment* for the client. This may involve contacts with family, employers, friends, and so on, in which explanations of the client's dilemma, emotional status, and the newly evolved coping style are provided. Such contacts also permit an evaluation of which specific individuals and situations are likely to be supportive and which will continue to be sources of stress. Thus the client can be guided to first attempt the new behaviors in *safe situations* and, after a period of practice and success, gradually expanding them into more difficult or unsure circumstances.

A last component of this implementation stage concerns the *preparation of the client to meet future stressors*. In addition to having mastered the disorganization and turmoil of the present crisis, supportive therapy has, in effect, also taught the client a general set of guidelines for dealing with life's problems. Rather than giving way to helplessness and disequilibrium, the client has come through a procedure involving a systematic and logical analysis of the stress, a careful evaluation of behavioral options, a problem-solving approach to developing new means of coping, and a graduated procedure for practicing and implementing new behaviors. These guidelines may profitably be made explicit and reviewed, with the aim of developing in the client a deeper, more flexible, and generalizable style of coping for the future.

Termination and Follow-up

Let us assume that the client has now embarked on a rationally derived course of action and that the crisis reaction has subsided considerably. It is important that the client not be suddenly dismissed from therapy at this point. Several issues remain to be considered.

First, it is likely that a relatively strong dependence on the therapist has developed, and a sudden loss of such support may prompt undue feelings of insecurity. Hence a *gradual decrease in therapeutic contact* is appropriate. Such contacts are also utilized to reinforce the client's sense of mastery and to orient the client toward sources of support that are available in everyday life.

Second, mutual assessment of the degree of success of the client's new coping behaviors may point up needed refinements or changes in adjustive behaviors. Embedded in such discussions are also considerations of what will happen should the coping behaviors ultimately prove to be ineffective. What backup strategies may be invoked? How does one fight off the tendency to panic or become disorganized again?

Finally, the therapist is faced with the issue of what to do about longer-range problems that may underlie the present crisis situation. Is the client in an emotional condition to even consider these deeper personal vulnerabilities or motivated to entertain the possibility of seeking additional help with them? These are delicate judgments for the therapist in view of the recent crisis in the client's life. However, if deemed advisable, raising the possibility of further therapy and arranging for referral to an appropriate agency may be of long-range benefit to the client. A summary of supportive techniques is presented in Table 5.1.

UNRESOLVED ISSUES IN SUPPORTIVE THERAPY

A word of caution is in order. The material in this chapter, representing the combined judgments and clinical experiences of many crisis workers who have written in this area, may convey the impression that supportive therapy is well documented and scientifically based. Unfortunately this is not the case. Careful research that evaluates the effectiveness of this therapy or investigates the processes involved is relatively sparse. Hence the reader should recognize that a great deal of future work is required in order to improve the treatment procedures, develop more precise evaluation techniques, and promote more effective training of crisis therapists.

Foremost among the unresolved issues is the question of whether supportive therapy does indeed have beneficial effects. One would think that such a fundamental question would have received considerable research attention; however, this has not occurred. In their recent review of this area Butcher and Koss (1978) point out that several major problems are encountered in doing adequate research: (1) the difficulty in locating treated patients at some later,

Table 5.1
Phases and techniques of supportive therapy

Phase	Techniques
Initial evaluation, stabilization, and protection	Evaluation: intellectual, emotional, and interpersonal resources, hope structure, motivation, severity of crisis, risk factors. Stablization: therapist presence, talking client down, muscular relaxation, diverting activities, focusing on reality, discouraging preoccupation with negative fantasies and emotions. Protection: removal from stressful circumstances, environmental manipulation, behavioral prescription and scheduling, direct supervision and protection.
Analyzing sources of stress and reestablishing inner controls	Mobilizing logical thought patterns: identification of main components of stress, clarification of details, analysis of implications, focusing on positive factors.
Analysis of coping behaviors	Review of ineffective coping strategies: self-evaluation of unrealistic goals, decision processes, and impulsive reactions. Teaching of problem-solving techniques: inhibition of impulsive behaviors, consideration of options, evaluation of possible outcomes. Development of new coping behaviors: direct advice, suggestion, modeling, encouraging independent discovery.
Implementation of new coping behaviors	Verbal and behavioral rehearsal, preparation of environment, practice in safe situations, application to stressful circumstances, generalizing to future stressors.
Termination and follow-up	Gradual decrease in therapeutic contact, refinement of coping skills, anticipation of future stress, possible preparation for treatment of underlying vulnerabilities.

follow-up period of assessment; (2) problems of specifying the diagnosis and other characteristics of the samples of patients being studied; and (3) variations in the types of measures used to evaluate therapeutic efficiency.

Among the few evaluation studies that have been conducted (Maris and Connor, 1973; Green, Gleser, Stone, and Siefert, 1975), the results generally indicate that anywhere from 60 to 76 percent of patients treated with brief, supportive therapy show improvement. These may seem like reasonable success rates, considering the usual severity of crisis reactions; however, in the absence of comparable, untreated control subjects, these figures are difficult to assess scientifically. It is of course understandable that researchers might not be prone to withhold therapy from patients in crisis in order to constitute an experimental control group; nevertheless, the absence of such comparison data leaves the question of therapeutic efficiency open.

Perhaps more provocative are research findings that as many as 15 percent of clients treated by supportive therapy may actually get worse (Green, Gleser, Stone, and Seifert, 1975). Here again, these data are difficult to evaluate in the absence of control group results. It may be that a considerably higher proportion would have deteriorated had they not received treatment. However, we are left with the uneasy possibility that therapy itself may have resulted in a deterioration of some clients' condition—an issue that has been raised regarding psychotherapy in general by Bergin (1971) and Strupp, Hadley, and Gomes-Schwartz (1977).

Given the possibilities of both improvement and deterioration as a result of supportive therapy, related questions are raised. Can we identify some of the factors within the therapeutic endeavor that contribute to success or failure of treatment? May some of these factors be related to therapist training, experience, or personality factors? Or do client variables (e.g., severity of the disorder, age, socioeconomic background) affect the outcome of therapy? Further, we can also ask if there are specific processes that take place in the day-to-day administration of therapy that play a special role in success or failure.

The answers to such questions are not yet forthcoming from the research literature. The few studies that have been conducted (see Butcher and Koss, 1978) have not amassed enough data to warrant conclusions; however, therapists and clinicians of the future face a challenging and interesting task of discovering the subtle factors that lead to successful supportive therapy.

CHAPTER SIX

BEHAVIORAL APPROACHES TO PSYCHOTHERAPY

In introducing behavioral approaches to therapy, permit me an analogy drawn from developmental psychology. The analogy is appropriate in the sense that behaviorism has some well-defined stages of growth; indeed, it continues to display a vigorous process of maturation. A beautiful and robust birth took place in the early decades of this century with the work of Pavlov on conditioned reflexes and of Thorndike on the law of effect. Pavlov's pioneering work (1927), in which he investigated the means by which a neutral stimulus (e.g., a tone) comes to elicit a reflexive response (e.g., salivation), forms the cornerstone of classical conditioning theory; and it probably has become one of the most widely known psychological demonstrations in this century. Thorndike's work (1932) on the rewards and punishments that follow behavior, and thereby strengthen or weaken that behavior, forms the basis for later work on reinforcement theory and the whole area of operant conditioning. Both of these theorists viewed such simple learning phenomena as based on associations between stimuli and responses (probably by establishing neural connections), and as such, these associations form the "building blocks" from which more complex forms of learning are constructed. These formulations were hailed because of their directness, clarity, and empirical, research base. A science of behavior was born.

The 1930s and 1940s may be described as the childhood years, with an orderly but slow maturation of this new science. The basic associationistic notions were extended into the more complex realms of verbal learning, memory, and motor performance. Not many practical applications were derived, for the main emphasis was on expanding basic theory and laboratory experimentation. Except among the researchers themselves, it was a relatively quiet and unpublicized time of growth.

In the late 1950s and 1960s a stormy and contentious adolescent burst upon the scene. As will happen during this exuberant era of development, nearly everyone got upset with this upstart science. No longer content to stay in the laboratory, some "behaviorists" were ready to try out their notions in practical settings—with psychiatric patients, with sufferers of mental retardation, with children who were behavior problems in school, and with clinic patients who suffered from specific fears. The adult world at the time—that is those who were comfortable with their traditional approaches and techniques—undoubtedly felt threatened by this gangly and aggressive "new kid on the block." Considerable opposition was voiced in the literature and in the classroom, to which the behaviorists reacted with occasional counteraggression and exaggerated claims. The confrontations often generated strong feelings as to which camp held the chalice of truth, and for a time they gave the whole era an ideological flavor that ran counter to dignified scholarship.

Traditional psychodynamic theorists hurled the charge that the behaviorists were mechanistic, superficial, and unconcerned with mental, social, and emotional aspects of human functioning. In turn, the behaviorists countered with accusations of vague and unsubstantiated theorizing by traditionalists, and took them to task for their lack of a research approach.

Despite the vehemence, each camp seemed to have a positive and motivating effect on the other. During the late 1960s and early 1970s there was a remarkable upsurge of research on psychodynamic orientations to therapy (Bergin and Garfield, 1971). At the same time, many behaviorists were attempting to extend their rigorous and objective research methods to the more private world of mental and emotional patterns. In the process, both sides had to give ground. The traditionalists engaged in some healthy self-inspection (as results of their research required), and they also began to recognize the value of many behavioral contributions to the field. Similarly, the behaviorists came to the realization that cognitive and emotional processes could not be ignored in building a comprehensive approach to human functioning. They also recognized that many of the relatively simple concepts (and laboratory research methods) that had been adequate in earlier decades were no longer sufficient to handle these new and complex areas of study (Mahoney and Arnkoff, 1978).

With these developments, the behavioral approaches seem to now be entering a thoughtful and challenging period of early adulthood. Ideological fervor and adolescent rigidities are being replaced by a more eclectic and flexible study of psychological problems and psychotherapy. However, firm commitment to objective research methods still remains, along with an awareness that many subtle and complex aspects of living have yet to be scientifically explored.

Behaviorism may be viewed as a broad movement within the social sciences. No single theory or treatment procedure captures the essence of this movement. If there is a unifying principle it is a commitment to a systematic, data-based approach to understanding human functioning. This empirical orientation applies both within the formal confines of the research lab and in clinical practice. In working with an individual client, for example, a behavioral therapist would likely proceed as follows:

1. Measure the frequency and intensity of symptoms and problem behaviors.

2. Carefully assess the conditions under which the problem behaviors and symptoms occur. Conditions here can refer to both environmental circumstances and internal stimuli such as thoughts and emotional reactions.

3. Try to develop hypotheses about the functional relationship between the problem behaviors and those conditions that elicit them.

4. Test these hypotheses by using specific treatment methods, logically derived from the "functional analysis," and measure their effect on the problem behaviors.

5. Revise and refine the treatment methods, as necessary, on the basis of their measured effectiveness.

In clinical practice, then, we can see several characteristics that distinguish behavioral approaches to treatment. Measurement and assessment of treatment effectiveness is an ongoing process. Specific therapy procedures are tailored to each client's needs on the basis of incoming data. And in most instances, the treatments that are utilized are derived from learning-theory principles that have been validated in the laboratory. In addition to this sytematic, empirical approach it should be noted that behaviorally oriented therapy shares with other treatment modes concerns about such issues as establishing client-therapist rapport, maintaining client motivation, and promoting a sense of mastery in the client (Marks, 1978).

With this brief overview it is apparent that presenting a cohesive and contemporary description of behavioral approaches to psychotherapy will be a difficult task. Not only is the field expanding and changing, but many issues remain unresolved and are awaiting research clarification. In addition, the area encompasses many different therapeutic procedures that singly and in combination have been applied to a wide variety of psychological disturbances. Thus, presenting a picture of a unified treatment process in this area is hardly possible. It would be more in keeping with the nature of this area to describe the basic principles upon which treatments are based and to try to convey the emergent character of the whole field. To accomplish these aims the material on behavioral approaches will be covered according to the following outline: (1) a review of the important changes in outlook and emphasis that have taken place in the last decade; (2) a survey of the principal therapeutic procedures that are in use, along with discussions of their conceptual bases; and (3) discussion of practical and theoretical issues related to producing lasting therapeutic effects.

RECENT TRENDS

Without having lived through it, the excitement and revolutionary zeal of the early 1960s is difficult to appreciate. As might be expected during such times of intellectual upheaval, positions were overstated, toes were stepped on, and the realities of clinical problems tended to be submerged by concerns over the purity of science. Imagine the following hypothetical conversation between a brash, young behavioral psychologist of that era and the director of a large state mental hospital:

Behaviorist: Dr. X, you've got over four thousand mental patients in this place. Over half of them have been here longer than five years, and the other half look like they're destined to stay here a long time also. You're running a human warehouse.

Dr. X: Now, young man, it's obvious that you do not understand the nature of schizophrenia, which is the disease that most of our patients have.

Behaviorist: Maybe I don't. How do you see it?

Dr. X: Well, schizophrenia is a lifelong, progressive psychotic illness that is probably hereditary or caused by severe, early trauma. The symptoms—unrealistic thinking, delusions, hallucinations, and bizarre behavior—usually get worse in adolescence and early adulthood. At a later age, these dramatic symptoms abate and are replaced by the kind of withdrawn and lethargic condition that you see in most of our patients. At any rate, the patients are too ill to survive without our care. We can't cure them, but with drugs and careful supervision we can control their symptoms and protect them from themselves.

Behaviorist: All of that is just your point of view, and my guess is that it's mostly old folklore and myth. A bunch of nonsense to justify this huge custodial institution and to excuse away the fact that you're not providing any treatment for these patients.

Dr. X: Now, now, young man. Don't go around making rash and insulting statements on matters you know nothing about.

Behaviorist: But I do know something about it. I have been collecting data on one of your wards, and the results are rather striking.

Dr. X: Data?

Behaviorist: Yes. Listen to this. It's just part of what was observed. First of all, it was found that almost every time a patient acts in a bizarre or psychotic way, one of the nurses or attendants gives that patient attention. They'll speak sympathetically, sometimes put their arm around the patient, and generally act in a reassuring way. On the other hand, when that same patient is behaving in a sane and normal way, he is pretty much ignored by everyone. And finally, if that patient acts in an assertive or independent way, the staff reacts punitively—maybe putting him in an isolation room or threatening him in some fashion.

Dr. X: So?

Behaviorist: Well, it's perfectly clear to me. It's the same as in our laboratory experiments. The staff is reinforcing bizarre behavior by giving it attention. They're extinguishing normal, healthy behavior by ignoring it. And they're punishing independence and assertiveness—the very qualities that the patients need to survive on the outside. It's no wonder your patients are acting in bizarre or lethargic ways. The hospital staff itself is producing, or at least encouraging, those kinds of reactions. We really need to make some drastic changes here.

Dr. X [*To himself*]: I've got to get rid of this joker. He just doesn't understand the nature of schizophrenia.

Scenes similar to this one most likely took place with school principals, directors of institutions for the mentally retarded, and the personnel in out-patient clinics at the time. Although often rebuffed, the behaviorists persisted and eventually were able to set up "experimental treatment programs" in which they could apply and evaluate therapies based on behavioral principles. Representative of these early and pioneering researcher-therapists were Ayllon and Azrin (1965), Lindsley (1963), Lovaas (1967), and Wolpe (1958). These researchers took great pains to use basic laboratory procedures (derived mostly from experimental work on animals) in applying these relatively simple operant and classical conditioning techniques to the treatment of chronic psychotic patients, autistic children, and phobic individuals. In attempts to preserve the "purity" of the behavioral concepts and to approximate the experimental controls of the laboratory, it is quite likely that "outsiders" viewed these treatments as artificial and mechanistic. Nevertheless, the results of these early studies were exceedingly promising and were historically significant in promoting the growth of present-day behavioral therapies.

In the years since these early, pioneering works a vast amount of clinical and laboratory research has been accomplished. As a result there has been a substantial broadening of the types of clinical problems to which behavioral techniques have been applied and some significant changes in theoretical perspectives. In the following sections these recent trends will be reviewed.

Trends toward an Interactionist Perspective

The early behavioral theorists tended to view people as passive responders to environmental stimuli. That is, behaviors were perceived as being largely under the control of reinforcers, punishers, and conditioned stimuli in the immediate situation. This early point of view had direct implications for the practical therapeutic procedures that were utilized. In the pretherapy assessments of clients, for example, considerable effort was devoted to identifying the relevant external stimuli and contingencies that "controlled" abnormal behaviors. What tended to be lacking, of course, was attention to "internal processes" in the client and long-range patterns in the individual's life. These limited perspectives often resulted in insufficient evaluation and understanding of the major factors operating in a client's personality. Single deviant bits of behavior became the object of study and the focus of therapy.

The intervening years have seen a marked loosening of this radical point of view. Although still firmly committed to an orderly and empirical development of the field, present-day behaviorism appreciates the complexities of person-environment interactions. Individuals are no longer viewed as merely passive reactors to the environment; rather, they are seen as actively selecting, appraising, and attributing meaning to the stimuli that surround them. Further, individuals are viewed as having an impact on the environment (particularly on other people). Thus behavior may be conceptualized as part of an ever-changing interactive process between the individual and the external world (Mischel, 1976; Magnusson and Endler, 1977).

These changes in emphasis have had corresponding effects on clinical practice. Prior to therapy, clients now undergo a thorough and wholistic evaluation, which includes not only careful assessment of deviant behavior patterns, but also an appraisal of styles of perceiving, modes of thought, emotional-motivational factors, and reciprocal influences between the client and the environment (Ross, 1978). Similarly, it would be relatively rare for a contemporary behaviorist to treat an isolated pattern of troublesome behavior. Rather, therapy concerns itself with the relationship between many related systems of behaviors and the cognitive processes that mediate them (Murray and Jacobson, 1978; Mahoney and Arnkoff, 1978).

Trends toward "Clinical" Research

The research base upon which behavioral approaches are constructed has also undergone significant changes in the last twenty years. The early work was conducted largely in the animal laboratory. The many well-conducted studies in this realm were aimed at elucidating basic principles of behavior that the early theorists thought would be applicable to all living organisms. Since laboratory animals were the subjects in this research, the focus was on readily observable motor responses and simple choice behaviors. Researchers were concerned, for the most part, in being able to apply their results to theory development, rather than to solving practical human problems. Taking an historical view, one can argue that perhaps this relatively narrow laboratory approach was a necessary stage in the systematic growth of a science of human behavior.

The laboratory emphasis on simple, observable responses to a large extent dictated the types of problems that were addressed when clinical researchers initially ventured into the world of human disorders. Clients with gross behavioral deficits (e.g., chronic and lethargic patients in mental hospitals, mental retardates, etc.) or those suffering with specific conditioned fear responses received considerable attention. As noted in the previous section, promising therapeutic demonstrations were carried out. Psychotic patients who had been vegetating in the back wards of mental hospitals began to show demonstrable improvement in such areas as self-care, the performance of routine tasks in the hospital, and general sociability in the ward. Mentally retarded individuals exhibited improvements in language skills, work performance and self-control of inappropriate behaviors. Likewise, applying principles learned from animal experimentation on the reduction of specific fears, human patients suffering from phobias seemed to display substantial improvement.

These early demonstrations, although applied to only a few areas of mental health, were nevertheless a great impetus to behavioral research. New areas of application were explored during the 1960s and 1970s—social skills deficits, shyness, test anxiety, aggression, obesity, depression, sexual deviations, alcohol abuse, high blood pressure—to name but a few. In contrast to the earlier research, however, most of this newer work was not a direct outgrowth of animal experimentation. Rather, the research of the 1960s and 1970s derived its principles directly from experiments with human subjects, primarily college student volunteers who, for the most part, displayed mild, nondebilitating forms of these problems. Occasional studies were carried out with clinical patients having more severe forms of these disorders, but many of these reports were of limited generality since they involved case studies of only one patient. To a large extent, then, by the midseventies behavioral therapy had expanded its horizons in a careful experimental fashion.

This more recent work, however, is not without criticism, even from within the behavioral ranks. Marks (1978), for example, is appropriately dubious of the clinical utility of the "analogue research" that was carried out on undergraduate volunteers. He argues that therapeutic principles derived from studies of mild forms of disorders probably do not apply to clients with more severe, clinical intensities of these problems. He urges that therapy researchers devote their energies to studying the actual populations to which treatments will be applied and thereby develop techniques that take into account the clinical realities of distressed clients.

We can see, therefore, over the past two decades, a discernible progression in the types of research conducted by behavioral clinicians: (1) controlled laboratory studies using animals as subjects; (2) application of laboratory principles to limited numbers of clinical patients to test their applicability; (3) a broadening of the types of problems under investigation, using college volunteers as the focus of study; and most recently (4) the beginnings of large-scale investigations of behavioral techniques with clinical populations.

Trends toward the Study of Covert Processes

As indicated in previous sections, the early workers limited their studies to readily observable behaviors and environmental factors. Mental events were considered off limits because they came from the private inner world and therefore were not directly measurable. To become involved with such processes as thought patterns, modes of perception, expectations of the future, and so forth, was considered as indulging in needless speculation and as a retreat from science. The movement toward incorporating such cognitive processes under the umbrella of behaviorism has been a slow, arduous development; yet, in contemporary work, the marriage of cognitive psychology and behaviorism seems to be firmly established (Mahoney and Arnkoff, 1978). The numerous historical trends that have brought this about offer a fascinating story of scholarship and scientific development.

Several prominent theorists provide the backdrop for the emergence of cognitive concepts within the behavioral tradition. The early work of Albert Bandura during the 1960s on observational learning, with its emphasis on perceiving and symbolically representing others' behaviors, seemed to open a door to cognitive and mental events. Similarly, the clinician-scholar, Julian Rotter (1954), emphasized the role of expectancies in the learning of social behaviors. And as will be seen in the next chapter, George Kelly's development (1955) of a psychology of personal constructs (perceptual and cognitive categories by which we interpret and organize our sensory impressions of the world) gave cognitive events a central role in his theory of personality. As a group these theorists cannot be considered as representatives of a strict behavioral tradition; however, their precise scholarship and commitment to research made them highly influential in the field.

Perhaps the most direct forerunner of current interest in cognitive processes from within the behavioral camp is B. F. Skinner. Although considered the father of radical behaviorism, he also theorized about the effects of mental events in governing behavior (1953). Suggesting that thought processes could be viewed as obeying the same laws as other responses, Skinner's germinal work served as the touchstone for numerous later investigations in cognitive-behavioral psychology. Mahoney and Arnkoff (1978) suggest that these developments can be subdivided into the topics of behavioral self-control, covert conditioning, and cognitive learning therapies. Let us briefly examine each of these areas as to their major concepts and, in a later portion of the chapter, return to specific therapeutic techniques involved.

Behavioral self-control Intuitively, self-control refers to a variety of human functions in which behavior is regulated (or inhibited) despite existing pressures to behave otherwise. The person on a diet who resists a tantalizing piece of cake is obviously foregoing immediate gratification in the service of long-term weight control and health. Similarly, the individual with an impulsive and troublesome temper who decides to walk away from a provoking situation is exercising self-restraint rather than giving way to immediate, emotional dictates. To be sure, the reader could think of many similar examples that indicate that much of our behavior is governed by internal mental processes — analyses of behavioral alternatives, decisions regarding short- versus long-term consequences, ethical considerations, and so on. It is apparent that a variety of human problems may be defined as resulting from deficiencies in such self-control processes. Those that have received the most attention in the literature are diet management and smoking, with some work also having been done in the areas of study habits and interpersonal relations.

Various therapeutic techniques have been developed to assist in the development of self-control. A basic technique in this area is that of *self-monitoring*. This term refers to training procedures that assist individuals in keeping accurate records of their behaviors — especially those related to problem areas. A fundamental dictum of effective personal control is, of course, regular and reliable self-observation. Such procedures permit assessment of rates of progress, recording of the occasions when undesirable behaviors are likely to occur, and monitoring of changes in alternative, adaptive responding. For example, a heavy smoker who is trying to reduce the number of cigarettes per day will probably not be able to assess how much smoking is actually taking place without careful self-recording. Relying on recollection or hazy impressions leaves too much room for bias or forgetting of such a well-ingrained and automatic habit. In the absence of accurate recording, such an individual may also fail to note those occasions when susceptibility to lighting up a cigarette is particularly high — for example, with the morning cup of coffee or when distracted by a challenging task.

Some of the early research on self-monitoring suggested that the very process of recording one's own behaviors has a beneficial effect in reducing unwanted responses. These findings, however, have apparently not stood the test of time, and it now appears that self-recording may be viewed as only one procedure — albeit a fundamental one — in a wide array of self-control techniques.

A second category of self-control procedures refers to training one's clients in the area of *stimulus control*, that is, regulating one's exposure to stimuli that ordinarily elicit unwanted behaviors. For example, individuals struggling to maintain a weight-control program may be encouraged to organize their daily routines so as to minimize contact with food cues — staying out of the kitchen except at mealtimes, studiously avoiding the bakery window with its tempting displays, and so forth. In this fashion, stimuli that arouse hunger pangs are minimized, with a resultant reduction of automatic or impulsive eating. As a corollary to this procedure, such clients may also be taught to increase their exposure to cues that prompt more adaptive behaviors (for example, those that arouse desires for physical activity, exercise, or sports in the case of an overweight client).

A third area related to the overall topic of self-control pertains to the notion of *self-reward*. We have all undoubtedly experienced occasions in our lives when we say to ourselves, "I did very well there. I deserve a pat on the back. I think that I will do something good for myself." Such instances of self-reinforcement may be reasonably common for most people, but often they occur in a haphazard manner. Considerable research has indicated, however, that self-administered rewards are as effective as external ones in strengthening the rewarded behaviors. In this regard, then, it is possible to teach individuals to regularly and systematically use self-reinforcement as a procedure to enhance desired behaviors and to reward appropriate restraint on unwanted reactions. As such, it is a therapeutic procedure of considerable importance in assisting individuals in the development of self-control.

The concept of self-reward, however, is more complex than might appear on the surface. Embedded in it are several component processes that are more difficult to pin down. The first deals with the notion that it is the individual who defines what is rewardable behavior. Thus self-reinforcement procedures often involve the monitoring and *evaluation* of one's own performance. But this evaluation may be gauged against either some externally defined standard or a self-imposed one, the latter frequently varying according to mood or other personality factors. Along similar lines, a person may have achieved a designated standard of performance on a particular target behavior, but for emotional reasons withheld the self-reward (as, for example, might occur with a depressed person). In addition, it is apparent that self-rewards (which are presumably freely available to the individual) need to be used discriminately; that is, they should be self-administered contingent on appropriate performance and not on a random, noncontingent basis. Finally, the type and magnitude of the reward itself is an area of wide latitude. Does effective self-reinforcement require the administration of tangible rewards (e.g., treating oneself to a special meal at a favorite restaurant), or is the internal emotional response of giving oneself praise sufficient to strengthen foregoing behaviors? As can be noted in the above discussion, the notion of self-reward encompasses a broad range of allied issues that need to be considered in the practical therapeutic application of this concept.

The last area to be discussed regarding self-control concerns *self-punishment*, the delivery of painful stimuli to oneself following the occurrence of unwanted behavior. This procedure shares many of the same complexities as mentioned with regard to self-reward (self-evaluation of undesirable responses, type and degree of self-punishment, etc.). Further, it involves the added complication of having an individual purposely administer an inherently obnoxious event to himself or herself — a state of affairs that produces understandable difficulties of motivation and consistency. Perhaps it is for this reason that the research literature on the clinical effectiveness of self-punishment is rather unpromising. Future experimentation may indicate some specialized uses for this procedure, but until such work is carried out, self-punishment remains the least important of the self-control techniques.

No discussion of self-control would be complete without mention of the area of *biofeedback*, a set of methods through which an individual may acquire skills in regulating a wide array of her or his own physiological processes. Stemming largely from the laboratory work of Neal Miller and his colleagues (1969), biofeedback procedures involve the recording (usually with a polygraph) of a designated physical system (e.g., heart rate, blood pressure, muscle tension at the back of the neck) and simultaneously converting the reading into an auditory or visual signal that is displayed to the individual being treated. Through this artificial means, the person whose system is being recorded receives clear and continuous information as to the level of activity in the system—information that is routinely difficult to sense within oneself under ordinary circumstances. Extensive practice with such biofeedback procedures affords the individual opportunity to learn to detect the status of physical activity and, in addition, allows practice in the self-control of these systems (through self-imposed relaxation, engaging in certain thought patterns, etc.). The obvious application of these procedures to the area of psychosomatic problems (e.g., high blood pressure, tension headaches) has prompted a great deal of research in the area of clinical uses of biofeedback, along with a flurry of interest in such related areas as relaxation training, meditation, and yoga.

Covert conditioning This concept refers to a wide range of conditioning phenomena that presumably can occur through the vehicle of thoughts and imagination (rather than via external, tangible stimuli or reinforcers). In essence, it is based on the assumption that private mental events (cognitions) obey the same laws of learning as other responses. The development of conditioning treatment procedures involving such covert events represents another of the major points of overlap between behaviorism and cognitive psychology.

Perhaps the earliest application of covert conditioning took place in the use of behavioral procedures to treat specific fears and phobias. The basic therapeutic approach, devised by John Wolpe (1958) involves exposing a phobic client in very small and graduated increments to imagined scenes of the feared stimulus or situation. This gradual approach presumably desensitized the client to the feared situation in small, tolerable steps, thereby permitting a slow and systematic reduction of fear. Later workers with this technique have suggested that positive therapeutic results could be achieved more efficiently by having the client undergo progressively closer exposure to the feared situation itself (Marks, 1978). Nevertheless, Wolpe's original use of imaginal processes represents an historically important venture into covert processes within behaviorism.

A comparable translation from external, tangible stimuli to imagined events has taken place in the area of aversion therapy as well. The essential behavioral form of this type of treatment involves the administration of an aversive stimulus (e.g., painful electric shock) after the occurrence of unwanted behavior. Extensive research literature indicates that this punishment technique can be effective in at least suppressing undesirable behaviors, if not totally eradicating them. Cautela (1973) has been most influential in developing a cognitive form of this treatment, termed *covert sensitization*. In essence, an individual is asked to imagine (via verbal directions from the therapist) an occasion at which the unwanted behavior is taking place (e.g., an alcoholic imagining drinking a glass of whiskey). As part of this imagined event, the client is also instructed into imagery in which an aversive consequence takes place (e.g., feeling violently nauseated). The association which presumably develops between these two imagined events is thought to suppress the undesirable behavior. Numerous case studies have been published that suggest the clinical value of such procedures; however, large-scale studies have not as yet shown impressive results.

Several other cognitive-behavioral procedures should be mentioned in passing, although they also suffer from meager research support to date. *Thought stopping* refers to techniques by which clients are taught to control repetitive, disruptive thoughts. In the simplest form of this procedure, the individual is first instructed to indulge in the unwanted rumination (e.g., repetitive preoccupations over minor money affairs). The therapist suddenly shouts the word *stop*, producing an emotional reaction and bringing the ruminative chain to an abrupt halt. Later in the treatment sequence, the client is instructed to shout similar commands, hence introducing the element of self-imposed control on disruptive thought patterns. With practice this self-command becomes covert, so that the client can now terminate ruminations by merely thinking of stopping them.

Similar mental gymnastics occur in a procedure called *coverant control*, in which imagined behaviors are followed by verbal self-commands indicating the desirable (or undesirable) consequences of those behaviors. A typical example here might involve an obese client who is taught to respond to hunger pangs by thinking, "Eating between meals will make me fatter. If I desist, I will become healthier and better looking."

In taking an overview of the procedures under the covert conditioning heading, several points should be noted. First is the historically important issue that these contributions represent significant expansions of traditional behaviorism into the realm of thought patterns and mental events. Further, these excursions into covert processes were attempted via a systematic application of known behavioral principles and with ample dedication to research evaluation and analysis. Such laudatory and creative efforts are not minimized by later research findings that suggest only modest clinical success with these techniques. It is entirely possible, for example, that each of the procedures described above is too specific or too narrow to be of clinical utility in the overall adjustment of most disturbed clients. Perhaps future work will demonstrate that various combinations of techniques are successful or that they may be useful adjuncts in more broadly based treatments emanating from learning theory. That such is probably the case is suggested by the material to be covered in the next section.

Cognitive learning therapies Cognitive learning therapies have the common feature of taking a wider and more general approach toward helping clients solve personal difficulties than the methods described earlier. Rather than attempting to treat very specific symptoms with focused cognitive-behavioral procedures, these approaches are aimed at improving the general problem solving that individuals use in their daily lives. Thus cognitive learning therapies may include many of the individual techniques described under the topics of self-control and covert conditioning, but their aim is to teach methods that are applicable to a wide range of actual and potential problems.

Although there is considerable overlap, cognitive learning therapy can be roughly divided into two areas of emphasis: those treatments that focus on *cognitive restructuring* and those that attempt to improve coping and *problem-solving skills*. The former base much of their work on the assumption that personal problems arise largely from faulty thought patterns, incorrect premises about the self and others, and irrational ideas and attitudes. The latter, as the title implies, view maladjustment as arising from the use of ineffective or deficient skills in managing stress or in handling life's problems on a day-to-day basis. Common sense dictates that these are not mutually exclusive approaches as to underlying assumptions, and in actual practice cognitive learning therapies may lean toward either cognitive restructuring or skills training, depending on the needs of the client. In the following paragraphs the major tenets of each area will be reviewed, along with discussion of their range of applicability.

Two of the leading proponents of the cognitive restructuring approach are Ellis (1970) and Beck (1976). Both share the view that psychological problems and maladjusted emotions often stem from maladaptive thoughts and that the principal aim of treatment should be the changing of these disruptive cognitive patterns.

In Ellis's rational-emotive therapy emotional disturbances are seen as being caused by a limited number of "irrational" ideas that are ingrained at the core of an individual's thought structure. Such absolutes as "One must be loved and accepted by everyone" or "It is essential to be perfect in everything that we do" inevitably lead to excessive feelings of frustration or anxiety; therefore they need to be modified and tempered into more reasonable form. Rational-emotive therapy attempts to bring about such changes by direct persuasion, the presentation of rational arguments, clear and forceful feedback regarding inappropriate ideas, and instruction and guided practice in using sensible, realistic thoughts.

Beck's "cognitive therapy" is based on a somewhat different perspective of cognitive malfunctions. He proposes that various clinical syndromes (for example, depression, paranoia, or anxiety states) develop from special patterns of irrational thoughts, each of which is relatively unique to each disorder. For example, problems of a depressive nature are seen as emanating from habitual cognitive patterns that emphasize loss, self-devaluation, and a negative, pessimistic view of the world. Paranoia, on the other hand, is characterized as a disorder in which thoughts of harm and malevolence from other people predominate. Such thought patterns are seen as being perpetuated and enhanced by unrealistic mental processes—by selectively perceiving those facets of the environment that support the irrational idea, making inaccurate inferences, and mentally magnifying trivial incidents.

Beck's treatment approach also differs in several ways from Ellis's. It is not as confrontive or as directly instructional as rational-emotive therapy. Rather, Beck relies on a more slowly paced dialogue between therapist and client in which the client is first encouraged to become aware of automatic and unrealistic thought patterns, followed by the development of more accurate cognitions. The last stage involves putting into practice newly developed modes of thought in order to receive feedback regarding their accuracy and effectiveness. The entire sequence may be described as a process of guided self-discovery in which the therapist's questions and urgings for logical analysis gradually prompt the client to develop more adequate cognitive processes.

Both rational-emotive therapy and Beck's cognitive therapy have enjoyed considerable popularity and empirical attention in recent years (see Hollon and Beck, 1978), with encouraging research results. The relatively wide appeal of these approaches is perhaps based on their directness, logic, and systematic analysis of an obviously important area of human functioning—thinking processes. The success may also be due to the attempts to treat broad-based cognitive problems—an approach that is not specifically symptom oriented, but that may have a generally positive impact on clients' attitudes, perceptions of themselves, and views of the world.

Cognitive learning therapies that emphasize the development of more efficient coping and problem-solving skills are represented by a wide variety of theorists, each with a slightly different emphasis. Goldfried (1971), for example, has expanded the standard desensitization procedures involved in treating specific phobias into a therapy program of learning how to cope with general feelings of anxiety. Basic to this treatment package is the idea that clients can learn to face anxiety-provoking situations, to tolerate the ensuing negative feelings, and then to develop personal methods (via self-relaxation) for the reduction of anxiety. The development of such strategies is thought to assist persons to cope more effectively with many potential stressors that are encountered in life; hence this approach presumably has greater generalizability than the treatment of specific fears.

A somewhat different perspective is provided by Spivack, Platt, and Shure (1976) and by Mahoney (1977), who view many emotional problems as stemming from inadequate skills in solving situational and personal problems as they arise in daily life. In such therapies, clients learn progressively more sophisticated skills in the systematic application of rational, "scientific" reasoning to personal difficulties. Such problem-solving sequences as specifying and analyzing the problem, collecting information, considering options, anticipating possible outcomes, experimenting with various behavioral solutions, revising plans accordingly to feedback, and so forth, represent typical cognitive skills that are taught. Once acquired, such strategies are considered to have applicability to a wide variety of situations, and hence represent a general enhancement of clients' adaptive abilities.

In many ways the cognitive learning therapies represent an interesting hybrid of diverse theoretical conceptualizations. Not only are they a blend of cognitive psychology and behaviorism, but also we can discern some theoretical legacies of psychoanalysis and humanism—the latter two reflected (although with different terminology) in attempts to (1) improve clients' abilities to accurately discriminate (become aware of) external and internal problems; (2) correct perceptual and mental distortions (defenses) that tend to perpetuate problems; and (3) generally enhance clients' capabilities for independent living and personal growth (self-actualization). It can be argued that such conceptual overlaps signify a maturing of the whole field of psychotherapy and a uniting of diverse traditions in the all-important task of providing effective service to clients.

The many historical trends that are interwoven in the fabric of the behavioral therapies are summarized in Table 6.1. This chart does not do justice to the multiple influences that crisscrossed the area during the past decades, but hopefully the reader will gain a rough overview of this maturing field.

BASIC THERAPEUTIC PROCEDURES

In the interest of accuracy, this section must begin with a description of two dilemmas, for which there are no ready answers, faced by present-day behaviorists. The first, at least, represents a major challenge to future therapists in this area, since it deals with fundamental behavioral theory. Behaviorism has always prided itself as being based on experimentally derived principles. These principles have been extensively evaluated in both animal and human laboratory experiments, and as we saw in the previous section, a great deal of research and theorizing has tried to extend them into the realm of mental events as well. Further, these principles seem to be reducible into several fundamental paradigms that form the basis for learning theory—classical conditioning, operant conditioning, observational learning (modeling), and cognitive learning. These basic areas of study thus represent the foundation for virtually all of the practical treatment procedures used by behavioral therapists.

This neat and systematic superstructure of theory, laboratory experiments, and practical application has begun to sway to an alarming degree in recent

Table 6.1
Historical trends in behavioral approaches

Focus	1950s	1960s	Current
Theory	Environmental control of discrete behaviors	Emotions, information processing, and interpersonal relations	Interactional approach: (1) personal perceptions of environment, (2) inter-related systems of behavior; (3) reciprocal individual-environmental effects
Research	Controlled laboratory research aimed at theory development	Case studies demonstrating applicability to clinical problems	Research on clinical populations with severe disorders
		Research on undergraduate volunteers with wide variety of mild disorders	
Therapy	Changing observable discrete behaviors	Reducing specific fears, changing expectancies, personal constructs, mental events	Changing cognitive-behavioral patterns via:
			Self-control: (1) self-monitoring, (2) stimulus control, (3) self-reward, (4) self-punishment
			Covert conditioning: (1) imagined fear situations, (2) covert sensitization, (3) thought stopping, (4) covert control
			Cognitive learning: (1) cognitive restructuring, (2) problem-solving skills

years. Many of the behavioral therapies indeed seem to work with clinical patients, but when current-day researchers try to investigate *why* they work, they come up with some disturbing results. It appears that the successes are not readily explained by the basic principles upon which the therapies were originally designed. Rather, the research results suggest that the success of these treatments is affected, to a large degree, by such nonbehavioral factors as (1) clients' beliefs about the effectiveness of therapy; (2) broad changes in clients' self-concepts and feelings of mastery; (3) clients' motivations to adhere to a treatment program; and (4) certain emotional aspects of the therapist-client relationship. What an embarrassment! Can it be that the learning principles are irrelevant (see Marks, 1978; Murray and Jacobson, 1978)?

Undoubtedly the truth lies somewhere in a middle ground. The basic behavioral principles must be involved at some level of the treatment process, since therapists' procedures are so directly derived from them. But it is also becoming apparent that raw behavioral techniques alone are insufficient to bring about lasting improvement in clients. Increased attention to the non-behavioral factors cited above may be necessary in understanding the treatment process in its totality. It is in this light, then, that the following sections are presented. The fundamental learning processes will be described, along with a discussion of the general, nonspecific factors which seem to contribute so heavily to behavioral therapies. It will be left to future researchers to weigh the relative contributions of each to the treatment process.

The second dilemma facing behaviorists involves the "purity" of the basic paradigms and principles themselves. This problem derives from the fact that when one attempts to translate simple and highly controlled laboratory procedures into real-world treatments of human problems there is an inevitable blurring and overlap among the paradigms. Thus, when later in this section we discuss therapies that are outgrowths of, for example, classical conditioning procedures, the reader should keep in mind that other paradigms may also be involved (see Kanfer and Phillips, 1970). For this reason most contemporary behavioral clinicians have gotten away from trying to identify the single, fundamental learning mechanism that underlies a particular form of treatment. Rather, the research emphasis has become one of refining and improving combinations of procedures that will lead to the best practical results (Ross, 1978).

Applications of Classical (Pavlovian) Conditioning Principles

Perhaps the best example of the classical conditioning paradigm as it applies to psychological problems can be found in the development of fears. In 1920, Watson and Rayner published their well-known demonstration in which a "phobia" was produced in a young child named Albert. They originally placed in front of Albert a small white rat, to which he showed no particular fear or aversion. After this, the presentation of the furry rat was accompanied by sudden loud noises, which did indeed startle and upset the boy. After several such pairings it was observed that Albert displayed signs of fear to presentation of the white rat alone, as well as to such similar stimuli as other furry animals. Evidently, because of the contiguous pairing of an originally neutral stimulus (the white rat) with an inherently frightening stimulus (the loud noise), the former acquired fear-producing properties.

As can be noted in this example, classical conditioning involves what has been termed the process of "stimulus substitution"; that is, by pairing a neutral event (the conditioned stimulus or CS) with an event that reliably evokes a response (the unconditioned stimulus or UCS) the CS eventually comes to elicit that response. We can also see in Watson and Rayner's demonstration the concept of stimulus generalization, in which neutral stimuli (other furry animals) that are similar to the original CS also have acquired fear-evoking qualities.

Much subsequent research on the classical conditioning paradigm has suggested that many specific fears (and other emotional reactions) in our lives may be learned in this fashion. This later research, however, has also demonstrated that the processes involved are more complex than is implied in the case of little Albert. For example, it is apparent that some types of "neutral" stimuli (those that are intense, easily perceived, or in some way related to a fear-producing situation) can more readily acquire phobic properties. In addition, behaviors that reduce fear (such as withdrawing from a frightening situation) are reinforced, thereby strengthening these defensive behaviors. We see in this last point an effect that is technically not a part of the classical conditioning paradigm. Rather, the strengthening of a response as a result of its fear-reducing effect is actually an instance of operant conditioning, an area of learning that will be discussed in the next section.

The fact that certain stimuli or situations can acquire fearful and aversive properties lies at the heart of most treatments based on classical conditioning. The essence of such therapies involves the production of negative emotional reactions (fear, revulsion, etc.) to cues that are normally associated with clients' maladaptive behaviors. For example, a habitual cigarette smoker under normal circumstances probably experiences pleasurable reactions to simply the sight, feel, and aroma of a cigarette even before beginning to smoke—pleasant little preludes, as it were, to actually inhaling and tasting the tobacco. Should this smoker desire to break the habit, a classical conditioning approach would attempt to change (recondition) the anticipatory reactions to cigarette cues from pleasurable to aversive. Thus the sight, the aroma, and even the thought of cigarettes might be paired with strongly aversive events (for example, painful electric shocks, states of nausea, fearful reminders of lung cancer, and so forth). Such therapeutically induced aversions presumably evoke tendencies to avoid the offending stimuli (or at least to interfere with their pleasurable effects) and consequently to interrupt the act of smoking itself.

This kind of "aversion therapy" within a classical conditioning framework has been applied extensively to two major disorders — alcohol abuse and sexual deviations. With drinking problems, as in the example of smoking, stimuli associated with alcohol consumption (the sight, smell, and taste of liquor) are systematically paired with strongly negative events (electric shock or drug-induced nauseous reactions). With sexual deviations such as fetishism or transvestism, the stimuli that frequently serve as the forerunners of the deviant behaviors (sight of the fetish object, aberrant fantasies, inappropriate sexual arousal) are likewise associated with aversive stimulation.

Several complicating factors are noteworthy in these procedures. Most obvious, perhaps, is the observation that after a course of aversive conditioning the client may avoid the maladaptive behavior for a period of time, only to experience growing difficulties in controlling these responses as the learned aversive reactions begin to subside. This necessitates occasional follow-up courses of treatment — a situation calling for sufficient client self-monitoring of impulse control and adequate motivation to actually seek out further help. At a more technical level, choosing the most workable aversive stimulation during such reconditioning procedures also presents problems. For example, if a nausea-producing drug were used, care must obviously be exercised as to appropriate dosage, possible negative side effects, and the time course involved in actually producing the aversive reaction. The use of electric shocks (say to the fingertips) also presents several problems, most notably selection of appropriate intensities, taking into account clients' changing sensitivities to electrical stimulation, and clients' possible reluctance to maintain motivation in such treatment. Selection of the most effective CS is yet another area of consideration. The therapist can choose some stimulus that is closely associated with the maladaptive behavior (e.g., the sight of a shot glass full of whiskey) or some component of the behavior itself (taking a sip of whiskey). No simple rule seems to govern such choices, and it is left to therapists to determine the most effective combination of procedures for each individual client.

Classical conditioning procedures have also been used extensively in the treatment of bed-wetting (enuresis), although in this context it would not be considered a form of "aversive therapy." Enuretic children may be viewed as having deficient control over the urinary sphincter muscle while asleep. Under normal circumstances the stimulation provided by a full bladder is sufficient to wake up a child and to produce sphincter contraction, thereby preventing untimely urination. The enuretic person, in effect, fails to wake up (and to contract the sphincter) and hence wets the bed. Based on such an analysis Mowrer (1938) developed a practical apparatus that could be used to help enuretic individuals acquire proper sphincter control — an apparatus that has proven to be reasonably successful and that is widely used. In essence, it consists of a special electrically conductive pad that is placed under the client while sleeping. When the pad becomes moist with urine, a circuit is completed, ringing a bell, that awakens the client and also produces sphincter contraction. Mowrer's reasoning concerning the success of this procedure is as follows. Stimuli from the child's distended bladder (CS) are paired with the ringing of the bell (UCS). In turn, since the bell produces awakening and sphincter contraction, the stimulation of a full bladder would eventually come to elicit these as conditioned responses. In effect, a formerly neutral stimulus for the enuretic child (a full bladder) now evokes the desired responses of sphincter control and waking up.

This description of treatment for enuresis may also serve as a vehicle for discussing some of the inevitable overlap among paradigms that occurs in practical situations. Under most circumstances the enuretic child may be a focal point for family concern and attention. Will mother be disappointed again at discovering wet, aromatic bed sheets in the morning? Will the taunts of siblings have to be faced yet another day? Threats to self-esteem abound. Using Mowrer's procedure with some success hence has implications that go beyond basic classical conditioning principles. The successfully treated enuretic child now awakens, proceeds to the bathroom, and can then return to sleep in a dry bed. The physical comfort of the dry bedclothes and sense of mastery at having avoided another "accident" surely serve as strong reinforcers for this sequence of appropriate eliminative behaviors. In addition, the reactions of praise or relief from family members and the avoidance of negative responses contribute substantially to the rewarding nature of this success experience. These social and personal outcomes, of course, go beyond a purely classical conditioning interpretation of what underlies successful treatment. These sorts of reinforcement effects are more closely associated with the operant conditioning paradigm, which will be discussed below. Later in this section treatments that are explicitly derived from such mixed models will be described. Suffice it for now to repeat the point made earlier that most behavioral treatments involve such combinations of factors, although many learning theorists may emphasize only one because of conceptual preferences or personal bias.

Applications of Operant Conditioning Principles

Operant procedures are primarily concerned with the control and manipulation of the consequences of behavior (that is, those events that follow behavior, such as rewards, punishments, the cessation of positive or negative stimulation, and so forth). A long legacy of laboratory research indicates that such consequences, which are contingent upon the preceding responses, can have marked effects on the future occurrence of the behaviors. Operant conditioning also focuses on the stimuli that precede or accompany behavior, because these may serve as signals as to whether certain consequences may occur. For example, an elementary school pupil may suppress desires to horseplay in class when the teacher is present, for she or he has learned in the past that punishment is likely to follow such behavior. However, the temporary absence of the teacher from the classroom may serve as a cue that it is safe to enjoy the pleasures of robust play.

The strong effects that consequences can have on behavior patterns has major therapeutic implications, and indeed operant procedures have probably had the widest range of application within psychiatry, psychology, education, and rehabilitation of all the behavioral paradigms. Operant conditioning represents a therapy approach that is rooted in scientific methods, careful analysis of each individual client, and a programatic dedication to solving practical problems rather than advancing abstract theory. With these aims it has come to be known as "applied behavior analysis" in contemporary usage.

As might be expected, the therapeutic manipulation of consequences in order to change maladaptive behavior may involve a multitude of procedures and variables. Thus, with each individual client, decisions regarding the use of rewards, punishments, or the nonoccurrence of any consequence are required. Similarly, issues pertaining to the type and magnitude of rewards, for example, come into play, as well as questions as to the most effective timing and scheduling of reinforcement. Finally, the operant therapist must consider the appropriate "target" behaviors on which to work and the most effective way of sequencing one's efforts when helping a client to negotiate a change in a complex array of behaviors. Because of these varied types of questions, practicing therapists rarely take a doctrinaire approach to clients, but more usually adopt a flexible, empirical stance in discovering what specific procedures will be most effective with each problem.

In order to illustrate the major concepts and procedures in this area, a composite description of operant techniques as applied to hospitalized psychiatric patients will be presented. It is hoped that this approach will be more meaningful than a mere listing of procedures and definitions. Applications to other types of clients will be described in later portions of this section.

Let us first examine some of the behavioral characteristics of a hypothetical patient who has been on a psychiatric hospital ward for a considerable length of time. First, this patient is largely inactive, spending most waking hours simply sitting in a chair in the hospital dayroom without reading, watching television, or conversing with fellow patients. Personal grooming is obviously at a low ebb, as judged from a generally unkempt appearance. Virtually no efforts are made by the patient to contribute to communal work, such as cleaning the dayroom, helping to serve food, making his own bed, and so forth. Occasional episodes of bizarre behavior (e.g., grotesque posturing, expressing the delusion that he controls the world) mar an otherwise vegetative existence. Finally, although this patient largely avoids interaction with the staff, at times he engages in brief, rational conversation with them and also seems to follow simple instructions regarding mealtimes, getting up in the morning, and so forth.

As is apparent in this thumbnail sketch, these characteristics would undoubtedly prevent this patient from maintaining an unsupervised life outside the hospital. By the same token, the aim of the operant treatment program to be described is to help this individual develop and utilize personal, vocational, and social skills that are sufficient to allow an independent and productive existence in the community. Obviously this cannot be accomplished overnight; however, through a systematic and gradual acquisition of skills, this patient's adjustive capacities will be progressively increased.

Several subprograms that focus on some basic behavioral issues might be used to begin with. Ward personnel (and perhaps a behavioral technician assigned to this patient) will be trained in strengthening the positive, adaptive behaviors already being displayed by this patient. Thus, each time he engages in appropriate conversation or displays self-care behavior a reward (positive reinforcement) will be given to the patient. Depending on what proves to be effective with this person (e.g., a piece of candy, a cigarette, praise, etc.), such reinforcement is carried out with little delay and reasonable consistency whenever such rudimentary but adjustive behaviors occur. At the same time, whenever a clearly maladaptive response is displayed (e.g., bizarre posturing) ward personnel will ignore or walk away from the patient, hence taking care to not even inadvertently reinforce such behaviors by giving attention or other social rewards. This nonreinforcement (otherwise termed extinction) is, of course, aimed at weakening inappropriate response patterns.

Throughout all phases of this operant learning program it is essential that careful observation and record keeping be carried out regarding the frequency and duration of the target behaviors. This permits assessment of changes in both positive and negative response patterns over time and can serve as an indication of whether the particular reinforcers being used are indeed effective with each patient.

As some of the basic self-care and social skills improve, new elements of adjustive behavior are addressed—those related to eventually being able to work at a job and maintain a steady income. Here again, the process of developing appropriate work habits is approached gradually, so that the client is not taxed beyond current abilities. Thus, to begin with the client may be encouraged to engage in a minimal task (e.g., spending twenty minutes each morning to help clear away the breakfast dishes in the ward dining room). Such "work" behaviors are also followed by appropriate praise and reinforcement, so as to establish them as a part of the patient's daily pattern. Thereafter, in a gradual fashion, more extended and complex work is urged (again, appropriate to the client's abilities and training), so that a vocational repertory is systematically expanded. In this fashion the manifold behaviors and skills that are required for eventual adjustment on a job in the community are slowly "shaped" (this is also termed successive approximation).

Needless to say, the therapeutic process described thus far sounds more simple and trouble-free than is actually the case. Our hypothetical patient is likely at times to become frightened or overburdened by these gradually expanding activities. New people are encountered; some tasks may be too difficult; old anxieties may be triggered. Each such episode may prompt a regression, which needs to be handled in a supportive, encouraging fashion. However, with an understanding and helpful staff, even these difficult occasions can serve as important learning experiences. That is, the client begins to associate the presence of people (even under anxious circumstances) with emotional support and helpfulness. Stimuli associated with people can thereby serve as cues (discriminative stimuli) for the receipt of help and social reinforcement. Thus, despite temporary setbacks, the overall treatment program can maintain a thrust toward rehabilitation and interpersonal adjustment.

Several months after the initiation of this treatment program some notable changes can be observed. The deadening vegetative patterns described earlier have now given way to a moderately active daily routine. The client works four hours a day in the ward cafeteria, spends a half-hour each morning and evening cleaning his living area, and devotes several hours to recreational activities. Social behaviors have also improved, with the most noticeable change having occurred in the client's relatively easy rapport and conversation with fellow workers and staff in the cafeteria. Incidents of bizarre behavior have declined, and when they do occur, they tend to take place in the more secluded areas of the ward rather than in public. In all, at this stage in treatment symptomatic improvement has clearly occurred, but as can be seen, this client has a considerable amount still to be accomplished before independent living can be achieved.

In terms of basic skills, our hypothetical patient still needs preparation in at least two major areas of independent living: (1) organizing free time and scheduling activities, and (2) earning and managing money. Let us briefly consider each of these issues and review the phases of an operant treatment program that attempt to deal with them.

Many disturbed persons seem to require a highly supervised and structured environment that provides guidelines for behavior. To a large degree psychiatric hospital wards provide such a setting, with, however, the unfortunate side effect that patients become unpracticed in self-scheduling, decision making, and the taking of responsibility for organizing work and leisure activities. Therefore, as advances are made toward eventual discharge from the hospital, the patient will need to acquire such self-regulatory skills as part of the rehabilitation program. As with the development of basic work habits, this more complex set of behaviors will also be approached in a gradual, stepwise fashion. To achieve these ends, the hospital wards can be organized so that patients may progress or "be promoted" to less and less structured environments as their skills improve. Along with the greater freedom and privileges that are afforded on the higher-level wards, there is also increasing responsibility on the patient for self-controlled behaviors—getting to work on time, contributing to communal activities, managing grounds privileges, making decisions about appropriate attire, and so forth. In operant terms, the patient's daily behavior is under progressively less stimulus control by external cues as advancement is made through the wards.

The issue of learning money management may be dealt with via the gradual imposition of a *token economy*. Here again, the intent is to systematically expose the patient, in manageable stages, to the same rigors of personal finance faced by most people outside the hospital. In the initial phase of such a program, the patient is paid (in hospital scrip) for the productive work he accomplishes—even though he may be working for only a portion of the day. At the same time, opportunities to spend this "money" for nonessential amenities are provided. As the patient's work capabilities (and pay) increase, the opportunities to acquire other items are likewise expanded. Eventually the patient will progress to a stage where he essentially gets "full" pay for a complete workday, and in effect, is managing a reasonably complex system of personal finances.

The tokens (or scrip) that constitute the pay in such a system may be defined as *conditioned reinforcers* in operant terminology. That is, since they can be spent for food and other delights, the tokens are consistently paired with primary reinforcers, and thereby they acquire value or reinforcing properties themselves. Amazingly, what is taken almost for granted by the average person needs to be carefully programmed for the long-term psychiatric patient. An important component of this training is learning to save and budget one's money and becoming aware of the consequences of failure to do so—skills that are obviously critical to success at independent living.

As we approach the final phase of the rehabilitation program, concerns shift to issues of leaving the hospital. Here again, a gradual process of adapting to the "outside" world is followed, so as not to suddenly overwhelm the patient with too many new stresses and demands. A part-time job in the community is gradually phased in as the patient continues to live in the hospital. Now being paid with real money, he also gains a gradual exposure to stores, restaurants, and so forth, in the community—activities that call forth important and basic behaviors in dealing with people at large. Throughout this phase, group treatment that includes other patients of comparable adjustment is carried out, involving tutoring, guided practice, and corrective feedback regarding basic social skills. Training regarding the higher level demands of applying for jobs, negotiating a lease with a landlord, and so forth, are also dealt with during this period.

As a last phase, the patient may move to a halfway house in the community. In this semisupervised setting the patient assumes far greater responsibility for self-management, independent decision making, and adjusting to the requirements of social living. Social skills are refined and methods for coping with interpersonal stress become the focus of treatment. From here, the transition to completely independent living brings the entire process to a natural conclusion.

The developing research literature on the application of operant techniques to a wide variety of adjustment problems is quite impressive. In addition to their extensive use with hospitalized psychiatric patients, they have also brought about improvement with the mentally retarded, autistic children, disruptive children in classrooms, delinquents, addicts, and alcoholics. This research literature needs to be interpreted cautiously, however, since many problems are typically encountered when trying to evaluate complex treatment programs. For example: (1) appropriate, untreated control groups are frequently absent in the research design; (2) in the complex social processes that occur on hospital wards or in the classroom, it is often difficult to pinpoint the precise factors which are responsible for behavioral improvement; (3) many of the research reports have too few subjects, or unrepresentative samples, thereby restricting the generalizability of the findings; and (4) too often, the research projects do not have adequate follow-up periods of evaluation by which to assess the permanence of changes brought about in clients. Despite these problems, however, the preponderance of evidence strongly suggests that the systematic and judicious use of operant procedures plays a central role in treatment (see Kazdin, 1978, for a more detailed critique).

Applications of Mixed Procedures

Conceptual analysis Laypersons and professionals alike view *anxiety* as a major emotional component of many psychological problems. This pervasive emotion, which can have dramatic physiological, behavioral, and psychological effects, has been studied extensively in the laboratory and in clinical patients. With this wealth of research, several behavioral treatments for anxiety-related problems have been developed that have achieved wide acceptance both within and outside the behavioral camp. As will be seen below, these treatments are based on learning principles derived from both classical and operant conditioning; hence they are presented here as "mixed procedures."

Basic conceptualizations of anxiety-related problems come from experimental work in the areas of escape and avoidance learning. A classic study in this field was performed by Solomon and Wynne (1953), and it is an appropriate example to highlight the operation of classical and operant conditioning effects. Dogs were used as subjects in this research and the apparatus consisted of an enclosure with two compartments separated by a low barrier. A subject was presented with a neutral stimulus (e.g., a white panel) in one compartment, and shortly thereafter, severe electric shock was administered. The dog could escape the shock by jumping over the barrier to a "safe" side of the enclosure. During the first few trials of this procedure the dogs displayed disorganization and distress, but then they learned to escape the shock within relatively few trials. During this early phase of the procedure the subjects usually waited to jump the barrier until they felt the electric shock (UCS), but in later trials it was observed that the dogs would cross the barrier upon seeing the white panel (CS). In this fashion they could avoid the electric shock altogether and reach the safe compartment before the painful stimulus occurred. In effect these subjects had now made the transition from *escape behaviors* to *avoidance responding.*

Some important characteristics can be observed in the avoidance learning portion of this research. First, of course, is the observation that the CS acquires fear-arousing qualities by virtue of its having been paired with painful electric shock. This fear response to the color white can be inferred from the obvious signs of distress displayed when it is presented and also from the observation that subjects will work hard and learn new responses in order to escape from it (even when no shocks are forthcoming). In clinical terms we might say that the subjects have developed a "phobia" to a previously neutral stimulus, in the same sense that little Albert showed phobic symptoms to furry animals in Watson and Rayner's work described earlier. Second, it is clear in the Solomon and Wynne research that when the dogs successfully jumped the barrier, this behavior was strongly reinforced because it was fear reducing. In this regard it is interesting to note that the speed with which the dogs made the avoidance response upon seeing the CS continued to increase even though they had not felt the shock for many trials. This leads us to a third important point — that is, that avoidance behaviors acquired in the fashion described above are notoriously resistant to extinction. The traumatic shocks may be successfully avoided for hundreds of trials, and yet the "phobic" escape behaviors (and fear) in response to the white color go on unabated. In fact, at this stage of the experiment the shock apparatus can be completely disconnected since the subjects can so successfully avoid it. Yet the barrier jumping goes on endlessly, presumably motivated by fear, in this instance, of the white color. Perhaps we have here an experimental analog of the persistent and often unrealistic fears that some maladjusted individuals carry with them for years and years.

Various interpretations have been given to explain the persistence of such avoidance behaviors (see Kanfer and Phillips, 1970). Two principal mechanisms seem to operate in concert to produce the enduring patterns. The first, based on an operant conditioning process, proposes that the avoidance behavior is reinforced each time it occurs because fear is reduced. In the subject's behavioral history, jumping over the barrier has proven to be an effective "coping device" with which to deal with fear, and in effect, it continues to serve such a purpose. The second interpretation relies on a classical conditioning viewpoint. Here let us look more closely at the configuration of stimuli that occurred when the animals first acquired the fear. The white color regularly preceded the electric shock by some seconds, so that white became a reliable signal for the forthcoming pain. Under these circumstances it is quite understandable that the white CS should come to elicit fear. In effect, a bond is established between the CS and pain stimulus. Many trials later, after successful avoidance responding has been established, *and the shock apparatus has been disconnected*, the experimental animal has no opportunity to learn that the conditions have now changed. By its very nature, the rapid and efficient barrier jumping removes the subject from the presence of the white stimulus and thereby prevents the new learning that shock is no longer forthcoming. Phrased somewhat generally, we can say that the very nature of many avoidance behaviors do not permit us to *unlearn* (extinguish) CS-pain associations that were formed earlier in life, because we do not remain to face the CS for a long enough period to discern that the "painful" stimulus will not occur.

Although the foregoing discussion has been somewhat abstract, it is important to consider some of its implications for notions of maladjustment and treatment. We might ask, What difference does it make whether the experimental dogs jump the barrier or not? What penalty are they paying for the persistent and unnecessary avoidance behaviors? Let us complicate the experiment one step further in order to deal with these questions. We have an animal who has gone through the escape and avoidance procedures and now is extremely fearful of the color white—who continually runs away and avoids the white compartment, even though the shock apparatus has long been diconnected. Let us also say that the two compartments in this apparatus constitute the total environment for the subject, and that the white compartment is the only place where food is available. Now the animal is faced with conflict: enter the fearful compartment or suffer pangs of hunger. Under some circumstances, for example, where the fear is exceptionally strong or the animal very timid, the dog may literally starve.

We can see here, perhaps, a microcosm of the penalties that operate in real-life human phobias. By persistently avoiding certain fear-provoking situations or places (crowds, elevators, public transportation, and the out-of-doors are some common examples), the phobic client is sharply restricted in being able to meet life's demands and, in some circumstances, to satisfy basic survival needs. Being unable to go to one's job or to get to the supermarket obviously places the client in an exceptionally vulnerable and dependent condition. A tragic element in such disorders is the fact that clients frequently admit that their fears are groundless, yet they feel completely at the mercy of the phobia.

Treatment implications The work of Solomon and Wynne is also a good point to begin a discussion of treatment issues in this area. At the heart of the dogs' persistent fear is the fact that the quick avoidance response prevents extinction of the association between white and the receipt of shock (after the shock apparatus has been turned off). Thus, as with many human phobias, avoidance behaviors that may have been appropriate at an early phase in life continue to occur in later stages, even though they are unnecessary and troublesome. In this light, a principal focus of treatment should be on arranging conditions so as to facilitate extinction of the association between the CS (white color) and pain; that is, to expose the animal to the white stimulus for a long enough period so that it can learn that shock is no longer forthcoming.

One obvious procedure here is to place the animal in the white compartment and to close the barrier, so that the usual avoidance response is prevented. Now the subject is, in effect, forcibly exposed to the fear-provoking stimulus and is also exposed to the fact that the shock is not occurring. The conditions are such that extinction of the white-pain association should take place, as well it does for a substantial proportion of experimental animals. However, an important issue to consider in this procedure is the observation that some animals become so fearful and agitated at this direct exposure to the feared stimulus that disorganized panic ensues, during which it is doubtful that any new learning can take place. The basic elements in this procedure have been translated by Stampfl and his coworkers (Stampfl and Levis, 1967) into a treatment method termed *implosion therapy*. Here the phobic client is exposed to the feared stimulus or situation in a direct and vivid way. This is usually accomplished by having the client imagine the fearful scene in fantasy, while the therapist verbally guides and elaborates on the imagery, or by having the client placed directly into the situation which provokes maximal fear (*in vivo* treatment). Clients initially report intense feelings of anxiety during such sessions, and the procedure is repeated until the fear and distress is diminished to a therapeutic degree.

Typical of this approach is a demonstration by Hafner and Marks (1976) in which clients with intense fears of crowds were taken to crowded stores and subways for three hours a day over a four-day period. In one phase of this study the accompanying therapist continually made comments about the lurking dangers and possible disasters that could occur in these settings, thereby actually maximizing the clients' fears. After this treatment (and indeed at a six month follow-up interval) considerable improvement was observed in these clients. Marks (1978) has also reviewed the research literature on implosion therapy and concludes that it has a demonstrated effectiveness with phobic clients and that *in vivo* exposure to feared stimuli appears to be more successful than imagery techniques. One important feature of this research literature, however, is an apparent underplaying of evidence that pertains to the risks and negative side effects of dramatic exposure to intensely feared stimuli. Just as some of the experimental animals who were locked in the white compartment developed grossly disorganized reactions, one wonders about comparable reactions among phobic clients who are confronted with the full force of their fears.

Let us use the experiments by Solomon and Wynne once more to consider a less risky therapeutic approach than the *in vivo* treatment just described. The basic aim is still to have the phobic animal unlearn the connection between white and pain and thereby diminish the avoidance pattern. We could begin by exposing the subject, not to the white-colored compartment directly, but to one that is very dark grey, that is, a stimulus that is far enough removed from the feared one so that no anxiety is aroused. At the same time we could also feed the animal some especially delectable food in the dark gray compartment.

On subsequent trials we would gradually lighten the shade of gray, in virtually imperceptible steps, and continue to feed the subject. In this fashion two interrelated processes would take place: (1) The subject would be systematically exposed to ever closer approximations of the originally feared stimulus, without avoidance behaviors being elicited. Thus extinction of the white-pain association would be progressively accomplished. (2) A new association would be learned to replace the original fear. Increasingly lighter shades of gray (and ultimately the white stimulus) would have been regularly paired with the receipt of food; hence white would become a signal for a positive, rewarding experience (one that is antithetical to the original fearful emotion).

The basic principles in this counterconditioning procedure have been adapted by Wolpe (1958) into a comparable method for treating human phobias. Patients are initially exposed to very weak and remote forms of the fear-provoking stimulus, which of course prompt little anxiety. Thereafter closer and closer approximations of the CS are introduced in a gradual fashion. At the same time a response that is antagonistic to fear is induced (for example, deep and pleasant muscular relaxation). By systematically pairing each of the graded series of stimuli with the relaxed state, a new conditioned reaction is established in place of the phobic response.

In actual clinical practice this conceptual scheme is implemented in three stages. The first is teaching the phobic client the techniques of deep muscular relaxation. Using methods originally proposed by Jacobson (1938), clients first learn to control and relax the large muscle groups of the limbs. In subsequent sessions, those of the trunk and extremities are worked on; thereafter, more subtle muscles of the neck, forehead, and so forth, become the focus of attention. The average client can thereby learn to enter into a state of complete relaxation in anywhere from three to eight training sessions. Second, using interview methods, the therapist attempts to discover all of the stimuli and situations that for the client are related to the phobia. These stimuli are then rated by the client as to the degree of fear elicited by each, and they are subsequently arranged in a hierarchical list of fearfulness. For example, a client who is phobic about crowds might rate being in a crowded and confined area, such as a subway car, as prompting maximal fear. A busy supermarket may rank a close second. Further down the hierarchy, walking on a moderately crowded sidewalk may receive an intermediate rating. At the low end of the rankings might be such situations as seeing a picture of crowds or standing at one's front door and looking at passersby. In the third stage, starting at the low end of the hierarchy, the client is repeatedly exposed to the least provoking stimulus while at the same time being in a state of deep relaxation. In effect, a process of counterconditioning is now being initiated. When the client can cope with the lowest ranking stimulus without experiencing fear, the procedure is repeated with the next higher stimulus. In comparable fashion the process is continued with each item on the list until eventually clients can face those situations that were rated as most frightening without feeling fearful.

A great deal of research has been conducted in evaluating the effectiveness of Wolpe's procedure, with results indicating substantial rates of improvement. Unfortunately most of this work has been done with college volunteers who suffer from relatively mild phobias. As cited earlier, Marks (1978) has criticized this line of research because of the populations that have been studied; others (e.g., Ross, 1978) have suggested that factors that go beyond counterconditioning principles are more relevant to clinical improvement. These factors will be discussed in a later section.

Marks (1978) has put forth a point of view that seems to incorporate the essentials of both Stampfl's flooding technique and the gradual counterconditioning approach. He suggests that the essential feature of treating specific fears is to expose the client to the feared situation as quickly and as directly as is practicable. Each client's situation is evaluated in terms of motivation, risk, commitment to change, and so forth, and then the client is brought into contact with the provocative stimuli as efficiently as possible. This therapy also tries to take into account such nonbehavioral factors as the effects of social pressures, the credibility of the therapist, and the client's abilities to follow through on therapy assignments. Basically, Marks seems to be expressing an approach that many contemporary behavioral therapists share—that is, the application of a wide range of techniques in a nondogmatic fashion in the treatment of disturbed individuals.

Applications of Observational Learning

Treatments that include the paradigm of observational learning rely on the notion that maladjusted individuals can improve their ability to live and cope effectively by observing desired behavior patterns in others (or in appropriate inanimate displays). A relative newcomer to the therapy field, these modeling techniques were historically overshadowed by those two competing giants of the area, behaviorism and psychoanalysis. However, extensive laboratory and clinical research over the past twenty years on observational learning have brought these procedures to an important status in contemporary work. Modeling therapy is firmly rooted in empirical research and behavioral observation, but as will be seen, it also has ventured into the realms of cognitive processes and self-perception.

On the surface, the idea that a person can learn more adaptive ways of coping with the world by observing a model is a deceptively simple one. However, through the pioneering work of Albert Bandura and those following in his tradition, a relatively complex network of procedures and factors has been identified. Let us first review the various types of effects that can occur when observing a model or exemplar.

First and perhaps most basic is the fact that models can play an *instructional* role for clients. New response patterns or novel ways to approach problems, which were unfamiliar to a maladjusted individual, may be directly taught by observation of someone else carrying out these behaviors. After such exposure many clients are able to produce these new patterns in their totality, without, for example, having to go through the gradual and time-consuming steps involved in behavioral shaping and reinforcement techniques. This type of modeling effect applies to the acquisition of complex behavioral sequences, new ways to organize and classify knowledge, and more adaptive problem-solving approaches.

Second, modeling effects can serve to weaken or strengthen restraints on existing behavior patterns. Clients who display impulsive and destructive responses may well profit from an exemplar displaying inhibition and control over such behaviors. Even temporary self-restraint may be of utility in that new and more adaptive patterns may be developed in the interim. By the same token, individuals who are overly inhibited or fearful show improvement after viewing models performing in a confident and effective manner. A greater feeling of optimism or a vicarious sense of personal effectiveness seems to reduce fears in the client. This reduction in fear can be used in conjunction with encouragement to carry out the inhibited behaviors, with a resultant growth in feelings of mastery and competence.

A third area of modeling pertains to the facilitation of existing responses. This effect is somewhat different from the reduction of inhibitions described above in that fear is generally not involved. Rather, it refers to enhancing the smooth flow of behaviors, improving sensitivity to cues in the environment, and facilitating entire classes of responses. For example, a client who has difficulty with general conversational skills may improve in overall verbal output, responsiveness to social stimuli, and the free flow of language after observing models in these activities. Many therapeutic applications of this area, as a matter of fact, lie in the area of interpersonal behaviors.

The last category of modeling influences deals with changing clients' internal standards and self-judgments. These internal standards constitute a sort of gauge against which current behaviors are regulated and evaluated. Psychological difficulties frequently arise when standards are too high (leading to chronic disappointment and self-castigation) or are lacking (resulting in lack of clarity in how to behave, faulty decision making, and so forth). The therapeutic use of models that exemplify realistic and appropriate internal standards thus can have dramatic effects in changing clients' self-perceptions and judgments about themselves.

Rosenthal and Bandura (1978) have summarized the principal factors that affect the occurrence of observational learning and hence the effective therapeutic application of these techniques. These factors are listed under several general categories. The first is presenting the modeling display in such a fashion as to capture the client's *attention*—that is, presenting the display in a coherent, well-paced, interesting fashion that is tailored to the client's perceptual and cognitive abilities. Included here are concerns about highlighting the important factors of a display, cautions about overloading the client with too much information, or using a sequence that may elicit undue fear and avoidance. Second, modeled displays must be presented so as to ensure adequate *retention* of the material. Again, thoughtful organization, sequencing, and summarizing of the material is important in this context. In addition, providing techniques by which the observer may encode complex material in memory (e.g., summarizing labels or pictorial images) is frequently made part of the display. Third, modeling effects are enhanced when the observational procedures allow for *reproduction* of the desired responses by clients, either in an imagined or actual fashion. Related to this point are the factors of *guided practice and corrective feedback*, in which clients rehearse newly acquired skills under the tutelage of the therapist. Finally, Rosenthal and Bandura suggest that therapists who utilize modeling techniques must attend to *motivational and incentive* issues. Simply having learned some new and potentially effective behaviors may not be enough. Clients must also be willing to now apply these behaviors in the routine of their daily lives. If threats or punishments surround a particular behavior, it may simply not be carried out, even though it has been well learned. On the other hand, if clients come to recognize that the newly acquired behaviors are associated with reward, goal attainment, and a personal sense of mastery, then the incentive conditions are present for effective application. Modeling procedures thus have two major areas of application in psychotherapy: (1) the reduction of fears and behavioral inhibitions and (2) the development of social and problem-solving skills (Bandura, 1977).

Nonspecific Factors

Extensive laboratory and clinical research indicates reasonably clear procedures (and combinations of procedures) for producing behavior change. To be sure, more refinement and sophistication are still to be achieved, but in essence, the basic technical aspects of treatment have been reasonably defined. It should also be recognized, however, that many of these treatment procedures place heavy demands on the client, such as exposure to fearful situations, undergoing aversive aspects of therapy, engaging in long periods of practice on new patterns of behavior, careful monitoring and record keeping, giving up habitual ways of gaining rewards and pleasure, running the risk of social embarrassment or censure as new patterns are tried in everyday life, and so forth. Quite clearly, then, successful behavioral therapy requires, as do other therapies, considerable persistence, courage, and dedication on the part of the client. Individuals in treatment are not merely "acted upon" by the therapeutic procedures. Rather, they must be active and motivated participants in the process, and it is this question of motivation that brings us to the next issue in this overview.

What keeps a client going in therapy? Why do a "homework" assignment when it would be so much easier to relax? Why show up for a therapy session when you know it is going to involve some aversive procedure? Obviously no single or simple answer can be provided to these questions, and yet they represent treatment issues that are as important as the technical, procedural ones described in this chapter. Here, then, we are getting into some of the nonbehavioral factors alluded to earlier. Let us take a closer look at some of the major factors that bear on clients' motivations.

First, *external pressures* to seek and continue in treatment refer to those urgings that come from family, friends, employers, and others who are concerned for the well-being of the client. Oftentimes enlisted as adjuncts to treatment, such individuals can play many therapeutic roles in addition to offering general support and encouragement. These adjunctive roles include behavioral record keeping, dispensing contingent reinforcements, helping the client to avoid provocative or tempting situations, providing corrective feedback, and so forth. The active involvement of others in the client's life thus can have direct treatment as well as motivational benefits.

Second, harder to evaluate and control are what might be called *internal pressures* coming from clients themselves. These pertain to feelings of dissatisfaction with one's current life-style, aspirations for a happier future, recognition that one is disappointing oneself and others, and just becoming plain "fed up" with being shy, fearful, overweight, or whatever. In the same sense that others in the client's life may be enlisted to provide motivational support, direct efforts can be directed toward prompting these pressures within the client as part of the treatment process.

Third, a variety of motivational factors can be identified as part of the *therapy setting* itself. Perhaps most obvious here are the direct rewards and incentives offered by the therapist, whether they be praise and encouragement or more tangible reinforcements, which are frequently used with more disturbed clients. In addition, clients' beliefs about the ultimate success of treatment also play an important role. Therapists who present therapy in a tentative fashion or who convey their own doubts as to its usefulness may be voicing a commendable scientific skepticism, but they are also likely to be undermining an important motivational system in clients. Also included in this category are issues related to the general client-therapist relationship. As described in earlier chapters, the communication of caring, respect, and interpersonal honesty by the therapist seem to be important ingredients in treatment, in part, at least, because of their positive effects on clients' motivation to work and persist in therapy.

Fourth, as clients begin to learn new skills or to overcome fears, a sense of competence also emerges, and this growth in feelings of mastery elicits the *inherent rewards* of personal growth and maturity. Although hard to define, we can surmise that such feelings play a major motivational role in maintaining clients' efforts in treatment. As individuals make some gains in the early phase of therapy, this inner reward system also prompts feelings of hope and confidence that continued work will result in more complete and general feelings of personal competence.

We can see, then, that behavioral therapists must concern themselves with more than just the technical aspects of treatment. Efforts to mobilize these motivational forces are of critical importance in bringing about sustained and active participation by clients (Marks, 1978; Rosenthal and Bandura, 1978).

As a last phase of this overview we must look again at the notion of personal competence. Bandura (1977) and Seligman (1975) assign this concept a major role in their views of adjustment and mental health, although they approach it from differing points of view. A sense of incompetence is frequently a central problem in maladjustment, because it imbues clients with feelings of pessimism and helplessness regarding their specific problems and life's demands in general. This helplessness contributes to reduced motivation to solve difficulties or to learn new methods of coping. Hence a disturbed individual tends to get "locked in" to patterns of inactivity or stereotyped repetitions of ineffective behaviors.

As progress is made in treatment, two classes of events take place: (1) improvement in specific behavioral and emotional patterns and (2) a general enhancement in feelings of competence. It is this second change that Seligman and Bandura view as critical for a sustained therapeutic effect. If, for example, a client is able to improve a specific behavioral pattern, but without feeling that she or he was responsible for that change, then future stresses in life are still likely to be met with a continued sense of helplessness and incompetence. On the other hand, when a particular problem is mastered in treatment and the client attributes this success to personal effort and competence, an inner sense of *self-efficacy* is generated (Bandura, 1977). Such a self-perception can dramatically improve one's overall morale, optimism, and abilities to meet new challenges in life in an adaptive and energetic fashion. In this light, the strengthened feelings of personal competence play a major role in allowing the specific gains in therapy to generalize to a wide variety of life situations, which, of course, would be the hallmark of successful treatment.

A summary of the basic learning paradigms that have been applied to behavioral therapy is presented in Table 6.2.

PRODUCING LASTING THERAPEUTIC EFFECTS

Therapists from virtually all schools of thought are concerned with the problem of producing only temporary therapeutic effects. Treatment may well produce some dramatic changes in behavior, but the client may slide back into maladaptive patterns once treatment is over. A glimpse at a better way of life is provided, which then tragically recedes as old fears and habits reassert themselves. Because of this vulnerability, behavioral therapists have paid particular attention to developing a technology for producing relatively enduring therapeutic changes. The various methods of this technology are frequently applied by therapists, singly and in combination, in the later phases of treatment in order to produce a smooth and effective transition to independent living.

Table 6.2
Summary of basic paradigms of behavioral treatment

Type of learning	Paradigm	Treatment applications
Classical conditioning	CS ——— CR Neutral stimulus Fear, aversion ⋮ UCS ——— UCR Aversive stimulus Pain, fear, aversion	Alcohol abuse, smoking, weight control, sexual deviations, enuresis
Operant conditioning	Response-consequence effects future occurrence of response	Hospitalized psychiatric patients, the mentally retarded, autistic children, those with behavioral problems, alcohol abusers
Mixed models	UCS ——— UCR ——— UCR Aversive stimulus Pain, fear, aversion Escape ⋮ CS ——— CR Neutral stimulus Escape, avoidance	Conditioned fear reactions, phobias
Observational learning	Observer - - - Reproduce model's behavior Model's behavior	Fears and inhibitions, social and problem-solving deficiencies
Cognitive learning	Cognitive restructuring, teaching problem-solving skills, guided practice, corrective feedback	Depression, rigid and unrealistic attitudes, behavioral and social deficits
Nonspecific factors	Positive incentives, external and internal pressures for change, acquisition of skills	Motivation for therapy, feelings of helplessness and incompetence

Many therapists assume (or hope) that behavioral patterns that are developed in therapy will be maintained later on by "naturally occurring" reinforcements in the client's everyday life. However, this reasonable expectation has not been verified by research in any substantial way (see Kazdin, 1978). It is difficult to determine the reasons for this failure, but one can speculate that a number of factors are operating. For example: (1) therapy may have been terminated too early to have the new behaviors firmly established; (2) the real-life situations faced by the client may be sufficiently different from the therapy setting, thus preventing transfer of the new behaviors; or (3) the client's everyday environment may have its own pathological or destructive characteristics that simply do not support these newly developed patterns. Whatever the reasons, it is clear that procedures in treatment itself are required to ensure relatively lasting effects.

One very basic technique in this realm is that of *environmental manipulation*. As part of treatment, the therapist can prepare key individuals in the client's life to meet these new behaviors in a reinforcing, supportive manner. Relatives, friends, teachers, and others can be enlisted and trained to act as extensions of the therapist even after formal treatment is finished. From another perspective, we can view such a procedure as more broadly based therapy in which the therapist is not only treating the client but also attempting to improve the supportive capabilities of important people in the client's life. In either instance the recruitment of such therapeutic adjuncts can be important in prolonging the adaptive behaviors developed in treatment (Kazdin, 1978).

Another important technique involves the use of *diverse conditions* and settings for training and reinforcements during treatment. If clients receive virtually all of their therapy in the same setting, they can readily discriminate that the conditions for reinforcement have changed when they leave therapy; hence, there is the risk that new behaviors will not be maintained. For this reason, using varied types of circumstances, a range of different reinforcers, and a variety of individuals to deliver reinforcement during treatment may aid in producing generalizable and long-lasting effects.

Several other procedures are also designed to reduce the sharp break between treatment and nontreatment conditions and thereby retard the extinction of new behaviors. In the latter phases of therapy, reinforcements can be made progressively more intermittent or given with longer delay after the desired response, thereby approximating the *irregularities of reinforcement* that may occur in everyday circumstances.

Treatment programs that in their latter stages emphasize the acquisition of *broad coping and problem-solving strategies* also seem to reduce the risk of rapid extinction. Although such programs may be composed of many small and diverse units of behavior change, helping the client to put them together into a unified and general methodology for meeting life's demands seems to promote retention and a wide range of applicability.

Training clients in techniques of *self-control* is yet another way to maintain behaviors after treatment has ended. As described earlier in this chapter, individuals can be trained in self-monitoring, stimulus control, self-reinforcement, and self-punishment procedures, which, of course, clients carry with them after treatment is terminated and which can be utilized in many different settings. Thus the maintenance for new behavioral patterns is not completely dependent on the vagaries of environmental reinforcers but rather is under the control of clients themselves.

The issue of self-control brings up again the notion of a personal *sense of competence*, which several theorists view as central to effective and lasting therapeutic results. This general feeling of mastery, which is enhanced through the learning of self-control techniques, provides a sense that clients can master their own fates. The perception that one is not at the mercy of environmental pressures or fear-provoking stimuli greatly strengthens the vigor and flexibility with which future life demands are met.

Finally, therapies that are aimed at bringing about changes in rigid, self-defeating attitudes, such as Ellis's rational-emotive therapy and Beck's cognitive therapy, also improve the chances for lasting treatment effects. As a result of such therapies clients alter their mode of interpreting the world and their own behaviors. Impossible self-imposed demands are made more reasonable, standards for praiseworthy behavior are tempered, and expectations of others become more realistic. Such changes in outlook and self-evaluation may be transferred to the activities of daily living and indeed can alter clients' very perceptions of their world.

A summary of these varied approaches to producing lasting therapeutic benefits is provided in Table 6.3.

Table 6.3
Retention of therapeutic effects

Arranging reinforcers	Environmental manipulation, training under diverse reinforcement conditions, making reinforcement progressively more intermittent and delayed
Strengthening personal competencies	Acquisition of self-control skills, learning general coping strategies, prompting a sense of mastery
Cognitive restructuring	Reducing excessive self-demands, tempering standards for self-reinforcement, making expectations of others more realistic

CHAPTER SEVEN

RELATIONSHIP THERAPY: CONCEPTS AND OVERVIEW

There are many ways by which an individual may lose faith in fellow human beings. The child who grows up with severely exploitive, abusive parents, uncaring teachers, and selfish and spiteful classmates probably loses it early in life. The adult who has undergone several disastrous marriages or love affairs, having felt taken advantage of and emotionally deceived, understandably develops a mistrust of being close to others. The person who lives in a family and subculture where the predominant values are "Take what you can get away with" and "Victimize others before they get you" would certainly have difficulty in understanding simple generosity or caring.

It has been suggested that we live in an era of "personal hedonism"—a sort of narcissistic atmosphere in which concerns for others are secondary to self-gratification. Thus individuals who have been hurt, rejected, or exploited in important relationships may have their alienation reinforced by the general social climate of contemporary society. The penalties for such cynicism and mistrust can be quite heavy. Loneliness, interpersonal strife, and constant vigilance are some of the obvious problems. At another level is the suppression of positive human values and a deterioration in abilities to experience affection, loyalty, personal commitment, and similar social emotions. In a sense, there appears to be a "shriveling up" of these emotional systems, and what remains may be described as a self-centered, detached, and philosophically depleted individual.

The central therapeutic task with clients such as this is the providing of a corrective emotional experience; that is, the therapeutic relationship itself is used as a vehicle by which the client can learn that not all human encounters need be exploitive and rejecting. For some clients, learning to relate to another in a positive, affectionate manner may be a new experience; for others it may represent a reawakening of emotional systems that have been dormant or suppressed. In either case, the underlying assumption of this type of treatment is that, once developed and experienced in the therapeutic relationship, the door is opened for caring relationships with others as well.

Naturally, relationship therapy is not as simple as this implies. Clients such as these frequently have developed obnoxious behavior patterns or openly express negative attitudes toward others. Indeed, the very ways in which they perceive and cognitively organize the social world may prevent the development of successful relationships. Hence, although a fundamental aim of treatment is the enhancement of positive emotional systems within the client, numerous other subgoals may also be considered. These frequently involve helping the client to become aware of the interpersonal effects of obnoxious behaviors and the learning of more successful social skills. Further, significant portions of therapy may be devoted to the clarification and change of perceptions, values, and interpersonal goals. In order to accomplish such multiple aims, relationship therapy encompasses a wide variety of treatment techniques that come from diverse theoretical backgrounds: psychodynamic, insight approaches; behavioral technology; cognitive psychology; and the humanistic tradition.

In this introductory section it should be pointed out that most contemporary theorists stress the importance of a positive client-therapist relationship as a fundamental aspect of all forms of psychotherapy. At the same time, however, most theorists do not portray relationship therapy as a distinct type of treatment; and where it is cited (e.g., Wolberg, 1967) it is not accorded the same status as, for example, supportive, insight, or behavioral therapies. This does not mean that relationship therapy is without a rich historical tradition. John Levi in the 1930s, Franz Alexander in the 1940s and 1950s, and Frederick Allen in the 1960s have all stressed the central importance of the therapy relationship as a means of bringing about a corrective emotional experience for the client. Wolberg (1967) emphasizes the principal aim of establishing a close relationship in working with aggressive adolescents and in treating detached, schizoid clients.

The point of view adopted in this book is that relationship therapy can be defined as a distinct form of treatment and, moreover, that it is worthy of elevation to the status of an important option in contemporary psychotherapy. The rationale behind these views is based on the general principle that, as our culture changes and as new psychological stresses begin to emerge within a society, treatment modes need to keep pace. In this light, one can argue that the problems of detachment, mistrust, and interpersonal cynicism mentioned earlier seem to be emerging as major psychological disorders of the 1980s. As increasing numbers of individuals become "victimized" by a mass impersonal culture, devastating divorce rates, trends toward temporary but intense relationships, and a general decline in communal values, one can reasonably expect a rise in what might be called syndromes of alienation.

In this chapter I will describe the major theoretical issues in relationship therapy. Then, I will present several case descriptions aimed at illustrating typical clients who are appropriate candidates for this form of treatment. Thereafter, an overview of the various stages of relationship therapy will be provided. In Chapter 8 I will describe the specific techniques that are involved, along with a summary of a treatment case.

THEORETICAL BACKGROUND

The introductory discussion to this chapter suggested that clients in need of relationship therapy have wide-ranging problems in the interpersonal sphere. The fundamental difficulty seems to be deficits in forming positive emotional *attachments* to others. The first portion of this section will therefore review theory and research in this basic area, with emphasis on the life stages during which attachment issues are particularly relevant. A second section will cover problems in the manner in which alienated individuals perceive and evaluate other people—that is, the distorted *cognitive processes* that form the basis for interpersonal mistrust and cynicism. Third, the ideas of humanistic theorists who focus on distorted perceptions of the self and problems of aimlessness in life will be reviewed. Finally, a review of *psychodynamic theory* as it applies to problems of detachment and alienation will highlight the central role of anxiety and hostility in this area.

Attachment

Our affiliations with other people generally extend throughout the entire life span, from the basic physical and emotional contact of the newborn infant with its mother to the mutual care and enjoyment of shared leisure activities among the aged. The nature of these interpersonal attachments obviously vary depending on age and social role; nevertheless, these relationships frequently form the cornerstones of an individual's existence. Several theorists (Erikson, 1963; Sheehy, 1976; Levinson, 1978) have intensively studied the various phases that one goes through over the life span, and their observations regarding stages of interpersonal development are especially pertinent to our discussion.

Childhood and adolescence Erikson suggests that a sense of trust develops during the first two years of life, largely as an outgrowth of consistent, warm, and affectionate parental care. The infant develops a general sense of well-being and fundamental expectations about the nurturance and responsiveness of others. This basic trust forms the foundation for internal feelings of security and emotional attachments to others that become elaborated in later childhood years as parent-child relationships become more complex.

The work of Harlow (Harlow and Harlow, 1966) involving rhesus monkey infants who were reared in isolation during this critical stage in development provides some indirect evidence of the importance of establishing attachments in the first two years of life. Such motherless monkeys developed in later life such profound deficits as isolation, social unresponsiveness, and sexual and parental apathy. Clinical observations of human infants deprived of similar parental experiences suggest that many comparable social deficits occur in later childhood and adolescence. Hence, we may be seeing here some of the fundamental processes involved in the forming and development of a basic emotional system—that of attachment and affection for others.

Some of the later work of Harlow (1969) also has important implications for therapy. These studies indicate that many of the social deficits described above may be reversed as a result of subsequent social experiences, notably contact and play with agemates during the older childhood years. What initially were thought to be irreversible losses resulting from basic deprivations during infancy turned out to be only temporary deficits that could be regained through later social contact. Certainly there are major difficulties in generalizing from research done on primates, but these observations suggest that human affectional systems that are frustrated during early stages of development may be aroused and nurtured through "therapeutic" efforts at some later stage of growth.

In discussing the middle childhood years, Erikson describes the processes involved in acquiring such personality attributes as a sense of autonomy, initiative, and personal competence. Although these are largely constructs related to one's self-concept, Erikson does not minimize the importance of interpersonal qualities as well during these years. Critical aspects of conscience, self-control, and relationships with others are formed that may have lasting effects into adolescence and adulthood. Considerable research has been done on social development in this era (e.g., Bandura, 1973: Sears, 1970), and some of the child-rearing factors that may lead to interpersonal difficulties have been reasonably well documented. These complex results defy easy summary, but general conclusions may be drawn: (1) parents who use severe physical punishment as a means of discipline are likely to have very aggressive children, and among boys such methods are correlated with delinquency; (2) parents who are permissive about their children's aggressiveness are likely to have aggressive children; and (3) parents who use physical discipline techniques and who are judged to be "cold" parents are likely to produce poor conscience development in their children.

We begin to see in these results some of the childhood factors that may form the basis for later problems with attachment and affection. Sawrey and Telford (1975) elaborate on the development of distrust and isolation among children in their discussion of more subtle parental influences. Homes in which children constantly witness quarreling, threats of separation, the use of affectional displays as a weapon, expressions of general cynicism about others, and so forth, quite understandably become aloof and indifferent to people. Growing up in such an atmosphere in effect teaches that it is dangerous to extend oneself to others, no matter how much one may be hungering for warmth and affection.

These childhood patterns of aggressiveness, detachment, mistrust, and weak conscience become critical with entry into the adolescent years. Complex and sometimes contradictory forces seem to operate during this tumultous period in life. On the one hand, it is a time when the young person is breaking away from parental influences, seeking new experiences and a more adult identity. Thus it is also a period when marked changes in personality may take place depending on the types of relationships and events that occur. This again has important therapeutic implications because this "openness to change" may be capitalized upon in attempting to reverse the detached, mistrustful pattern described above. On the other hand, children who have undergone especially severe childhood years and have developed well-ingrained systems of aloofness and alienation may in effect have closed themselves off from potentially therapeutic relationships during the adolescent years. A continuation of unsatisfying interpersonal experiences and a focusing on the negative side of the world only seems to establish their cynicism more firmly. Consider the following commentary by a seventeen-year-old, who speaks of his attitudes during group therapy:

People are out for themselves. Everybody is self-centered. Nobody really understands or cares about anyone else. Someone may come on to you like a friend, but you know it's false. It's just a game, or they want something from you. Look at politics, religion. They're all the same, out for power, money, you name it. The whole world doesn't have a drop of sympathy or compassion.

One can appreciate the virtual impossibility of this individual to form a genuinely close and affectionate relationship with another. We can also perhaps appreciate the enormous task faced by therapists in attempting to change such a grossly negative world view in a client. And yet this is the essential aim of relationship therapy.

The adult years Although the bulk of research and theory on emotional attachment has concentrated on youth, several important analyses of adult developmental stages have recently been published (Sheehy, 1976; Levinson, 1978) that point out many further areas of living to be mastered on the road to full maturity. A number of these developmental tasks concern vocational and economic issues and contending with the problems of retirement. These need not concern us for now. However, of great importance are several adult stages that directly relate to the issue of attachment.

The first of these occurs in the early adult years and involves developing a sense of intimacy with another person. Usually seen in the context of courtship and marriage, such interpersonal qualities as the sharing of values and goals, open communication, mutual satisfactions in physical intimacies, and assuming responsibilities for the other's well-being reach full maturity. It is apparent, however, that achieving such intimacy also involves considerable risk. Openness with another implies exposing one's weaknesses as well as positive attributes. The expression of love seeks affection in return. The communication of deeply held values calls for an understanding, compassionate listener. In sum, the emergence of intimate feelings also ushers in a period of emotional vulnerability. Thus, as might be expected, this critical period of adult development is also a time when problems of attachment may take place. Extending intimate feelings to another, only to be exploited, ridiculed, or rejected, most likely produces a degree of caution in future relationships. If this happens several times more serious forms of emotional reticence—detachment, reserve, or variations of the alienated pattern described earlier—may well be engendered.

The middle adult years may also present problems of attachment, although perhaps not as dramatically and acutely as in earlier phases. Individuals have now "settled in" to the long-term tasks of raising a family, earning an income, maintaining a home, and so forth. Two interrelated areas of risk at this stage have been identified by investigators: (1) assuming the fallacy that one's personal development is now complete, with a resultant sense of stagnation, as life is perceived to be routine and unexciting; and (2) emerging feelings of being constrained by marital and family responsibilities, with a consequent withdrawal from intimacy and a turning to self-indulgence.

To complete this discussion of periods of vulnerability during the adult years, some commentary on the retirement period is necessary. Often romanticized as an era of leisure and freedom from work, Sheehy (1976) and Levinson (1978) inject a note of reality concerning some of the interpersonal problems faced by the aged. They theorize that a sense of estrangement and isolation seems to lie at the heart of these problems and moreover that the isolation is frequently seen as being *imposed* by loved ones, the culture, and indeed, by fate itself. Often, moving to a retirement home is interpreted as a convenience for one's children and relatives rather than a positive assertion of choice and independence. Retirement from a lifetime of work produces a dramatic reduction in the interpersonal satisfactions derived from coworkers. A widowed spouse not only must deal with the cruelties of fate, but also has to contemplate one's own death alone. Rightly or wrongly, the perceived injustice of these events enhances personal feelings of alienation and the aura that somehow one has been "put aside" by the world. The tragedy of such alienation in the elderly strikes home when we consider that a retiree may still live another ten, twenty, or even thirty years—a virtual lifetime of possible isolation and loneliness.

Summary We can see that problems in forming and sustaining emotional attachments with others may develop across the entire life span. The early childhood years and adolescence seem to be times of special vulnerability because of the important interpersonal influences that normally occur at these stages of development. It also appears that the emergence of a sense of intimacy during early adulthood is a time when emotional traumas may have serious effects. Being interpersonally exploited or abused, especially during these vulnerable phases of one's life, seems to increase the risk of producing a widespread reaction that may be termed an alienation syndrome.

Interpreting the Social World

An important component of the concept of alienation concerns the manner in which the behaviors and motives of others are perceived and interpreted. If such cognitions are distorted or too limited, the possibilities for a sound and realistic relationship are reduced. In the present discussion, then, we will be focusing, not necessarily on the actual interpersonal events that occur, but rather on how those events are filtered, organized, and understood by the alienated individual.

General theory The conceptual background for this material comes from the extensive work of George Kelly (1955) and Carl Rogers (1959). Although these theorists approach the issues from different perspectives, they share the fundamental view that understanding an individual's behavior requires an analysis of the unique personal constructs and internal frame of reference by which the person interprets events in the world. Both theorists also agree that such personalized perceptions govern reactions to oneself (thus forming the basis for self-concept), as well as determining how we understand the behaviors of others and events in the world generally.

A central concept of this point of view is that of "personal constructs" or "perceptual categories." Information that is detected by our senses is organized, interpreted, and made meaningful by an internal classification system that is largely developed through prior experience. Thus, for example, a child who grows up in a stimulus-rich environment and who learns a complex language and conceptual framework pertaining to these varied stimuli becomes capable of making subtle distinctions among events in the world. One often hears the illustration of Eskimo children, growing up in arctic climates, who develop as many as fourteen distinct perceptual-verbal categories that refer to different qualities of snow. Their particular learning experiences thus permit an exquisite, fine-grain analysis of this critical phenomena in their physical environment. By the same token, a child growing up in Miami Beach may understandably develop only a two-category cognitive system with respect to snow—that is, it's either snowing or it's not—with no discrimination among sleet, slush, powdered snow, and so forth.

Cognitive constructs pertaining to the interpersonal world also develop on the basis of prior experience and learning and in general provide a basis for understanding the motives of others, evaluating their personal characteristics and deriving expectations about their future behavior. Such category systems are usually multidimensional, and this complexity stems from a variety of sources. First, perceptual categories pertaining to people develop as a result of direct experience and from what one is told (by parents, friends, the media, etc.) about the nature of the social environment—two sources of information that do not always agree. Second, since interpersonal affairs are frequently associated with emotional and attitudinal reactions, such category systems often also involve deeper systems of needs, fears, resentments, and so forth, in the personality. Third, the inherent variety and diversity of the interpersonal world itself seems to require a multifaceted and flexible system of personal constructs through which to appreciate the uniqueness of others.

Personal constructs and alienation Rudimentary category systems about the interpersonal environment undoubtedly begin to form in early childhood. As the person matures and experiences an ever-widening array of social contacts, the internal personal constructs pertaining to people take on added dimensions and distinctions, achieving great richness and subtlety in the socially mature adult. However, a number of problems that prevent the full development of such elaborate cognitive systems may arise. Obviously, individuals whose social contacts have been limited, because of either living circumstances or self-imposed isolation, are likely to acquire only a few, gross categories by which to organize their perceptions of others. Persons who are chauvinistic or prejudiced, for example, are frequently described as functioning with such simplified systems, for example, "They're either one of us, or they're alien." Stereotyping and discrimination of this sort (Allport, 1960; Brigham, 1971) often are reinforced by prejudicial attitudes that are communicated through political demogoguery, simple-minded media presentations, or everyday social intercourse.

More ominous developments seem to occur with individuals who have undergone emotional trauma at the hands of others. The child who is chronically exposed to cold, hostile parents, having only rare contacts with warmth and gentleness, probably evolves a system of personal constructs in which a major category might be labeled "dangerous, hurtful, and uncaring." This often-used way of categorizing people at home is also likely to generalize to new encounters as well, thereby impeding the possibility of forming future relationships on a positive basis.

The effects of emotions, particularly anxiety and stress, are also noteworthy in this area. In fearful situations, the fine discriminations among perceptual categories tend to break down as the individual reverts to such basic constructs as "dangerous" versus "safe." Under emergency conditions in which rapid decisions are required for one's physical safety, such all-or-nothing classifications may certainly be necessary; however, were individuals to function at this rudimentary level over the long term in their lives, even routine interpersonal perceptions and sensitivities would be sorely lacking.

These cognitive deficits seem to be characteristic of many alienated individuals. The hardened delinquent may categorize most people as either "dangerous exploiters" or "suckers to be easily victimized." The young woman who is ridiculed and spurned in a love affair may keep potential suitors at a distance by viewing them as "smooth operators," "too pushy," or "immature and self-centered." In each case, the limited categories for classifying people are all-inclusive; that is, every new individual that is encountered is, in essence, forced into one of these niches, usually on the basis of limited or even incorrect evidence.

Personal constructs and behavior Both Kelly and Rogers propose that behavior is determined by one's perceptions and interpretations of situations. In this light we can see in the examples cited that alienated individuals to a large extent perceive others as being malevolent, untrustworthy, or uncaring. The social behaviors of the alienated thus appear to be consistent with these perceptions and in effect serve to protect them from anticipated hurt. The aggressiveness of the alienated delinquent, the social withdrawal and isolation of the schizoid personality, and the verbal games played by the detached intellectualizer all function to keep others at an emotional distance.

An unfortunate outcome of these behaviors is the likelihood that they will arouse negative reactions in others (fear, counteraggression, frustration, etc.), thereby precipitating the very behaviors they have come to expect from people. Thus the limited and malevolent perceptual categories of the alienated receive frequent confirmation—a sort of self-fulfilling prophecy that gets reinforced in each new encounter.

Therapeutic tasks Our discussion of personal constructs and perceptual categories would not be complete without some reference to specific therapy aims in this area. In the section dealing with attachment issues we saw that the major aim of therapy was to develop a relationship such that the client comes out from behind a wall of alienation and forms a positive and close emotional tie with the therapist. We can now see that an important component of that goal involves a change in the personal constructs that the client employs in perceiving others. The essential tasks here are to: (1) increase the number of the client's cognitive categories concerning people so that finer and more accurate perceptions can take place; (2) improve the client's skills in attending to a wide range of social information, rather than selectively focusing on information that conforms to preconceived biases; (3) help the client to develop cognitive categories through which positive behaviors and motives of others can be classified and understood; and (4) help the client become aware of the effects of his or her own behavior in provoking negative reactions in others. At the heart of such goals is the simple adage that one must be able to conceptualize the possibility of affection from others before it can be experienced within.

Concepts from the Humanistic Tradition

The humanistic tradition in personality theory is difficult to define. At a general level it refers to theorists who focus attention on three interrelated issues: one's relationship with oneself, one's sense of community with fellow human beings, and the philosophical meaning that one develops for one's life. Viewed in this broad perspective, humanism encompasses such theorists as Alfred Adler, Abraham Maslow, Carl Rogers, and Victor Frankl. Although these theorists focus on somewhat different aspects of human problems, they share one basic viewpoint—that people have to search within themselves for personal identity and meaning. This emphasis on the inner world (the private phenomenology) of the individual has prompted criticism from theorists dedicated to an objective and empirical study of human functioning. However, such criticism may be tempered by two trends within the humanistic tradition: (1) it continues to have wide popular appeal, suggesting that its ideas are touching upon important issues in contemporary culture; and (2) considerable research, particularly by Carl Rogers and his students, has been conducted in attempting to explore the personal phenomenology of individuals.

Adler (1927) viewed the maladjusted individual as "striving for isolation and lusting for power" in order to overcome feelings of inferiority. Strivings for power, in Adler's view, are not necessarily reflected in isolated interpersonal maneuvers, but rather become a central part of the neurotic's whole style of life. Organizing one's existence to gain superiority and prestige for their own sake was viewed as preventing the very qualities that Adler considered to be the essence of humanity—logic, creativity, sympathy, cooperation, love, and meeting the responsibilities of a communal life. For Adler, then, the aims of psychotherapy were to orient the client toward a life of social usefulness and a sense of positive feeling towards others. Adler felt that the process of therapy must be intimately bound to a deep and sincere relationship with the client in which the therapist transmits his or her own sense of community feeling to the client.

Rogers (1967) and Maslow (1968) focus on the individual's relation to him- or herself. Maladjustment is seen to occur when significant portions of experience or aspects of personality are not incorporated in one's self-concept. Probably resulting from a long-term process of automatically accepting external definitions of the self (e.g., from parents, from the culture), the maladjusted individual in effect loses touch with his or her unique inner potentials and personality processes. In the attempt to preserve an essentially invalid or superficial view of oneself, this individual is seen to deny or distort experience, to restrict interpersonal relations, and to pursue a rigid, robotlike existence (Rogers, 1959).

Important aspects of Rogers's theory are also concerned with the interpersonal process. Indeed, he views certain qualities of the therapist-client relationship as essential to successful treatment. As we have seen in earlier chapters, these qualities involve the communication of unconditional positive regard, empathic understanding, and personal genuineness by the therapist. Under these "facilitative conditions," the theory suggests that a client's own potentials for growth and a deeper experiencing of him- or herself will be fostered. Although formulated in vague terms, a considerable amount of research evidence suggests that Rogers's views about treatment have validity (see Truax and Mitchell, 1971).

Frankl (1965) is perhaps the most philosophical of this group of therapists. He views the problems of people in contemporary culture as largely spiritual in nature. Many maladjusted individuals may be seen as aimless, bored, and uncommitted—essentially progressing through life without direction or meaning. Frankl states that mental health workers are frequently confronted by clients who suffer from this "existential vacuum." Specific symptoms or identifiable behavioral abnormalities do not appear to be prominent in these individuals. Rather, Frankl focuses on a general "inner state of emptiness" to characterize this class of present-day neurosis. In essence this condition prevents the maladjusted individual from becoming emotionally attached to other people or to spiritual values. Frankl's approach to therapy (logotherapy) is thus oriented toward helping clients develop goals and responsibilities in their lives, especially responsibilities toward fellow human beings. It is a therapy aimed at helping clients discover the "why" of their existence.

We can see in the ideas of all these humanistic theorists a broader view of our notion of alienation. It refers not only to detachment from other people but also, and perhaps more fundamentally, to a detachment from oneself. While such concepts are vague, they have an intuitive appeal to many therapists who see a substantial proportion of clients who appear to suffer from bleak, superficial, and meaningless life-styles—who are emotionally unconnected with either themselves or others.

Psychodynamic Theory

A somewhat different conceptual perspective on problems of alienation is provided by psychodynamic theory (Wolberg, 1967). Here the emphasis is placed on the defensive function of detachment and emotional isolation from others—defense against strong, underlying anxiety or anger that threatens to erupt should the individual get close to someone else. By maintaining emotional distance, one is thereby protected from the risk of being overwhelmed by debilitating internal forces that threaten the integrity of the personality.

According to the psychodynamic view, children who are rejected and abused experience severe anxiety and rage, which become fundamental emotional systems in their personality structure. As the maturing child withdraws from affective ties with others and develops a hardened, cynical view of the world, these threatening emotions become more manageable. This process eventuates in a habitual style of dealing with the social environment—detachment, mistrust, restricted perceptual categories, and various behavior patterns designed to keep people at a distance. These character defenses may take various forms, depending on specific learning factors in the individual's environment. Aggressive, delinquent patterns are one possibility. A passive, shy, and withdrawn character structure is another. Yet a third might be represented by individuals who chronically approach others in a rigidly intellectual, businesslike fashion, never allowing their feelings or a sense of affiliation to enter into their dealings with people. Whatever the surface characteristics of such alienated individuals, at the heart of the syndromes is the maintenance of a fundamental defensive apartness from others.

The notion of conflict also enters into the psychodynamic perspective. While alienated individuals are attempting to control infantile sources of anxiety and rage, they also may be driven by hungerings for nurturance and affection. These basic human needs, though frustrated and suppressed in earlier social relationships, nevertheless exert pressures for gratification. Occasional fantasies about a more congenial world, needs for physical intimacy, and labors with the pains of loneliness may surface. However, the anxiety and anger that accompany these slight relaxations of protective armor will likely prompt a resurgence of defenses to keep others at a distance.

Therapy implications Psychodynamic theory adds two important aspects to our considerations of relationship therapy. First is the notion that motivations toward affiliation and positive human feelings may still exist, however suppressed and disguised, in the personality makeup of alienated individuals. Such a conceptualization thus provides the therapist with at least remote emotional systems within the client upon which to build a therapeutic relationship. Needless to say, some clients may have been so abused and may have erected such rigid defenses that these positive emotions are inaccessible. However, with younger clients generally, and with those whose histories have not been overwhelmingly severe, working toward establishing such emotional contact is a central task of relationship therapy.

The second therapeutic implication pertains to the defensive function of alienation. If strong anxiety and rage indeed lurk beneath the surface, then inviting the client into a close relationship poses a degree of risk for the client (and perhaps the therapist as well). The beginnings of positive emotional ties in effect represent a weakening of critically important defenses in the alienated individual, defenses that in the past were literally essential for psychological survival. Lowering these defenses will likely unleash strong fear, confusion, anger, and perhaps exaggerated attempts to prevent a positive relationship from developing. Such psychodynamic considerations highlight the importance of careful management of anxiety and anger in the client as well as the necessity for regulating the tempo of the emergent relationship in this form of treatment.

Summary

The various theories presented in this section were intended to provide a set of converging perspectives on a group of disorders that may be termed *syndromes of alienation*. While such syndromes may differ in their surface manifestations (e.g., aggressiveness, passivity and withdrawal, or intellectualization), they have a common core of interpersonal deficits. It is the core problems to which relationship therapy is aimed. A summary of the theoretical areas, the related core problems, and the therapeutic tasks associated with each of these complementary viewpoints are presented in Table 7.1.

CASE EXAMPLES

One of the negative consequences of human ingenuity is the many varied ways in which people hurt each other. Physical harm, deception, unfulfilled promises, and the withholding of affection all produce a store of different negative emotions in the victim. Furthermore, diverse life circumstances and societal forces dictate the many ways that these hurts are expressed. Hence, when we talk about syndromes of alienation, a wide variety of symptoms and interpersonal styles may be involved. What groups them together is the common underlying disenchantment with fellow human beings.

In this light, the following case examples are not intended as a formal typology of alienation problems. Rather, they are offered merely as examples of the various directions that such interpersonal difficulties may take.

Aggressive-Antisocial Developments

Joey is under the care of the juvenile court in his small community. Only twelve years old, he communicates a deep sense of anger and suspiciousness toward all who have dealings with him. He has a long history of truancy, incorrigibility, and fighting at school. Recently he set fire to his uncle's barn and was caught evidently trying to run away to another part of the country. When first apprehended by the police he seemed to be petrified with fear. When he discovered that he was not going to be physically harmed, however, the fear was quickly replaced by a surly, uncooperative, and withdrawn demeanor.

Joey is the only child in a family whose financial situation fluctuates from poverty to modest success. His father was described as a small-time operator in the community who is always working on one "deal" or another—partial ownership of a tavern, leasing farm implements, taking commissions for arranging government subsidies—enterprises that all collapsed through mismanagement and lack of attention. His mother works as a waitress and was variously described by people who knew her as beautiful, immature, quarrel-

Table 7.1
Theoretical perspectives, core problems, and therapy tasks associated with syndromes of alienation

Theoretical area	Core problems	Therapy tasks
Attachment theory	Withdrawal of affection from others. Fear of interpersonal hurt.	Establishing a positive therapy relationship.
Cognitive theory	Limited perceptual categories. Negative expectations of others. Overgeneralization based on minimal information.	Increasing the number of perceptual categories. Building positive constructs. Making accurate discriminations.
Psychodynamic theory	Character defenses that contain infantile anxiety and rage. Interpersonal behaviors that keep others at a distance.	Gradual replacement of defenses with positive social behaviors. Insight into sources of inner stress.
Humanistic theory	Denial of inner experience. Alienation from oneself. Absence of meaning and communal responsibility in life.	Using the therapy relationship to facilitate self-discovery, the development of goals, and prompting social feelings.

some, always seeking a good time, and waiting for her husband to "strike it big."

Joey never had a chance with his parents. He was unplanned and unwanted—a major inconvenience to their life-styles and ambitions. Of course, there were some good times, particularly in his early years. He can remember happy occasions when he was four or five years old. When his father had just gotten some money, he would walk hand in hand with him down the street: jovial, exchanging greetings, displaying their new outfits, parading the recent success. Joey felt especially proud on these occasions because it seemed as if his father were "showing off" his son as well. Happy times with his mother are kept in more murky corners of Joey's memory. He can dimly remember evenings when the two of them were home alone. She seemed in some ways to be upset—agitated, impatient, and depressed. She would hold him, almost enveloping him in sorrowful embraces. He recalls an almost breath-taking joy when this would happen in his younger years, but later, when he was eight or nine years old, his reaction was something akin to revulsion and anxiety. When he broke away, his mother would just sit there and cry.

For the most part, Joey's daily existence while growing up was marked by loneliness, fear, and yearnings for warmth. His parents seemed too busy or involved in their own disputes to even acknowledge his presence. He was not an easy child to raise, being undisciplined and frequently demanding attention. Sometimes, when he was especially obnoxious, one or the other of his parents would lose control and beat him in a sustained and violent way. This would usually shut him up, and he pulled within himself, trying to imagine ways of getting back at them.

Teachers in the early grades described Joey as a disruptive influence in school. His high activity level, constant attention seeking, and inability to work conscientiously on class materials prompted a great deal of irritation. Methods of discipline escalated from extra work on tedious assignments to frequent paddlings by the principal. Joey also seemed to have little sense of personal property, and on occasion he would simply take someone else's notebook, pair of gloves, or lunch money. When informed of these incidents, Joey's father, evidently fearful of his own reputation in the community, would be harsh in his physical punishments.

By the fifth grade, Joey had acquired the label of an incorrigible trouble-maker among teachers and fellow pupils. He had the reputation of a fierce fighter in the school yard and of someone who was adept at driving teachers to distraction. Openly disrespectful and rebellious, he would, for example, challenge a new teacher on the first day of class to test his or her mettle. If the teacher reacted quickly and severely, he knew his stay in this grade would be a long, arduous struggle. If the teacher ignored the challenge or tried to reason with him, he "knew" equally well that this class would be a push-over.

When Joey was twelve years old his father left home. There were, from Joey's perspective, no unusual forerunners to this departure. The habitual bickering and recriminations had not noticeably increased. There had been no discussions of possible separation or divorce. One day he just left, apparently never to return. Joey felt a knot of remorse for a brief time, but for the most part, he reports, "It really didn't matter." His mother's reaction did not surprise him either. Her flight into drinking and casual affairs only seemed to be an exaggeration of patterns that had been developing over the past few years. He completely lost what little sense of allegiance he had felt for both parents.

Joey was sent by his mother to live with an uncle who had a farm in a neighboring county. Her reasoning was that she could no longer provide proper discipline to her son and that perhaps a new home and school environment would settle him down. The uncle, a rather austere, remote man, had for years belabored Joey's mother for having married an ineffectual and immature man. He saw all of Joey's problems as stemming from his father's lack of firm discipline, and he was determined to mold his nephew into a law-abiding and industrious person. Hard work, no frivolity, and immediate retribution for even the smallest transgression prevailed in the environment that Joey now faced.

Joey was not strong enough to fight back directly, but little things started to go wrong on the farm. A tractor was improperly greased, and thereby needed repairs. A gate was left open on the way to school, so that his uncle had to spend the morning rounding up stray cattle. Each similar incident resulted in heavy punishment, but at least Joey felt that he was holding his own. Beneath it all, however, Joey could sense a complex of emotions that were mounting to extreme levels. Anger seemed to be at its core. Fear and an aura of being overwhelmed were intimately mixed in. More remote were vague hungerings for stability and closeness, but these feelings were dismissed because he knew the world just was not that way. His inner turmoil was approaching a critical point. Was he going crazy? He had to do something to get relief. One last act of retaliation, a final assertion of selfhood, had to be done before he ran away — and so Joey set the barn on fire.

The juvenile court decided to place Joey in a foster home and also to have him enter into counseling. It was made clear to him that he would be sent to a juvenile institution if further problems developed in his new home or if he failed to participate in therapy.

Adult Affectional Problems

Ms. W, thirty-four years old, has been divorced for three years. She has two daughters, aged ten and eight, whom she cares for dutifully. Since her divorce she has worked her way up from clerk-typist to administrative assistant in the accounting department of a large business firm. Her life is well organized and encapsulated in earning a living and raising her daughters. She has a few female acquaintances in her apartment complex. They occasionally share an evening meal, go shopping together, or take their children to some activity; however, none of these friendships are deep. Ms. W feels that her life is sensible and safe. When pressed, she sorrowfully admits to a deep sense of barrenness and a foreboding that the future holds very little of meaning for her.

Life was not always this way for Ms. W. She grew up in a rather strict working-class family. She felt herself to be an integral part of the family group, although both she and her sister always knew that they were not as highly esteemed as their brothers. So be it. These were old-world views of her parents, and Ms. W was comfortable with their affection and guidance.

Ms. W describes herself as having been "average in every way" in high school—in academic work, in extracurricular activities, and in popularity. She "went steady" for three years with a quiet, well-mannered boy. Although Ms. W hesitatingly admits that they "did some heavy petting," she indignantly denies ever having had sexual relations with her boyfriend. Their relationship broke up quite naturally upon graduation from high school, because, as she recounts it, "we each just seemed to go our own way."

Ms. W was the first female in her extended family to attend college. It took some pressure from her and her mother, but her father finally relented, half-jokingly condemning the ambitions of "modern women." She enjoyed the easy rapport of the dormitory, and even more the sense of intellectual adventure in class. Her world was a series of ever-widening horizons—it was challenging, exciting, and optimistic. A new dimension was added when, during her second year, she met a young man who shared her enthusiasm. She and Jim would sit for hours talking about modern music, philosophy, poetry, and gradually, themselves.

A deep affection developed between the pair. Ms. W describes her junior year in college as the happiest in her life. Everything was shared. She and Jim studied together, exchanged new ideas, developed a robust sexual life, and spent hours excitedly planning for their future. Toward the end of the year they moved in together. When Ms. W's parents learned of this, they stopped all contact with her. Although she was hurt by their extreme reaction, she felt that they would eventually come to accept her role as a "liberated woman."

Ms. W dropped out of school and began work as a typist at the beginning of her senior year. Jim had received his B.A. and was entering a graduate program, and they both agreed that this arrangement was an investment in their future. Her boring job, coupled with many lonely evenings while Jim studied at the library, made this a trying time for Ms. W. Although she tried to be supportive of him as he suffered the tensions of graduate work, she also had a vague sense of being an outsider, of not really being able to share fully in his life. She held on to her optimism, however, secure in the vision of better times to come when he finished school.

Ms. W and Jim were married the next year on the same day that he received his master's degree. Although it was a happy occasion, somehow it did not have the emotional impact on Ms. W that she had anticipated. Jim was to start a job as a junior executive in a business firm almost immediately. Finances also dictated that she continue with her job rather than return to school. Perhaps, she reasoned, once they become more established, she could continue with her education. In the meantime, her life did not change very much.

When the first of her children was born two years later, Ms. W entered the realm of motherhood with a profound joy and a sense of oneness with nature. It was a time of emotional and philosophical rebirth, in some way touching deep chords of creativity within her. She could not help sensing, however, that Jim did not experience the same depth of feelings about parenthood. He played the role of the dutiful father and did his part of the new household chores. But he also seemed a bit too anxious to get back to the office or to work on a report that was due. Try as she might, she could not get him to fully understand or share in the profundity of her feelings.

The next several years saw family life proceed in a rather comfortable routine occasionally interrupted with times of celebration—his first big promotion, the purchase of a house, the birth of a second daughter. Ms. W's daily life was centered around caring for her children, decorating the house, reading, and waiting for her husband to come home. Most of the couple's conversations revolved around everyday happenings, office gossip, a planned new purchase for the house, and so on. Ms. W treasured and hungered for the occasional times that they went beyond the routine into deeper, personal communications or had an uninhibited, romantic sexual encounter. Although she did not particularly like the growing sense of dependency within her, she could do little to prevent it. She reasoned that such was the nature of family life, gradually acknowledging that her personal identity and sense of womanhood was totally centered on her roles of wife and mother.

When Ms. W was thirty-one years old, her husband announced that he was leaving home and would be seeking a divorce. In a burst of candor he admitted that he was involved with another woman, with whom he had been having an affair for over a year. He felt that it would be best for all concerned if they were both to start their lives over again with someone new, while they were still young enough. Ms. W's disbelief turned to anger, then to fear, then to a childish pleading, in rapid succession. Jim's excessively rational and business-like approach to this catastrophic event frightened her most of all.

After several months of emotional confusion, attempts at reconciliation, and well-meaning but conflicting advice from friends, it became clear that Jim was not going to return. As her inner turmoil began to subside, Ms. W could recognize that some basic changes had taken place in her personality. As she describes it, a kind of hardened shell had formed around her tender emotions. A deep feeling of personal insult and of having been used came to the fore. She began to see the world, perhaps more realistically, she thought, as mean and deceitful. She developed a resolve that her principal goal should now be to protect herself and her daughters from further hurt by an essentially selfish and untrustworthy environment. At the core of this resolve was her belief that she could never again allow tender and intimate feelings to be extended toward anyone but her children.

Schizoid Adjustment

"You want me to tell about myself? Just like that? Lady, I'll try. But there's not much to tell. [*What a bullshit thing. Social workers. Fill out dumb-ass reports. Shit. Might as well. Play the game.*]

"I'm twenty-seven. I signed myself in because I had an attack of nerves. Getting real tense. Jumpy. Things closing in. The medicine helped the last time, so I figured. . . . [*Look at the bitch write it all down. Shove it in her file. Shove it. Probably run home and screw her old man as soon as she can.*]

"Yeah, I've been in this place before. Three, four times. Yeah, a few other places too. Omaha, St. Pete. I got shook up real bad in the Army, and they've been giving me medicine ever since. I've been working here and there. Do okay for a while, then the nerves start acting up. . . . [*Like that bullshit job in the diner. . . . Don't see no ring. Maybe she's not married. Probably screwing the whole hospital. Tough old bitch. If she comes on to me, I'll . . .*]

"What? Well, I worked in a diner. And before that, cleaning windows. Whatever I can find. I guess I'm what you'd call a drifter. I like to move around. I get tense, kind of, if I'm hemmed in. [*Whoee, look at her write. Free as a bird, man. No shit from nothing. . . . Who did she think she was? Fat old waitress. Boffed her once and she thought she owned me. I'd end up supporting her and her brat kid forever.*]

"Yeah, I was thinking maybe someday I'd settle down. I never had a real home, you know. Don't know what it's like. Are you married? Grew up in the county home, and then the army, then, like I said, just drifting around. [*Oh, you old slut, if you only knew. . . . 'Get up, you skinny little bastard, nobody sleeps late here.' 'Yes sir. YES SIR!' Oh shit. What the hell did they want from me? I was just a kid. . . . She didn't answer me. I knew it. The bitch is on the make.*]

"And man, it wasn't easy. I never knew my folks. Killed when I was a baby. But that's the way the world is, I guess. Never thought of marrying. Oh, I've been around a little, you know, but never found the right girl. . . . [*Up yours, lady. Lap it up and get your ass in gear. . . . Funny. . . . That's what that runty sargeant used to say. 'Shape up sonny. You better get your ass in gear.' Queer as a three dollar bill. Just waiting to get you in his bunk. . . . Come on, you bitch, it's getting close to supper time.*]

"So maybe that's why I get so tense sometimes. Heh! Heh! Never found the right girl. What time is it? Oh, nothing. I just like to keep track of time. Like in the army. Everything by the numbers. Right on schedule. I had a hard time there. Couldn't get it in gear. But I had this old sargeant who kind of took care of me. [*Jesus, I got to get out of here. This bitch is getting on my nerves. Come on lady, make your move.*]

"Just like I guess you're going to take care of me. You know what I mean. . . . [*What the hell is the matter with her? She's just leading me on. Gets it off this way? Why does she keep bitching at me about taking care. . . . Oh shit, here we go.*]

"Do you think they'll give me some more medicine after supper? Yeah, I'm feeling real tense right now. I guess all this talk about being took care of is getting to me. [*They all took care of me, you dumb bitch! Took care of me! That's what it's all about. They screwed me every mother_____ chance they could get. Same as you, sitting there with a mother_____ smile on your face.*]

"Isn't it time for supper yet?"

OVERVIEW OF STAGES IN RELATIONSHIP THERAPY

In the case studies described in the previous section, an attempt was made to portray several typical clients with problems of alienation. These descriptions do not, of course, represent a comprehensive survey of all the possible difficulties of attachment that could be mentioned. Rather, these three cases, with different surface characteristics, were intended to illustrate the underlying themes of isolation, defensiveness, and emotional detachment that seem to be common to alienation syndromes.

In the same sense, it would be impossible to describe a series of regular, lock-step stages that are characteristic of relationship therapy. There are too many variations, too many unexpected twists and turns that occur as therapist and client intertwine their personalities. What can be described are a number of issues and problems that are typically encountered, what is likely to happen when these problems are resolved, and in what directions the therapist is trying to move the relationship. Hence, the material in this overview section is intended to provide a general summary of the issues to be faced. Although they will be presented in an approximate sequential order, the reader should bear in mind that they may surface in therapy at any time.

General Considerations

Going back to the theoretical and case materials for a moment, let us review the underlying dynamics of clients—dynamics which, in effect, they also bring with them into the therapy relationship. A history of having been psychologically hurt and abused by others seems to lie at the heart of these problems. Such interpersonal traumas were presumably severe or persistent enough to bring about a generalized emotional distancing from people, which in large measure serves as a protection against anticipated future hurt. This alienation may also serve as a defense against strong, historically rooted systems of anxiety or rage that threaten to erupt in emotionally provocative situations. Finally, an important part of clients' protective armor is their style of perceiving and thinking about people, that is, viewing and pigeonholing others into very limited, usually malevolent or noncaring, categories.

The task facing the therapist is an understandably difficult one. The essential aim here is to have the client come out from behind the protective armor and eventually form a deep, honest, and mutually satisfying relationship. From the client's perspective, the risks can be enormous. To be close and affectionate with someone means vulnerability. To open one's feelings exposes a storehouse of earlier agonies, fright, and anger. In a sense, the relatively safe mode of adjustment that alienation provides now becomes threatened by the therapist's invitation into a meaningful and emotional relationship.

Clients will undoubtedly resist the formation of such a relationship. If the status quo is safe, why should they risk a change? What insurance do clients have that they will not be hurt again? After all, the therapist is just another person, and the client is already reasonably convinced that people in general are untrustworthy. Many of the issues and problems encountered in treatment thus pertain to coping with the ways in which clients resist the formation of a relationship with the therapist. Once resistance is overcome, additional issues involve the management of strong negative emotions associated with earlier trauma, the learning of more realistic and refined ways of perceiving others, and the development of positive relationships outside of therapy.

In successful treatment, the development of a positive therapist-client relationship becomes the "important exception" in the client's social life. Coming in the context of a history of interpersonal strife, this critical relationship becomes an emotional learning experience that opens up new possibilities for the future. Being a partner in such a pivotal experience in the client's life places an extraordinary burden on the therapist. Not only must the therapist negotiate the technical requirements of overcoming resistance, managing debilitating emotions, changing cognitions, and so forth, but the therapist must do all this as part of a genuine, open, and honest participation in the relationship. Technical competence is not enough. Playing the role of a concerned therapist is equally insufficient. Indeed, to the degree that the therapist remains "outside of the relationship" or simply "acts the part," the client's cynical view of people may actually be reinforced.

A final point in these general considerations concerns the length of time involved in relationship therapy. The amount of time needed for successful therapy may be anywhere from several months to several years. It is conceivable with Joey, the twelve-year-old case illustration, for example, that six months may elapse before "emotional contact" is established. Thereafter, another half-year may be needed to implement emotional and behavioral changes in Joey's daily life. Following this, there may be a long period of progressively declining contact as the client establishes new and satisfying relationships outside of therapy. However, during this time the teenager may need to "keep in touch"—checking out new issues as they arise, seeking occasional advice, or simply relating to an old and important friend. Other clients, who are perhaps less "beaten down" by the world or are at a different age, may progress through therapy more quickly; in essence, however, these same broad phases of treatment seem to take place. A more detailed description of the phases is presented below.

The Initial Phase of the Relationship

Clients with alienation problems frequently enter therapy with many characteristics that work against successful treatment: suspicion of the therapist; a lack of commitment to change; traits designed to keep others (i.e., the therapist) at a distance; and, on occasion, participation in therapy under duress. Consider again Joey, the twelve-year-old in the first case illustration who was directed by the juvenile court to receive therapy or face institutionalization. It is quite likely that this troubled boy will perceive therapy as a form of punishment, and will view the therapist as the court's agent of punishment. These unfortunate interpretations only serve to strengthen this client's already existing fear, anger, and negative expectations of others generally, and of the therapist specifically.

The second case example, that of Ms. W, presents another, perhaps more subtle, pattern that is antithetical to therapy. For quite a few years she saw herself in a successful marriage in which she was emotionally open, loving, sacrificing, working for the future, and dedicated to the family. She believed that her husband shared these same feelings. Sure, the marriage had its ups and downs over the years, but these, she reasoned, occur with any couple. She "knew," at a basic level, that the marital relationship was firm and secure. When the abandonment took place, with the announcement that her husband had been having a secret affair for a long period of time, the emotional blow was double-barreled. Not only did the major relationship in her life disintegrate, but in addition, she was faced with the realization that the closest person in her life was a sham. Some new rules about people were learned: people's communications and behaviors are not to be trusted; people's appearances are deceiving; and in the final analysis, people are self-serving and uncaring. From this perspective, we can anticipate mistrust of the therapist, no matter how warm or supportive that therapist might be. The warmth and friendship extended by the therapist are likely to be seen as a "good act," cleverly portrayed but ultimately also a sham.

The schizoidlike person in the third example probably enters therapy with an even less coherent and less realistic set of expectations than the other clients. One gains the impression from his monologue that life is perceived as mean and chaotic. Social encounters are a series of photographic images, stark and inhuman, in which cruelty and exploitation abound. He meets the world with a lifeless mask, while underneath he is immersed in a private torrent of ugly memories, misperceptions of the present, and pressures for immediate need gratification. The therapist here is likely to be seen as another transient individual, devoid of human feeling — at best, a mere convenience upon whom to spin a web of fantasies; at worst, a diabolical force bent on malevolence and destruction.

From these examples we can begin to appreciate the difficulties faced by the therapist right from the start of treatment. The aim of therapy is to develop a strong, positive relationship; yet the very nature of the problems experienced by alienated individuals serve to defeat this aim from the outset. It is apparent, then, that reaching this goal will have to take place in gradual, sometimes agonizing steps. The opening phase of therapy is merely the first move in this direction. Its aim is both modest and critically important: to initiate the relationship, within limits, on virtually any basis that the client finds tolerable and that will keep him or her in therapy. The specific approaches and techniques open to the therapist in this initial phase of treatment will be described in Chapter 8.

The Testing Phase

The therapist is under scrutiny by the client from the onset of therapy, almost as if she or he were an adversary. From the client's point of view, the therapist is a person who is trying to move close emotionally, to establish contact, to open up the client's inner life. The therapist is therefore a threat to an established way of maintaining safety. As described earlier, the client most likely has some strong preconceptions about the essential untrustworthiness of people in general (including the therapist). Once therapy begins, the client, in effect, sets out to confirm these preconceptions and to find out the details of just how this particular therapist will show his or her failings.

In the theory section of this chapter, the notion of perceptual categories into which people get classified was discussed. This frame of reference may serve as a convenient way to consider the testing process that the therapist undergoes. Recall that alienated individuals were described as usually operating with a limited number of such categories, so that others may be easily and quickly assigned to one of these (negative) cubicles of the mind. Once such a cognitive assignment is made, the client can feel justified in behaving toward the classified individual as if the qualities of that category were true about the person. The client's conception of the world is thereby again confirmed, and the pattern of alienation remains intact. Thus the major task facing the therapist at this early stage of treatment is to prevent such a premature categorization of him or her from taking place. If it should occur, the hope for an emotional breakthrough in the therapeutic relationship would be seriously impaired.

The testing phase of therapy, as well as the categorizing process described above, can be conceptualized in several steps. First, the client enters treatment with strong preconceptions that the therapist is essentially an unworthy individual, just like others who have been encountered in life. However, the client may be unsure of just how this unworthiness will display itself, that is, into which of the client's "person categories" the therapist may be assigned. Thus the client initially searches for evidence that will aid in this categorization. "How does this person come across in our first meeting? Hostile? Dictatorial? Frightened? Phony? Pompous? What have I heard about this person from others that will help peg him or her? Who does this person remind me of in the past?"

Second, if no clear evidence is forthcoming, the client may begin to probe. "Let's see what kind of answer I get to this question," or, "I wonder how he or she will react when I do this?" In a sense, a "diagnostic process in reverse" is taking place in which the client is trying to gather enough evidence by which to label the therapist. In contrast to therapeutic diagnosis, however, the client's aims seem to be a confirmation of the conception that people are unworthy and a detailing of how that unworthiness will be manifested. Ultimately, the client is expecting to find that, as in past relationships, the therapist will in some way be rejecting and uncaring.

Let us assume that after these initial tests and probes the client still cannot clearly categorize the therapist, nor has the client received confirming evidence that the therapist is rejecting. Under these circumstances we can anticipate some degree of impatience, confusion, and anxiety on the part of the client. A neat and safe conclusion to the relationship is not taking place. In some fashion, the therapist is not readily falling into the predesignated categories; moreover, there are even some hints, unbelievable as they may be, that this person may actually care. Prompted by the confusion, anxiety, and need to maintain stable perceptions of the world, we can anticipate an escalation of the testing. Consciously or unconsciously, the client begins to function under a strategy such as, "How far do I have to push this person before he or she will show their true colors and reject me?"

The progressive increase in the severity of tests can be an especially trying time for the therapist. One's patience gets strained, vulnerabilities are exposed, defenses are aroused, and perhaps most serious, the therapist's dedication to helping the client may weaken. The testing may proceed for a long period of time (perhaps for months) and may indeed bring the therapist to the point of "giving up" on the client. Should this happen in a serious and permanent way, with its attendant withdrawal of emotion and interest in the relationship, the possibilities for successful treatment are virtually nil. The client has successfully sabotaged the process, confirmed his or her preconceptions about people, and can retire again into the relative safety of alienation. The successful management of the testing process and keeping perspective on one's own emotions are therefore critical aspects of relationship therapy.

The Weakening of Defenses

As the testing phase is successfully negotiated by the therapist, new elements of the treatment process emerge and take precedence. These pertain to a loosening of the client's perceptual categories and interpersonal defenses, with accompanying increases in anxiety, hostility, and self-doubt. It is a period of heightened feelings of vulnerability that require special attention from the therapist.

The inability of the client to classify the therapist into a preexisting malevolent category represents a major challenge to his or her view of the world. The developing therapeutic relationship opens the possibility, however remote, that some people may possess basically positive qualities and may be willing to extend those qualities to the client. This in turn prompts the need to reconsider the system of categories that has been used, and possibly to expand these classifications to include benevolence, caring, friendship, and so forth. From the client's perspective, such possibilities can have staggering implications, because to admit to them means a negation of a whole style of living—a style that in the past represented safety, protection from exploitation, and in some cases, one's very survival.

The developing therapeutic relationship also serves to prompt a variety of emotional reactions within the client. Most pronounced are feelings of anxiety, which seem to stem from several sources. Perhaps foremost is the anxiety associated with the weakening of the perceptual and interpersonal defenses described above. Again, to contemplate the possibility of a close relationship (with the therapist) engenders risks of new emotional hurt and abuse. Second, opening to the prospect of interpersonal closeness will likely rearouse memories and feelings of prior relationships in which the client was frightened, over-whelmed, and powerless. Taken together, these wellsprings of anxiety serve to produce remarkably heightened levels of tension (almost paradoxically) as the therapeutic relationship seems to be improving.

Along with heightened anxiety, this phase of therapy may also witness dramatic increases in hostility. Here again, there seem to be several sources that combine to produce angry episodes of considerable intensity. Perhaps most striking is a pervasive rage surrounding the client's interpersonal history — deep anger and indignation prompted by memories of cruelties of the past. Second, the increased tension and lack of certainty in the therapeutic relationship pro-duces a sense of frustration and impatience. The client seems to be caught in a dilemma, vacillating between desires to move closer in the relationship and fears that prompt withdrawal and continued isolation. Unable to resolve this approach-avoidance conflict, unpredictable outbursts of anger, blaming of the therapist, and generalized rage against a faithless world may erupt.

We can see then a highly volatile period of treatment that requires special sensitivity and support by the therapist. Emotional outbursts are very likely, and they seem to serve as indirect signals that the client is in the process of change. Although not fully committed, the client is at least contemplating the prospects of emotional closeness with the therapist and is desperately struggling with the emotional implications of such a breakthrough.

This period of treatment, involving the weakening of defenses, may also partially uncover an awesome and frightening system of reactions regarding the client's self-concept. One can speculate that these feelings and self-percep-tions may indeed be the most difficult for the client to face; hence, during this phase of treatment, they may at times temporarily surface, only to be disguised and avoided in quick order by the client. To a large extent these feelings operate with a perverse type of logic. The client, in effect, reasons, "If the important people in my life have abused, exploited, and rejected me, I must basically be a very contemptible person. How could anyone possibly respect me or have affection for me when I am so fundamentally unworthy?"

This inner core of self-doubt seems to be doubly threatening for the client. Not only does it expose basic deficits of self-acceptance and personal worth, but such concerns seem to inevitably prompt long-dormant hungerings for warmth, closeness, and stability. These, of course, are the very need systems that are especially dangerous for the client to recognize. To give free rein to such yearnings once again places the client in a vulnerable, dependent position relative to others. Little wonder, then, that during this difficult phase of therapy the client rigidly tries to suppress any fleeting impulses in these areas.

Emerging Closeness and Possible Crisis

The many conflicting trends described in the previous section seem to gather strength as therapy continues. The client begins to consider the very real possibility that the therapist is trustworthy, and she or he begins to experience a growing emotional closeness with the therapist. The emerging relationship may bring anxiety, anger, and self-doubt to intense levels, producing a very unstable therapeutic situation. Under the pressure of these strong emotions, there is risk that the client may seek relief in some impulsive and inappropriate manner.

Several possibilities may be considered here. The client may unexpectedly quit therapy and thereby escape from the threatening relationship. Along similar lines, he or she may focus on a minor flaw in the therapist, exaggerating this deficiency to the point that it provides a rationale for emotionally withdrawing from the relationship. Even more dramatically, the client may manufacture "one last, big test" for the therapist—one that under ordinary circumstances would almost guarantee rejection. If this were to happen, the client could safely return to an alienated pattern, feeling that, once again, his or her cynical view of people has been confirmed.

One way to consider this critical time in therapy is to view clients as being at an awesome emotional point of choice in their lives. On one hand, they have come to the brink of letting down defenses and extending positive emotions to another person, but they find the prospect too frightening. Thus clients consider taking the safe route, closing up feelings, and returning to a withdrawn, detached pattern. The other alternative is to commit themselves to the relationship, face the risks involved, and in essence, take a major step toward changing an alienated way of life. Although therapists are not always able to control events during this time of intense conflict, quite clearly their task is to help tip the scales in favor of an emotional commitment to the relationship.

Emotional Commitment

Let us assume that the relationship survives the client's impulses to leave or subvert therapy. The period of testing and indecisiveness has been surmounted, and a surge of new emotions is directed toward the therapist. The breakthrough has occurred, bringing with it a markedly changed atmosphere in therapy and a range of new problems and issues to be faced.

Perhaps fundamental to these changes is the fact that the client has found an ally and confidant with whom she or he can relate openly and nondefensively. Emerging from a chronic sense of aloneness, one can anticipate an emotional release and commitment to the relationship that is in sharp contrast to the earlier reserve and wariness. The client has accepted the invitation to form an attachment with the therapist; now the therapist must be prepared to meet the responsibilities of this attachment.

Recall that in an earlier stage of therapy, when defenses were weakening, the client worked hard to suppress underlying yearnings for affection, care, and nurturance. These long-frustrated needs may now surface dramatically and be directed toward the therapist. The form and intensity with which these needs are expressed may vary considerably from client to client. In the case example of Joey we may witness a period of strong identification and modeling of the therapist, a desire to be with the therapist as much as possible, and a frank dependency on the affection and warmth of this newfound friend. In the case of the divorced woman, these needs may be manifested in an outpouring of pent-up emotions and intimate disclosures to be shared with someone who is close and understanding. The third case illustration, the schizoid client, presents the least predictable pattern during this phase of therapy. The possible eruption of infantile dependency, cravings for physical contact, or overt expression of sexual impulses require special care and delicacy on the part of the therapist.

This phase of relationship therapy also ushers in, for the client, a period of direct exposure to inner questions of self-worth. Doubts about one's general value as a person and acceptability to others may be communicated to the therapist. As part of such discussions the client may agonize over injustices of the past, as he or she struggles to determine the reasons for others' rejection and exploitation. Was it because of some deficit in the client's personality? Or was the client simply the unlucky victim of others' shortcomings and lack of caring? Such questions may plague the client for a considerable time, and they seem to inject a melancholy, unsettling note into the newfound relationship.

The new rapport with the therapist may also evoke questions concerning the client's present life. She or he may voice strong dissatisfaction with current relationships and life-style, but at the same time express confusion as to how to change a long-standing way of living. Along similar lines, doubts arise about habitual ways of perceiving other people. Are others really as unfeeling and negative as was originally thought? Are there possibilities for closeness in the client's social world? The relaxing of defenses in the therapeutic relationship seems to have generalized beyond therapy, and the client begins to at least contemplate the possibility of a richer future.

In sum, this can be a very dramatic phase of therapy. A rush of positive emotions is directed toward the therapist, along with a strong dependency and needs for affection and reassurance. Some raw nerve endings are also exposed, particularly those involving self-doubts and where to place the blame for tragedies of the past. Defenses are down, and the client is taking the first steps toward an honest self-evaluation and a more realistic perception of the world. Despite these many struggles, however, this seems to be a profound and challenging period of therapy for the client. The initial impact of a "corrective emotional experience" is taking place, and the client gradually begins to be oriented toward the future to consider the implications of changes.

Reevaluation and New Goals

The emotional rebirth described in the last section leaves clients with both a sense of amazement about their good feelings and an aura of doubt regarding many aspects of themselves and their environment. An intuitive feeling exists within the client that a new and satisfying direction in life is taking place, along with the recognition that many specific aspects of this new direction have yet to be worked out. Thus the client enters a period of therapy that involves reevaluation of oneself and others, learning how to manage needs and feelings, and searching for meaningful interpersonal goals.

An important component of this process concerns a change in the way clients have habitually perceived other people. Their former style of expecting the worst of others and of classifying people in an "all-or-nothing" fashion now comes under serious question. Having found at least one person (the therapist) who does not fit preconceptions, the client begins to reconsider the nature of the social world. Part of this process may entail a review of prior relationships, with attempts to gain a deeper understanding of others' motivations, conflicts, good and bad characteristics, and so forth. Similarly, individuals with whom the client is currently interacting come under discussion, again with the aim of helping to develop a more flexible and multidimensional view of people. Ultimately the client comes to recognize that the former perceptual style played a defensive role in prematurely shutting others out and that now it is worth the risk and effort to gain a more realistic and deeper view of people.

Considerably more difficult and threatening are clients' attempts to evaluate the role of their own social patterns in relationships. Many clients "see" their behaviors (be they aggressive, withdrawn, detached, etc.) as merely reactions to the negative actions of others. They fail to recognize that in many instances their behaviors actually contribute to or (in some cases) are entirely responsible for deteriorating relationships. Recall in the case of Joey, for example, that his conduct with teachers was challenging and provocative. Teachers who may have been initially friendly and supportive were thereby put on guard and were very likely irritated—almost assuredly instituting a pattern of interaction that made the relationship progressively worse. With Joey, then, gaining an understanding of such patterns, particularly as they may be operating in current relationships, is an important component of the self-evaluation process. These kinds of insights, appropriate to the age and ability to understand of the client, seem to be essential ingredients for later attempts to change such ineffective behavior patterns.

During this phase of therapy, clients may also need guidance in managing their impulses and emotions. If indeed the breakthrough in the therapeutic relationship has, as it were, unlocked many long-dormant needs for affection and closeness, these needs may now get expressed in rather blatant or inappropriate fashion outside of therapy. In a sense, others in the client's world may not be ready for such expressions and may themselves become confused or defensive by the sudden change. Considering the vulnerability of clients at this stage in treatment, attempts to guard against these kinds of upsetting experiences are of considerable importance.

Discussions of emotional needs in therapy, however, serve an essential function: that of helping the client to start formulating both short- and long-term interpersonal goals. Questions arise concerning the types of relationships that would be satisfying to the client. How can they be achieved? Are these realistic expectations? What are the risks and pitfalls? As might be expected, an individual who has spent many years hiding behind a wall of alienation may be quite naive about the day-to-day give-and-take of close relationships. The client may harbor unrealistic or overly romanticized fantasies of friendship and intimacy. Or the client, still feeling vulnerable and unworthy, may see the future in pessimistic terms—proclaiming that the relationship they have found in therapy could never be replicated in their everyday lives. The therapeutic task, therefore, is to assist in the development of realistic goals, along with an appreciation of the interpersonal work involved to achieve them.

Implementing Goals and Current Adjustment

The next phase of treatment, implementing goals and current adjustment, has many of the same characteristics as those faced by parents (or older sisters and brothers) in helping young people in their search for a place in the world. A delicate and ever-changing balance is sought between giving protection, guidance, and support and encouraging independence and personal decision making. As the formerly alienated client takes the first tentative steps into new and meaningful relationships, considerable direction and encouragement may be needed. New realities are shared and discussed. Anxieties and temporary letdowns may be smoothed. Tendencies to withdraw or to use old defensive tactics can be pointed out. During these difficult times, an active and directive therapist can be of great help in initiating a new life-style. However, once the process is under way, and once the client begins to derive support and satisfaction from new relationships, the therapist begins to play less and less of an active role. New friends and intimates not only provide for the client's affectional needs, but they also offer corrective feedback when relationships start to go astray. A transition takes place wherein the spontaneous give-and-take of everyday relationships gradually replaces that provided by the therapist. In a sense, the chemistry of normal social exchange and emotional rapport with others continues to broaden the processes that were begun in therapy.

The Close of Therapy

To continue the family analogy cited in the previous section, relationship therapy does not have a well-defined end point. Rather, just as one's grown child (or younger sibling) continues to relate to family, even from afar, the socially maturing client may keep contact with the therapist. The knowledge that the emotional connection continues, though direct contact may be minimal, serves as a source of support for the client—sometimes for many years.

This model relationship, the one that served to reverse the pattern of alienation, remains as a cornerstone in the structure of the client's social life.

A summary of the phases and principal therapeutic tasks in relationship therapy is provided in Table 7.2.

Table 7.2
Phases of relationship therapy

Phase of therapy	Therapy tasks
Initial sessions	Getting a resistant, unmotivated, and suspicious client started in treatment
"Testing" of therapist	Preventing premature categorization of therapist by the client; maintaining commitment to client
Weakening of client's defenses	Managing escalating tests and heightened anxiety and hostility; encouraging and supporting the developing relationship
Emerging closeness with therapist and possible crisis	Providing emotional support; preventing dropping out of therapy; managing severe testing of therapist
Emotional commitment	Responding to client's attachment and dependency on therapist; assisting client in self-discovery and self-evaluation
Reevaluation and new goals	Actively attempting to change client's perceptions, expectations, and behaviors
Implementing goals	Encouraging and monitoring new relationships; gradually decreasing the intensity of the therapeutic relationship
Close of therapy	Further decreasing therapeutic contact; maintaining occasional communication

CHAPTER EIGHT

RELATIONSHIP THERAPY: TECHNIQUES AND CASE STUDY

TECHNIQUES OF RELATIONSHIP THERAPY

Technique may not be the proper word to use when discussing relationship therapy, for it implies something impersonal and artificial. These are the very characteristics that work against successful treatment. In the place of *technique* we should invoke a long list of interpersonal qualities that the therapist must possess in abundance—sensitivity, warmth, firmness, honesty, awareness of the client's plight, personal security, and patience, to name but a few. The key here is the ability to communicate these qualities to the client and to have them work in such a way that a therapeutic relationship can get started and nourished.

Successful treatment is also dependent on the therapist's awareness of what the client is going through at the various stages of therapy. As was seen in the previous chapter, the client's emotional status, for example, during the first few weeks of therapy may be radically different from that after the "break-through" has occurred. Thus the interpersonal skills and the emotional responsiveness required of the therapist must be finely tuned to the needs and defenses of the client as the treatment process unfolds.

Perhaps fundamental to the therapist's approach is the recognition that the obnoxious or unlikable surface characteristics often displayed by clients are merely defenses that they have erected to ward off a threatening environment. To be able to deal therapeutically with these defenses and at the same time not be repulsed by them may be the ultimate test of the successful relationship therapist.

General Characteristics

As implied earlier, therapy does not always take place in the formal confines of an office or on any rigidly set schedule of meetings. The nurturing of a relationship with a resistant, alienated client is tough enough without the added burdens of an artificial schedule or a sterile office. Reaching out to such clients therefore also means a willingness to have contact, within limits, in settings and at a pace that fosters the relationship and provides a degree of comfort and safety to the client. The possibilities are quite varied and are, of course, dependent on the age, sex, interests, and circumstances of the client.

We can again use the case examples in the previous chapter to illustrate this variety. Contact with the twelve-year-old Joey may be as varied as a simple walk to the corner drugstore for a soft drink, shooting baskets at a neighborhood schoolyard, going fishing, helping with school assignments, and so on—in effect, using whatever vehicles for establishing the relationship that are appropriate to the client. The middle-aged divorcee, with different needs and perspectives, may find the therapist's office a suitable setting much of the time. On occasion, however, shared experiences outside of the office, such as a shopping trip, going on a picnic with her children, or visiting an art gallery may also aid in establishing emotional contact. With the example of the schizoid client who had signed himself into the hospital, the choices may be more limited, but not totally restricted. Visits to the hospital canteen, a game of pool in the recreation room, going on patient excursions, and visiting potential jobs all represent activities that permit an opportunity to relate in a direct and concrete fashion.

The sex and age of the therapist also bears comment in these general considerations. Obviously, no hard and fast rule can be stated on these issues. The central factor again seems to be the potential compatibility between therapist and client in being able to initiate and foster a therapeutic relationship. Thus, commonality of interests, enjoyment of similar activities, and a reservoir of shared experiences are more important than sex or age per se.

The scheduling of therapeutic contacts is a matter of considerable delicacy and judgment on the part of the therapist. A number of contending forces are operating, particularly in the beginning of therapy, which makes these scheduling decisions especially important. From our earlier descriptions, it is likely that most clients, because of their defensive, alienated style, would prefer to minimize contact with the therapist. Hence, in the initial stages of treatment, the therapist may have to be reasonably assertive in setting up enough meetings and activities to ensure that she or he will have an impact on the client. At the same time the upper limit of the client's tolerance for what may be perceived as a disturbing intrusiveness needs to be appreciated. As therapy progresses this balance between sufficient contact to make a difference in clients' lives versus how much clients can tolerate will undoubtedly shift. Thus the therapist makes continual assessments regarding the frequency and intensity of meetings and adjusts the schedule to maximize the growth of the relationship.

Finally, considering the relationship aims of this type of treatment, there may be little of a proscribed agenda for therapy contacts. The discussion of particular topics, attempts to change certain patterns of behavior, or efforts to resolve conflicts within the client, while important, all take a second seat to the principal aim of therapy: that of nurturing and developing the relationship itself.

Procedures at the Beginning of Treatment

How on earth do you get a relationship started with an individual who is anxious, angry, mistrustful, and skilled at keeping people at a distance? The answer, quite simple, is that very frequently it is impossible. Many alienated individuals suffer through their entire lives alone, their detachment an impregnable fortress, their armor more than sufficient to drive the average intruder away. However, circumstances that make an intrusion possible and appropriate occasionally occur, and it is at these times that the relationship therapist may devote his or her skills and good will to a humane purpose. Let us investigate these circumstances with an eye toward the means of initiating a therapeutic relationship.

Three general classes of procedures are available during this crucial time of treatment: responding to client openings, managing clients' attempts to alienate the therapist, and defining the reasons for therapy. The first two refer to styles of interviewing that, although not necessarily dramatic, produce a gradual coming together of client and therapist, setting the stage for the development of a relationship. They are also procedures with enough generality so that they may be utilized in later stages of treatment as well. The third procedure, defining the reasons for therapy, is an attempt to negotiate an acceptable rationale that the client can employ to justify continuing in treatment. As will be seen, the therapist may not always be able to bargain for the best possible contract, but with a resistant client, some compromises have to be struck occasionally in order to keep the client in therapy.

Responding to openings In previous sections of our discussion, in order to convey an understanding of alienated patterns, the lines were perhaps drawn too starkly. For example, the impression may have been communicated that alienated individuals are constantly on guard against others and never let down defenses, admit to loneliness, or contemplate a better way of life. Such a total and rigid alienation may occur in only the most hardened individuals. A more realistic perspective portrays these clients as experiencing occasional lapses in their defenses and at times as being at least minimally responsive to interpersonal overtures from others. This was best exemplified in the case illustration of the divorced woman who sought therapy on her own because of a gnawing recognition that her current way of life left her empty and unfulfilled. Her active initiation of treatment and her quest for a more satisfying life-style provides the therapist with at least a toehold in beginning a relationship. Though subsequent stages of therapy may be filled with turmoil, this client has offered a slight opening upon which to build future contacts.

A first principle of initiating therapy, then, may be stated as follows: The therapist searches for, and remains sensitive to, any expressions (however slight) by the client that offer a reason for continuing the relationship.

- "I don't do much except hang around."

- "Sometimes I wish that my life was better."

- "I guess I need some help with my math homework, even though I hate it."

- "Don't know what the judge plans to do with me."

- "What do you think of that dumb-ass waitress wanting to marry me?"

These openings by clients, though elusive and brief, represent movement *toward* the therapist. To let them pass is a lost opportunity. To respond to them in an appropriate and genuine way keeps the interpersonal process going—makes the slight opening in the armor perhaps a little larger. Moreover, they are initiatives by the client and therefore hold the promise of fostering the relationship on a note that is immediate and meaningful to the client. They could, for example, be responded to with such statements as: "I'd be interested in talking to you about that," or "It looks like there are some things in your life you want to change. I'd like to help."

By remaining sensitive to such openings, and responding with interest and concern, the therapist may make small but progressive inroads into the client's life. Channels of communication are slowly opened, and if the client does not become too upset or anxious, a relationship gets started.

Managing hostility and distancing Despite the occasional openings provided by clients, most of their behavior at the beginning of treatment may be described as wary and defensive. Indeed, should they feel that the therapist is making inroads too quickly, the wariness may convert to open hostility, threat, or other measures to maintain distance from this intruder. Thus we may expect a degree of vacillation in the client's behaviors—an occasional, brief, and sometimes disguised lowering of defenses, followed by more open and persistent efforts to drive the therapist away.

A second principle in initiating treatment hence involves the therapist's recognition of and resistance to these distancing maneuvers. Remaining steadfast during such onslaughts and establishing more contact when openings occur communicates to the client that here may be a unique individual who does not readily retreat in the face of the client's pathology.

Several specific procedures are available for managing clients' hostility while at the same time maintaining or even strengthening the threads of a beginning relationship: reflection of feelings; defusing the emotions; and confrontive expressions of the therapist's reactions. *Reflection of feeling*, borrowed from Carl Rogers' client-centered therapy approach, refers to the sensitive tuning in on a client's emotional communication and then restating these emotions in an accepting, nonjudgmental fashion. This procedure, in essence, communicates the therapist's understanding of the client's current feeling state and an acceptance of its validity. In interpersonal terms it represents an affective movement toward the client, regardless of the emotion being expressed. For example:

Client: I don't know what I'm doing in a place like this. Ugh! A head doctor. This place gives me the creeps. You, you with your damned superior attitude and phony concern, you give me the creeps too.

Therapist: Yeah, I know. It is kind of a strange place to be. And I can see how I might come across to you with a holier-than-thou attitude, and not really caring. It is irritating when you see it that way.

The defusing of emotions may be used during periods of exceptional tension when both client and therapist suffer extreme discomfort or when the situation threatens to get out of hand. This procedure invites both participants to step back from the raw edge of intense emotions and gain some intellectual perspective (or even a lighthearted view) of the situation.

Client: Scum, yellow-bellied scum, that's what you are. How in hell's name can you ask me a question like that? [*Clenching fists*]. I'll wipe up the _____ floor with you.

Therapist: Whoa! Hold on! Let's not blow your cool. I asked if you were still living with your family, and you're ready to wipe me out. What's going on? Fill me in, will you? My Blue Cross isn't paid up.

Confronting techniques refer to direct expressions of the therapist's reaction to the client's hostile displays. They may vary in intensity and emotional content, but in essence, they provide direct and genuine feedback to clients concerning their impact on the therapist. As such, these procedures involve emotional movement toward the client, but they also may be perceived as threatening or argumentative. Some caution is therefore required in that escalation of defensiveness and hostility are occasionally elicited.

Client: I'm afraid you couldn't possibly understand the situation, my dear. So young. Inexperienced. I just can't understand how Dr. _____ recommended that I come here. Are you a student, or just what are you? I'll have you know. . . .

Therapist: Right now I'm feeling awfully put down. Aren't you being kind of overbearing with me?

Client: What? Over what? . . . I'll have you know that in my department I supervise fifteen girls, and not one of them has ever said anything like that to me, ever.

Therapist: I just said it. I said it because I felt it very strongly, and I want to be honest with you right from the start.

Client: Perhaps, my dear, we should discuss the difference between honesty and insult.

Therapist: Okay.

Defining the reasons for treatment Early in the therapy process it is important that client and therapist come to an understanding about the reasons for treatment. In a sense this understanding serves as an initial, unwritten agreement that provides a basis for their continued contact with each other. Sometimes this contract is direct and apropos, as for example with a client who seeks treatment because of felt loneliness and isolation. In this instance the agreement in general terms may be to explore the reasons for loneliness and to seek ways of overcoming a detached style of life. The purposes of therapy are explicit and mutually agreed upon.

With other clients, however, agreement on such directly relevant aims may not be possible. Unable to admit to problems in their lives, feeling uncommitted to any change, or simply engulfed in cynicism and anger, such clients may require an "interim contract"—one that is somewhat removed from long-range purposes of therapy but that nevertheless serves to keep the client in therapy. Take for example, Joey, the twelve-year-old who is coerced into treatment by the juvenile judge. His present psychological state does not permit expression of his needs for stability and security. Rather, he is tangled in a web of anger and suspicion, feeling caught between the judge's "punishments" of either entering treatment or being sent to a juvenile institution. Perhaps the only contract that is possible with him at the beginning of therapy is one that merely acknowledges the reality of his situation.

Therapist: Look, Joey, I know you're in a tough spot. The judge doesn't fool around. He's put it to you straight. Either you keep coming here to work with me, to see what we can work out to get things together for you, or he'll send you to _____. Maybe it doesn't look like much of a choice to you right now, but I'm willing to give it a try.

Client [*Angry stare*]: Shit!

Therapist: It maybe looks like a bum deal, but Joey, it's the only game in town.

Client: It's always the same. Somebody screwing me over. . . . Oh, what the hell, you can't be as bad as that other place.

The "agreement" reached with this client is clearly insufficient for the long-range purposes of treatment. The therapist is using what little leverage is available to keep the troubled child in contact. Embedded in the therapist's statements of the current realities, however, is an offer of a better way of life ("see what we can work out to get things together for you"). Though not a guarantee, and not met with enthusiasm by the client, perhaps such an appeal strikes a remote chord and hence also assists in Joey's decision to continue in therapy.

Managing the Testing Phase

As described in a previous section, the testing phase can be a harrowing time in treatment. It is almost as if therapy is proceeding at two levels: a surface discussion of such topics as everyday events, the client's history and current adjustment, future therapy activities, and so on; and at a deeper, largely unspoken level, evaluation and testing of the therapist by the client. It is clear that the latter is the critical process that requires careful management.

Recall that most clients enter therapy with the preconception that the therapist, just like everyone else, is untrustworthy and uncaring. The unresolved question for the client concerns which malevolent category best fits the therapist. Once able to so label the therapist, the client's expectations are confirmed and alienation can be maintained. Many of the client's behaviors are therefore designed to evaluate and test the therapist; moreover, these tests may escalate in intensity until there is indeed risk that the therapist will become so defensive that rejection does take place, thereby subverting the therapy.

Several management aspects of this difficult phase of treatment require comment. The first is the important aim of not allowing clients to classify the therapist into one of their limited categories. Instead, the therapeutic purpose here is to have clients begin to revise and expand their category systems—to make them more flexible, more fine tuned, and more appropriate for positive interpersonal encounters. In thus revising the clients' perceptual and cognitive framework several techniques may be utilized: *rational analysis, clarifying misconceptions*, and *interpretation*. Since the therapist's personality is also an important vehicle through which clients will learn to expand their perceptions of people, a great deal of honest and detailed *self-disclosure* is also required. By coming to appreciate the complexity and depth of the therapist, clients begin to question their rigid and limited view of people.

The second, interrelated aim during this phase is to manage the testing process, that is, to prevent it from escalating to levels where the relationship is threatened. The principal procedure here is the *setting of rational limits* on clients' behaviors early in treatment and enforcing these limits in a firm and consistent manner as therapy continues. Although not guaranteed to be effective, such a procedure will tend to keep the tests within reasonable bounds, not allowing them to spiral to outrageous levels.

It is unlikely that any one of these procedures alone will suffice for a successful opening of treatment. In combination, however, they help negotiate a critical phase of therapy and set the stage for a positive relationship that may emerge in later periods. For now, let us review some of the components of this complex group of treatment procedures.

Weakening rigid categories It is the third therapy session with Ms. W, the middle-aged, divorced client. She has been talking in quite a bit of detail about her former husband's infidelity and his dishonesty in hiding it from her for so long. She concludes one portion of her lament with the following:

> **Client:** . . . So it proves one thing I've always suspected. People are cheap, self-centered. They're always watching out for themselves. Maybe it's out of weakness, or for some, it's just plain malicious, selfishness, but in the end, they don't give a damn about you. I finally opened my eyes, and maybe that's why I've been pretty successful in business. I worked myself up to a supervisor position, and I did it by not trusting anyone. It's a dog-eat-dog world—in business, in marriage, in everything. . . .

Using the combination of tactics cited earlier (rational analysis, clarifying misconceptions, interpretation, and self-disclosure) the therapist attempts to raise doubts about this all-encompassing negative view of the world. No single exchange is likely to produce dramatic changes, but consistent efforts, over time, may eventually loosen the client's rigidities.

> **Therapist:** That seems like a pretty extreme point of view. Do you really believe all people are like that?
>
> **Client:** Oh, some can put on a good act, for a while. My husband did. But don't let it fool you. They're all for number one, underneath it all.
>
> **Therapist:** I guess I've got my share of suspicions about people too. I've had some disappointments and heartaches, but I can't believe that it's that way with all people, all of the time. Have you always seen things this way?
>
> **Client:** Well, er, no. I, I just came to my senses when my husband left. Before that, I, it was, I, I . . . You have the damnedest way of asking questions. I'm not sure if you're a nasty person—or just a very shrewd one.
>
> **Therapist** [*Laughs*]: Neither. I want to be a friend. But not one who'll just say yes to all your pronouncements. Some of them are pretty extreme, you know. I just feel that you've really closed yourself off from people, and you expect the worst from them. It's understandable in a way. I know you've been terribly hurt, but being this pulled back, you seem to see everybody on just one dimension.

Client [*Sarcastic*]: Lovely, sweet words, my dear. Very touching, coming from someone so young and inexperienced.

Therapist: Hm! . . . When you put someone down, you know, it really hurts. I guess I sounded trite just then, but I really meant it, about the way you see things and about being a friend.

Although the therapist is not apparently producing any remarkable changes here, she is firmly and logically raising questions about the client's perceptual style. In addition, she injects some aspects of her own views and emotions while attempting to build the relationship. Even when the client becomes defensive and hostile, the therapist maintains her self-disclosing and friendly stance. Projecting this approach over many sessions, we can perhaps anticipate three processes of change within the client: (1) a gradual weakening of rigid perceptions as a result of the rational and interpretive analysis provided by the therapist; (2) a developing appreciation of the complexity and depth of the therapist's personality; and (3) a gradual acceptance of the therapist's offers of friendship and support.

Setting limits Imposing boundaries on clients' behaviors is especially important with cases where the possibility of "acting out" aggressively is suggested by background information. Setting such limits early in treatment, along with a specification of penalties should these limits be broken, thus reduces the possibility that the tests imposed on the therapist will escalate to extreme levels. Both participants are thereby protected. The client is not left in an ambiguous condition as to how far she or he can go in trying to prove the unworthiness of the therapist. At the same time, clients, frequently driven by anxiety and generalized anger, have some external restraints on behavioral patterns that they ordinarily may not be able to control. From the therapist's point of view, such limits protect them from behaviors that may indeed provoke rejection and "giving up" on the client—a reaction that brings effective treatment to an end.

The limits that are imposed will of course vary from case to case, depending on the type of client, his or her behavioral history, and the present circumstances. Common to all cases, however, are the essential features that the limits and penalties are fully explained early in treatment, that the rational basis for them is communicated, and that once imposed, they are enforced with regularity. For many clients such clear and predictable rules in a relationship may come as a welcome contrast to the chaotic and ever-shifting way of life in their background. The client also comes to understand that within these protective boundaries there is ample room to develop a free and wide-ranging relationship with the therapist.

The penalties that are invoked when the rules are broken also vary depending on client and setting. For example, with a client being seen at an inpatient facility, extra privileges (canteen, special recreational events, etc.)

may be temporarily reduced. With outpatients, where less control is possible, cancellation of a planned excursion, a shortening of some desired activity, and so forth, may also be invoked. Once clients have progressed in treatment to a point where they derive some positive affect and support from the relationship, the abrupt termination of a session when an offense occurs may serve as a reasonably strong penalty. Again, when a client, on occasion, goes beyond a predesignated limit, care is taken to explain the reasons for the penalty to be invoked, along with a reaffirmation of the solidity of the relationship.

Since we are considering here the control of extreme behaviors, some clients may also require clarification regarding legal penalties imposed by outside agencies. For example, a delinquent under probation by a juvenile court may make the false assumption that being in treatment somehow exempts her from judicial punishment. Thus this juvenile, motivated to see whether the therapist will go so far as to rescue her from the police, may engage in some illegal act and get caught. Under most circumstances such extreme tests obviously go beyond the control of the therapist, and the entire treatment process may be destroyed. To such clients, therefore, it is essential to explain the legal consequences of their behaviors and the restrictions imposed on the therapist in being able to protect them.

To illustrate the setting of limits let us return to the case of the schizoid client who signed himself into a psychiatric hospital. After several days on the ward, it was noted that he seemed drawn to the occupational therapy department, which provided training in carpentry and machine shop procedures. After several brief and casual conversations with the occupational therapist, the client expressed the wish that someday he might have a steady job that could provide good pay and security and said that gaining some technical skills might help him achieve this goal.

As part of the ward treatment team, the occupational therapist reported this "opening" to the team, and after review of the client's history it was decided to offer him the opportunity for a program of vocational training. An important component of this training program would be the development of a therapeutic relationship with the occupational therapist. It was recognized that this would not be an easy task in view of the client's unstable history, record of strife and fighting on previous jobs, and generally suspicious attitude toward supervisors and coworkers.

At the first formal meeting between client and therapist, a proposal for training on a daily basis was made, along with an offer of the therapist's guidance and friendship. As part of this meeting the limits were also communicated:

Client: Yeah, that sounds good. I know I've always had a thing with machines, but I never got a chance to use it.

Therapist: Well, I'm glad you'll be joining us. Six guys have been coming pretty regularly, and I think they're making real progress. It'll be good to have you coming into the group.

Client: Yeah. Okay. Can I start today?

Therapist: Yes you can. But I want to explain some things to you first. Now we both know that things have been rocky for you in the past — you've been fired from a lot of jobs and had lots of hassles with people, and you've even done some county time. Now all that tells me is that you've had some hard knocks, you've been kicked around some, and you've been fighting back. And I respect you for trying to get some things straight now. But with all that, there are some rules here that I want you to understand. There are just a few, but they are important.

Client: Oh, man! Here we go. . . . Let's have em.

Therapist: First of all, we've got a lot of equipment here. It's expensive, and the hospital can't replace it. And it's stuff that is helping a lot of guys. So we do a lot to take care of it, maintain it. Sometimes when you're learning and things don't go right, you get frustrated, and next thing you know, you're breaking one of the pieces. Don't do it. It'll mess up things for a lot of people. If it happens, I'll have to keep you out of the shop for at least a week.

Client: That's no problem [*Laughs*]. I won't tear up your place.

Therapist: Okay. The only other rule has to do with hassles in the shop. If you're not getting along with someone, or if you don't like the way I'm handling things, then I want you to talk to me about it. Straight out. Just let me know, and we'll try to work it out. But there's a firm rule about no physical stuff, no threats or intimidation of the others, no purposeful trying to mess up their work. Some of these fellows are pretty withdrawn and shook-up as it is, and it's important they get a chance to make a comeback without extra hassles. And with me, it's just not part of the job, and not my way, to fight things out, when things go wrong. We can talk, work it out that way, but any fighting, and you'd have to stay out of here again, for at least a week. We could still talk things over, but outside of the shop.

Client: No sweat on that one either.

Managing the Developing Relationship

As the client proceeds in therapy several concomitant processes that produce a complex array of new issues for the therapist take place. Formerly rigid preconceptions about people (and the therapist) are beginning to weaken, leaving the client feeling anxious and vulnerable. Contributing to the tension may be a resurgence of anger about past injustices as well as the surfacing of long-suppressed needs for care and security. Amidst this general loosening of defenses is a growing awareness that perhaps the therapist is someone with whom an emotional relationship can be formed, and we see the initial stages of a reaching out to the therapist. Taken together these many trends may produce sharp fluctuations in mood, reduced controls on impulses, and a generally volatile atmosphere in therapy.

Requirements for effective management of this phase are equally complex. Therapeutic procedures and perspectives will be discussed under several sub-headings, and although these procedures are described separately, the importance of a consistent and integrated approach should be emphasized. The individual procedures are a shift in perspective by the therapist, supportive techniques, and coping with personal emotions.

Shift in perspective We can summarize the therapist's overall approach in the opening phase of treatment as follows: offering friendship, firmly keeping clients' behaviors within reasonable bounds, and rather directly challenging clients' defenses (ways of categorizing and warding off people). In the present phase we begin to see the fruits of these efforts. Clients are indeed "opening up," are less sure of their attitudes about people, and are more responsive to inner needs and feelings. As with anyone who is tentatively giving up a particular way of life and embarking into new psychological territory, clients may become anxious and confused during this period of treatment. The therapist's approach shifts to meet these new issues.

Fundamental to these changes is the therapist's recognition of the fact that the client is entering a vulnerable time of therapy. A client, for example, who has been surly and withdrawn during the first six weeks of treatment may not display any dramatic changes in these characteristics. However, increased signs of tension, vague expressions of confusion, or disguised hints that new emotions are emerging provide clues to the therapist that processes of change are taking place. Sensitivity to such signs of weakening defenses dictates a rebalancing of the therapist's approach in the following areas:

1. The therapist increases expressions of personal friendship, understanding, and rapport. In earlier phases of treatment such feelings were, of course, also expressed, but usually in milder, less intrusive form. In the present period of therapy these invitations to a relationship are put forth in stronger terms and thereby represent a major source of interpersonal support for the vulnerable client.

2. Direct challenges to the client's defenses are curtailed and are replaced by more subtle encouragement of the changes taking place within the client. In a sense, the therapist has already prompted a process in which clients themselves are beginning to question their alienation mechanisms; now, the task is merely to keep that process going.

3. Firm limits on the client's behaviors are maintained. As indicated earlier, the weakening of defenses may produce tendencies to act out extreme behaviors impulsively. The affirmation of the behavioral rules that have been in force in the relationship hence provides some external restraints that aid the client in controlling these impulses.

Continuing with the case of the hospitalized client, the following excerpts illustrate the occupational therapist's approach one month after the start of treatment.

Client [*Angry*]: You know, you've been bugging me to hell the last couple of weeks. Look at things this way. Don't look at things that way. Don't do this; don't do that. Get the _____ off my back. What is it you really want from me?

Therapist: I know it's been a hell of a time for you, but you've been doing really well. I give you a lot of credit for hanging in there.

Client: You keep giving me all this hogwash about improvement, but all I can see is my mind getting _____ up. . . . And what do you get out of it? You get extra points or something? Or do you get your kicks by getting someone under your power? Sometimes I could just punch you out.

Therapist: Well, remember the rules. Nothing physical, but as far as talking goes, the sky's the limit. You still don't trust me, do you? . . . The kicks I get are seeing you getting yourself straightened out. And I, er, I get good feelings from, that we're becoming friends.

Client [*Tense, nervous*]: Damn! You say that. But I don't know. I don't believe you. I never had a _____ real friend in my life. I don't know. You've got to want something more.

Therapist: Like what?

Client: I don't know. . . . Shit! . . . Maybe you're another _____ queer, or something [*Angry, agitated*].

Therapist: Come off it, will you. You've had some bad experiences as a kid, and in the army, but don't go around seeing queers around every doorway.

Client: I don't know. I'm all _____ up.

Therapist: Come on, lighten up a little. Don't get all tense and everything. You've been doing real well, in the shop and all. I'll try to lighten up too. Let's go get a cup of coffee.

Supportive techniques In Chapter 5 procedures for helping clients in crisis were reviewed. These techniques may be called upon, in a temporary way, during this phase of relationship therapy as well. Recall that one of the circumstances under which supportive therapy was indicated involved the sudden breakdown of psychological defenses and the consequent eruption of frightening and overwhelming emotions. Such debilitating conditions could occur in relationship therapy when, for example, clients' alienation defenses are too rapidly dispelled. The anguish of past tragedies and unfulfilled needs suddenly are confronted. The impact may produce crisis conditions, with the attendant risks of panic, severe depression, uncontrolled rage, illogical thought processes, and so forth.

Therefore, during the phase of relationship therapy when clients' defenses are weakening, it is important that the therapist carefully monitor the degree to which crisis conditions are being approached. While it is true that most clients will inevitably go through a phase involving heightened tension and emotionality as their patterns of alienation are disrupted, for some the transition may be too severe. At these times the therapist shifts to such supportive techniques as relaxation procedures, active and directive guidance, focusing on factual, realistic aspects of the situation, deemphasizing discussion of emotions and fantasies, and instituting controls on impulsive acting out. (See Chapter 5 for a more complete discussion of these techniques.) Once such temporary crises subside, the therapist returns to the central task—that of encouraging and nurturing the developing relationship.

Coping with personal emotions Almost paradoxically, the period in treatment when a relationship is beginning to form is also a time when tests of the therapist may escalate. It is as if clients need to be sure of the safety and genuineness of the relationship before a full emotional commitment is allowed. If rejection or exploitation is going to occur, the client seems to say, let it happen now, rather than later when it could really hurt. This testing also occurs at a time in treatment when the client has had opportunity to gain knowledge of the therapist's weaknesses, areas of sensitivity, and so forth, so that frequently the challenges that are imposed strike hard at personal vulnerabilities. Therefore therapists must be prepared to manage these tests in a nondefensive, nonpunitive manner. At the same time, such tests may be recognized as representing clients' anxieties and needs for reassurance and as preludes to a deeper relationship.

Several techniques may be utilized to negotiate such testing episodes: (1) open acknowledgement of the emotional impact of the client's behavior, thereby providing feedback to the client of the effects of her or his behavior on others; (2) frank disclosure of personal vulnerabilities and their roots, hence keeping the relationship open and honest; (3) encouragement of self-exploration by the client as to the motivations for the provocative behavior; (4) mild interpretation of the client's emotional and motivational state; (5) continued enforcement of the predesignated limits on the client's behavior.

Several such tests occurred in the treatment of the divorced woman described earlier, and they provoked some strong reactions in the therapist. During the third week of therapy, the following exchange occurred:

> **Client:** Have you read _____'s new book on emotional adjustment to divorce?
>
> **Therapist:** No. I've heard of it, but I haven't had a chance to read it.

Client: Oh. I see. . . . Well, in it she discusses the importance of ventilation and catharsis in getting rid of pent-up feelings about the divorce.

Therapist [*Somewhat sarcastic*]: That's interesting. What else does she say?

Client: Maybe since you're supposed to be the expert you can read it for yourself, and then tell me. And then maybe you can also tell me why we haven't tried that here.

Therapist [*Suppressed anger*]: I've tried the proper things with you, believe me. I've even . . .

Client [*Interrupting*]: Tell me. Where did you get your degree?

Therapist: I received my masters at _____ University. I told you that when we first met.

Client: Oh yes, I'd forgotten. And how long ago was that?

Therapist: Last year, in June. . . . And I had a six-week postgraduate workshop in marital counseling with Dr. _____.

Client: Yes, of course.

Therapist: Well, I see that our time is almost up for today. I'll look forward to seeing you on Thursday.

This excerpt reveals a therapist caught off guard, who is defensive, petulant, and obviously eager to finish the session. An area of vulnerability has been touched upon, and the client presses her advantage. The nontherapeutic handling of this episode raises further questions for the client about the possibility of forming a meaningful relationship with the therapist. Toward the end of their next meeting, the same theme is introduced by the client in stronger terms. The tests are escalating.

Client: Oh, by the way. You can expect a word or two from the clinic director. I sent her a letter requesting a change of counselor.

Therapist: You what?

Client: I just don't think you're experienced enough or old enough to handle my case.

Therapist: Damn! I thought we had an agreement to talk over any problems between ourselves.

Client: Well, I suppose we did, but we never seem to get anywhere, so I thought it best to go right to the top.

Therapist [*Angry*]: You've been an absolute horror, ever since we first met. Holier than thou. Prim and proper, but underneath it all, a nasty, mean person. . . . Well, who needs it. . . . I feel sorry for the next one who gets you.

Client: You mean you don't want to work with me anymore?

Therapist: That's exactly correct. I've had it.

Client: Hm. Just as I thought.

Contrast this unsuccessful management of a client's testing with that which occurred between the hospitalized patient and the occupational therapist. This incident took place during the fifth week of treatment.

Client: Where the hell you been all morning? I been working on this band saw, and I can't get the _____ cut right.

Therapist: I had to spend some time with Hansen. He's been having a bad time. We took a walk.

Client: For the whole _____ morning? First it's that other freaky guy. Now it's Hansen. I don't count for shit around here. Just like it's always been.

Therapist: Hey, man, that's not right. You count a lot with me.

Client [*Getting angrier*]: Bullshit! Words! Bullshit! [*Screaming*]. Why the hell are you staring at me? You're always staring.

Therapist: I'm not trying to stare, but you're so worked up and angry, I'm startled and upset.

Client [*Screaming*]: Upset, huh? I'll show you upset [*Picks up a piece of wood and menaces the therapist*].

Therapist: Now listen. Put down the stick. You're shook some right now, and so am I. I don't want a knot on my head, and you don't want all the hassle that will go with it. . . . Come on. Spill it. Something's eating at you. What is it? It's something with you and me.

Client [*Lowers the wood*]: I don't know. I need to take a walk, cool down.

Therapist: Take a walk?

Client: Yeah. Walk around. Get my head straight. . . . Like you did with Hansen.

Therapist: I'd like to go with you. Maybe when you cool down a little, we can get to the bottom of it. Is that okay?

Client: Yeah, I guess so.

Therapist: I'm sure doing a lot of walking today.

Managing the Emotional Commitment

As described earlier, the transition from the period of weakening defenses and testing of the therapist to that of an emotional commitment to the relationship may be dramatic. Having lowered the barrier of alienation clients now seem to depend on the newfound rapport and also have to contend with a surge of previously suppressed emotions. Feelings of affection, dependency, self-doubt, and heightened vulnerability seem to be the principal emotions that now come to the fore.

The task facing the therapist during this transitional period of treatment is quite directly to respond to this emotional commitment with warmth, sincerity, and support. Since this is a time in therapy when clients have made a first, major step in extending positive feelings toward someone else it would be premature to do more than simply reciprocate and solidify the relationship. The responsiveness required of the therapist may be taxing in that, previous to this phase, he or she had to deal firmly with challenging and conflicting behavior by the client. Now the therapist is faced with many tender and vulnerable feelings that call for sensitivity and a lighter touch.

In specific terms, the therapist often finds it appropriate to increase the frequency or length of sessions, to offer praise and encouragement of the client's new sense of attachment, and to provide support in the face of self-doubts and anxiety. Since this is the period of therapy that, in a sense, represents the first major impact of a "corrective emotional experience" for the client, it is incumbent on the therapist to make it as positive and rewarding as possible.

The emotional changes taking place also raise many new questions for the client, and these questions are frequently posed in rapid order to the therapist. Many of them may be merely informational, and as such may be answered factually and directly. Others, however, represent deeper personality conflicts, ambiguities about long-range goals, or ethical-philosophical questions—all of which defy easy answer. For issues of this complexity, therapists should obviously resist the temptation to give casual or trite answers. More appropriate here are open acknowledgements of the importance and depth of such questions, and the assignment of them to an informal agenda for future exploration and discussion.

Finally, during this period of sometimes intense client dependency and vulnerability, limits of a different sort from those imposed earlier need to be considered. On occasion, a client, prompted by a surge of strong emotional needs, will explicitly or covertly pressure the therapist to react in ways that go beyond therapeutic or ethical bounds. For example, demands to usurp all of the therapist's time, to become involved in new living arrangements, or to engage in sexual contacts all have to be met with firm, but understanding, refusals.

Techniques for Reevaluation and Goal Setting

As an outgrowth of the emotional breakthrough with the therapist, clients can now entertain the possibility of far-reaching changes in their interpersonal lives. However, a number of important tasks are faced before such a transition can be fully accomplished. Clients are motivationally ready to change old ways of perceiving, categorizing, and behaving, but now they have to learn new and more appropriate ways of reacting to others. In addition, there may remain many areas of self-doubt and anxiety that could inhibit new learning; hence, some resolution of this inner turmoil is required. Finally, although clients may have acquired a general sense of optimism about the future, the development of specific social goals helps to define the direction of further therapeutic work.

Two general classes of therapy techniques are utilized during this phase of treatment: (1) methods that prompt self-exploration and insight and (2) active guidance and social learning procedures.

Exploratory techniques Some degree of self-analysis seems to be requested by clients themselves during this period. Unresolved questions concerning why they were rejected and abused earlier in life call for answers. Similarly, confusion about what sort of impact they have had on others prompts clients to evaluate their own behavior patterns. In addition, clients are likely to be concerned about an uncertain future and may seek answers in this realm. Thus, during this phase of treatment, the therapist may not have to urge such exploratory activity; rather, it is a matter of flowing with the naturally occurring questions that arise and aiding in the process. In this sense, insight techniques that can be described as "mild" are used. These procedures are generally nonconfrontive and noninterpretive. To the contrary, they are relatively nondirective, merely supporting and encouraging clients' efforts to untangle the past and their own emotional reactions. The following techniques are useful during this period.

1. Nondirective leads—verbalizations that urge the client to continue on a line of exploration already in progress. For example: "You seem to be on to something important. Can you tell me more about it?"

2. Open-ended questions—somewhat more directive invitations to explore a particular issue. For example: "You seem unsure about why you did that. What were you feeling at the time?"

3. Reflection of feelings—restatement of emotions communicated by the client. For example: "If I sense what you're saying, you were kind of relieved when she didn't show up.

4. Response to nonverbal cues—comments on information communicated by body language or facial expressions. For example: "I couldn't help but notice that you were wringing your hands pretty hard when you were talking about that incident in the restaurant, even though it seemed to be a happy one. Is there more there than we've spoken about?

5. Exploration of long-term patterns—descriptions of similarities of response across different situations. For example: "You got a kick out of bugging that teacher. Kept her on her guard, as you say. Kind of reminds me how you made me feel when we first met."

6. Encouragement of summary analyses—requests for the client to integrate material into a meaningful pattern. This procedure is usually deferred until the latter stages of self-exploration. For example: "We've talked about lots of different times when people made you nervous and upset. Do you have a usual way that you react to these situations?"

7. Analysis of daydreams or nocturnal dreams and ruminations about emotional needs—invitations to the client to report and analyze emerging motivational and need systems, as reflected in fantasy productions. Special emphasis is placed on those that may reflect hopes and goals for the future. For example: "From the way you describe it you've really been dreaming about being the football hero in junior high, getting congratulations from the team, being a part of the group, and all that. What do you think those dreams are telling you about yourself?"

Guidance and social learning procedures As clients explore the past and gain some perspectives on its debilitating effects on their behaviors, perceptual style, and emotions, they become prepared for some new approaches to people. For many clients whose alienation problems have been chronic, this change leaves them facing a void. They have known no other way of life, and as such they may require considerable guidance in learning to relate. For others, whose detachment and withdrawal are of more recent origin, the therapeutic task is to rekindle earlier, more positive modes of social behavior. In either case, active efforts to establish more satisfying interpersonal skills in three interrelated areas are usually required: expansion and increased flexibility in the perceptual categories through which people are viewed and classified; replacement of obnoxious and defensive interpersonal behaviors with more personable and open reactions; learning to manage and express personal needs in appropriate ways.

The focal point for much of this learning is, of course, the therapy relationship itself. The client has progressed from the early stages of treatment, where the alienation problems were fully displayed in the relationship; hence, he or she is in a position to concretely review many of the distortions, false expectations, and inappropriate behaviors that occurred. In addition, having now developed emotional rapport with the therapist, newly emerging perceptions and behaviors can be strengthened and elaborated. Within the relative safety of therapy, entirely new skills can also be developed through modeling, practice, and active role playing. Consider the following excerpt during the fourth month of therapy with Joey.

Client: I don't know, . . . I guess I really do want to try out for the team.

Therapist: Yeah?

Client: But, well, I've only been in the school a couple of months, and I know the coach will say no.

Therapist: Why is that?

Client: I don't know. I just know he will.

Therapist: You remember when we first met? What did you expect from me?

Client [*Laughs*]: I figured you were going to be the meanest, ugliest guy in town. . . . Yeah, I didn't give you much of a break, did I? . . . You figure I'm thinking the same way now?

Therapist: Well if there's no real reason why he should say no, aren't you?

Client: I guess I am. He don't know me, so why should he say no right off the bat?

Therapist: Okay, let's take it a step further. Here's a junior high football coach. He's also a gym teacher, so he does this in the afternoons, after work. Now, tell me, what are some of the things that *might* be going through his mind when a new guy comes up to him about joining the team?

Client: I don't know. That's hard to figure.

Therapist: Try it. Let your imagination go, and see what you come up with.

Client: Well, let's see, maybe the school forces him to do it, but he really hates it. . . . Another player would just be a pain.

Therapist: Yeah, I guess that's possible. What else?

Client: Maybe he's got the team already set, and there's no more room.

Therapist: Okay.

Client: Maybe he's some kind of football nut, and he's looking for a superstar to make his season [*Laughs*]. He'll take one look at me and send me home.

Therapist: Could be. What else?

Client: I don't know. . . . That's all I can think of.

Therapist: How about just an average guy, who enjoys football and enjoys working with kids. Someone who might say for you to come on and join the group.

Client: I just never thought of that, until you said it.

Therapist: That's been part of the problem. You still kind of expect the worst from people, instead of thinking about all the possibilities.

Client: Same as when I started with you. . . . Yeah, I've got to give him more of a break.

Later in the same session, the following conversation takes place:

Client: You know, I'm scared to admit it, but . . . I don't know how to ask him. . . . I never ask people for anything.

Therapist: After our talks, you pretty much know where that comes from, don't you?

Client: Yeah, I know . . . but that doesn't help in talking to this guy.

Therapist: I don't know if you realize it or not, but for the last couple of weeks you've been talking real good with me . . . open, natural, right on, with some complicated stuff.

Client: Yeah, I know. But that's with you. I don't know this coach. No telling how it will come out with him.

Therapist: Well, I've got confidence in you. But if you want to practice some, why don't we give it a try right here? I'll be the coach, you be you, and we'll give it a few run throughs. I'll help you to smooth it out if you need it.

Managing the Implementation of Goals and Termination

At this period in the treatment process clients begin to broaden their interpersonal horizons. Emotions that heretofore have been focused largely on the therapist also seek expression outside of therapy. New relationships are developed and old ones are restored as the client attempts to fulfill interpersonal goals. These goals may be relatively simple and immediate, as in the example of Joey wanting to be a member of a school team, or they may be well-formulated changes in life-style, as for example, the divorced female client planning to seek a new romantic partner. Management of this phase involves assisting the client in making a smooth transition into new relationships and then receding into the background of the client's life as successes are encountered outside of therapy.

The initial portions of this phase frequently require active and directive tactics by the therapist. Understandable reserve and hesitancy about forming relationships may be countered by encouragement and modest pressure. Advice on how to handle novel situations and how to cope with new feelings may serve as temporary props for the client. Dicussion and analysis of other people's behaviors and motives continue the improvement in clients' sensitivities and judgmental abilities. Therapy sessions are also used to provide corrective feedback when clients' behaviors or perceptions show signs of regressing to former, inappropriate styles. Finally, during this implementation phase, the therapist prepares the client for the possibility of future interpersonal disappointments and hurt. It is obvious that not all new relationships are going to succeed for the client, and it is also possible that exploitive or rejecting individuals will be encountered. Advanced preparation for such unfortunate encounters may reduce the possibility of a return to alienated patterns.

Involvements in new relationships produce a natural decline in dependency on the therapist, and as these become established, further changes in therapeutic approach are appropriate. Progressive reduction in the frequency of contact, less active and directive methods, and a general relaxation of emotional intensity in therapy are the most notable alterations. The therapist slowly fades out of the picture, remaining available if needed, but in effect gradually becoming an important and warm memory in the client's life.

Summary of Treatment

The complexity of relationship therapy should not be underestimated. As is obvious from the previous sections, merely being a "good friend" is insufficient to accomplish treatment goals. Multiple tasks are faced, each dependent on the emotional status of the client at that particular stage of therapy, and the therapist must be prepared to change techniques and perspectives as these transitions occur. As stated in the last chapter, these stages may not always follow one another in an orderly fashion; thus the therapist must necessarily remain acutely sensitive to changes in the client. A summary of the various phases that clients may go through, along with the principal therapy strategies, is summarized in Table 8.1.

CASE ILLUSTRATION

To aid in summarizing this material, a review of the treatment of Joey, the twelve-year-old juvenile described earlier, will be provided. Although we have seen excerpts from later periods in therapy, in this illustration we will return to the start of therapy. Recall that Joey had been referred by the court, and had been given the option of participating in therapy or being sent to a juvenile facility. In an earlier excerpt, the therapist initiated treatment with this resistant client by posing the realities of the current situation openly and directly: taking part in treatment or being sent away by the judge ("It maybe looks like a bum deal, but Joey, it's the only game in town."). Joey angrily and grudgingly accepted this alternative.

In reviewing Joey's history, the intake staff made note of several features: chronic inconsistencies in affection and discipline; eventual abandonment by both parents; a long-term pattern of aggressive, rebellious behavior in school; a chronic history of social isolation from both adults and agemates; and most recently, attempting to run away from an intolerable situation (his uncle).

Table 8.1
Summary of stages of relationship therapy

Phase of therapy	Client characteristics	Therapist's approach
Initial sessions	Suspicious, expecting rejection, detached, angry	Responding to occasional "openings"; clarifying realities of client's situation; defining reasons for therapy
Alienation and testing	Seeking evidence to classify therapist in malevolent category; increases in provocative behaviors; suspicious, detached, angry	Setting firm limits; controlling of personal emotions; rationally and openly confronting responses to tests; defusing intense emotions; challenging defenses
Weakening of defenses and emerging closeness	Escalation of tests; heightened emotionality; anxiety and confusion; initial questioning of own perceptual style and self-concept	Increasing expressions of friendship and rapport; confrontive techniques replaced by encouragement to relax defenses; occasional supportive techniques
Emotional commitment	Reduction in provocative behaviors; initial change in perceptual style; change in relationship to closeness, dependency; anxiety, self-concept problems	Reciprocated emotions, support, and establishing new limits
Reevaluation and discovery of new goals	Quest to analyze life — background, impact on others, identity, continued change in perceptual style and behavior, search for new directions	Mild exploratory techniques; active guidance in changing perceptions, behaviors, and attitudes
Implementing goals	Seeking new relationships; attempting new behaviors	Encouragement, support, corrective feedback, refining new behaviors
Termination	Natural relationships outside therapy provide rewards, corrective feedback, and need satisfaction	Gradual fade out

Relationship therapy was the recommended form of treatment, with the expectation of a reasonably optimistic prognosis in view of Joey's age. Several areas of risk were also noted: difficulties in managing his aggressiveness; the possibility of running away if stress approached severe levels; and the likelihood that he would initially be an uncooperative client.

A young male therapist who had considerable experience with adolescents and delinquents was chosen to work with Joey. It was hoped that his relative youth and street-wise background would aid in establishing rapport and eventually a firm relationship with the client. A tentative schedule was proposed involving two afternoon meetings a week, along with having Joey attend a general recreational and sports program on Saturday mornings, which the therapist supervised.

The intake staff also recommended the following: (1) that early in treatment firm limits be placed on Joey's potential for physical aggression and destructiveness; (2) that the penalties for breaking these rules be a curtailment of recreational activities and cancellation of planned outings with the therapist; (3) that the client understand that failures to attend would have to be reported to the juvenile court; (4) that regular contact be established with Joey's foster parents and school; (5) that biweekly summaries of therapeutic progress be forwarded to the juvenile court; and (6) that the client be made aware of these arrangements.

The first two afternoon meetings, which involved lengthy walks through a nearby park and a refreshment stop at a soda fountain, produced somewhat of a surprise for the therapist. Although Joey was largely uncommunicative, his behavior was reasonably polite and formal. The expected signs of surliness and anger were not apparent. The therapist speculatd in his progress notes that perhaps the client had decided to "play the game" and at least "go through the motions" of therapy for the time being.

Toward the end of the second meeting Joey casually asked the therapist if he would "lend him" two dollars for carfare. The therapist again speculated that this was an initial test through which he was being evaluated. Handing over the money too eagerly might be interpreted as a sign of an "easy mark"; a curt refusal might be interpreted as a sign of an "uptight," unsympathetic person. The therapist decided to handle this incident by explaining to Joey that he could not ordinarily give money because of his rather restricted budget. But since they were becoming friends, he would be willing to share what he could with Joey when the need arose. Of the three dollars he had in his wallet, he "loaned" Joey one dollar.

Joey continued his generally reserved demeanor for the next two weeks. Talk was restricted to nonpersonal topics—the latest baseball standings, the relative merits of different brands of cars, and so forth. During the Saturday morning sessions, he remained apart from the group activities and refused invitations from the others to participate. His "tests" of the therapist continued with relatively minor incidents: requesting to leave early at one meeting because he was "bored"; accusing the therapist of favoritism in his umpiring of a Saturday morning game; relating that he had cut a math class at school.

At the third Saturday morning meeting, Joey became involved in a game with a group of younger children. During this activity he became verbally abusive and threatening to a nine-year-old boy, to the point where the therapist had to intervene. A small crowd of youngsters were gathered around, and the therapist asked Joey to accompany him to a more private sector of the field. Joey refused, and the following exchange took place:

Client: No, man. I won't go. I've got just as much right here as them.

Therapist: That's right. But things need to cool down. Come on with me. Let's talk.

Client: Shit, man. I told you no. I'm not going to let this little runt get away with cheating. . . . Who are you anyway to tell me what to do.

Therapist: Wait a minute, I'm not finished. Playing over here makes me think you're a little scared of the older group. That's okay for now, but that doesn't give you the right to take it out on kids half your size.

Client: Oh, shoot. I'm not taking anything out on anybody.

Therapist: There's more. I don't try to be bossy around here, and I guess I don't appreciate your trying to make it out that I am [*Chuckles slightly*]. Makes me look bad. Ruins my image with the rest.

Client: Aw, what the hell, I wasn't enjoying this anyway. Let's go.

Joey and the therapist walk away.

Client: I guess that does it with us, huh?

Therapist: What do you mean? We're just getting started [*Laughs*]. You don't get rid of me that easy.

Client: Man, I can't figure you out. I really put it to you back there, and all you do is laugh and say we're just getting started. Where you coming from anyway?

Therapist: That's one of the good things about getting to know each other. You can't always go by first impressions, either way. We've got a lot to find out—some good, some bad—about each other. . . . I think we're on our way. What do you say?

Client: Yeah, . . . I don't know. . . . Do you really think I'm chicken with the older guys?

At the next meeting, Joey was somewhat less reserved than usual, and he asked if they could attend a professional baseball game that was scheduled for an evening later in the week. The therapist was pleasantly surprised when Joey volunteered to pay for his own ticket. During the game the following excerpt occurred:

Client: Those umpires, they're something else.

Therapist: How do you mean?

Client: I mean they could make you or break you. What they say is *it*. I mean you can yell all you want, but they got the power.

Therapist: Yeah. I guess you're right.

Client: I mean they're just like everybody who got power. It's not fair.

Therapist: You're getting into some deep ideas. That's interesting. Where are you going with it?

Client: I'm not sure. I just know I hate them, so high and mighty. Big man. . . . Shit. . . . They're all the same. Nobody who got power is ever going to give you an even break.

Therapist: What if I were to tell you that the one behind the plate is just a sad old man—a widower who lost his wife two years ago to cancer. He's just trying to make it from day to day. . . . And the guy calling plays behind first is a pretty well-known musician—jazz piano. Real cool. Loose guy. The only power he's interested in is on the keyboard.

Client: Is that right? You putting me on?

Therapist: No, I read the sports a lot. Keep up with it, you know. They had a column last month about their private lives.

Client: That's funny. I didn't even figure they had private lives. . . . Hey, look at that cracker. He's stealing second.

Therapist: Having a good time?

Client: Yeah, It's great.

The therapist's progress notes indicate that over the next three weeks, Joey's behavior in therapy became erratic. Often moody and withdrawn, he spent several afternoons barely acknowledging the therapist's presence. At other times, he appeared to be exceptionally anxious and tense but could not identify the source of these emotions. Apart from these vague feelings of dread, he also talked about many specific conflicts at school, for example, his detestation of math and his confusion as to how to react to the math teacher's offer of extra help. Throughout this period the therapist maintained a close, supportive role, with few attempts to probe or challenge the client's behaviors. Arrangements for several special outings were made, along with an increase in the length of each contact.

Late on a Monday night, approximately a month after this moody period had begun, the therapist received a phone call from a police sargeant in a city about eighty miles away. Joey was in custody, having been found wandering and disheveled in the bus terminal of that city. After much hesitation, he had given the therapist's name to the police. No charges were pending, but the officers were concerned that this runaway be properly supervised.

The therapist drove to the neighboring city to pick up the client, and on the return trip the following conversation took place:

Client [*Nervous and withdrawn*]: What are you thinking?

Therapist: I'm not sure what to think. What happened?

Client: Aw, I don't know. . . . What's the use. . . . It's all a pile of crap.

Therapist: You really seem down. Feel like talking?

Client: No.

Therapist: Come on, give it a try.

Client: Christ! You don't give up, do you [*Angry*]. I stole some money, all right? I lifted it and just took off.

Therapist: What the hell!

Client: I knew you'd be upset.

Therapist: Damn right I'm upset. Tell me about it. What happened?

Client: I took about fifty bucks from the people I'm staying with. It was right there—in the bureau drawer. I just picked it up and hopped a bus.

Therapist: Why did you do it? They been bugging you, or something?

Client: No. They're okay, man. . . . I don't know why I did. . . . I just been all tensed up and everything. Needed to get away.

Therapist: From them?

Client: No.

Therapist: From school?

Client: No.

Therapist: From me?

Client [*Long pause*]: What are you going to do with me now? Turn me over to the judge? Send me away?

Therapist: What do you think I should do?

Client: If you had any sense, you'd kick me in the ass and send me back to the judge. . . . That's what my old man would have done. That's what my uncle did [*Starts to weep*].

Therapist: Joey, I don't want to do that. . . . I love you . . . like a son, or a kid brother, or whatever the hell you are. I don't want to lose you . . . into that jungle.

Client [*Crying*]: Oh, Jesus. Do you really mean that? You're not just saying that?

Therapist: No, I mean it. I was hoping you could feel the same way.

Client: I do.

For the next several weeks, Joey was at the clinic almost every afternoon. When the therapist had other appointments, he would wait patiently, reading or doing schoolwork. At their regular meetings, he was alternately cheerful and serious but obviously felt close to the therapist. He maintained a constant barrage of questions and was very insistent about obtaining answers. The questions covered many issues that apparently had been plaguing him for some time, such as the reasons for his father's abandonment of him, why most of his teachers seemed to hate him, if the therapist really considered him a coward, if masturbation makes one insane, and if he could ever be a successful person like the therapist.

Toward the end of this period, Joey obtained a part-time job so that he could begin restitution to his foster parents. It was with considerable pride that he could now also offer to treat the therapist to a baseball game at the stadium. He also made what appeared to be a serious commitment to work seriously at school. The progress notes indicated that he seemed to be very eager to please the therapist and to live up to the therapist's expectations.

The next two months were a time of hard work in school, at his job, and in therapy. The client seemed to thrive on these newly discovered motivations. He still expressed much confusion about his life, but felt optimistic that he was "clearing things up." The following two excerpts typify his efforts at understanding some major issues in his life and illustrate the therapist's attempts to encourage this self-exploration.

Client: I don't think I'll ever understand. How could he [his father] just take off that way?

Therapist: Tell me about him. What you remember. Maybe we'll get some clues.

Client: Well, he was big. Good looking, I think. Sharp dresser. He seemed to know everybody. We'd be walking down the street, and it would be, "Hi Sam, hello Bill." You know, that kind of thing.

Therapist: Sounds like he was popular and successful.

Client: Well, I don't know. . . . Maybe. I'm thinking maybe, he needed to, you know, seem that way. Like, putting up a front. . . . Yeah, because there were times when I'm pretty sure we didn't have any money. Really scrounging. . . . But there he was, smiling, sharp, giving a big hello to everybody.

Therapist: You don't sound so angry now when you talk about him. Maybe more like sympathetic.

Client: Yeah. . . . I don't know if I'd call it feeling sorry for him. But I guess he had his problems . . .

At the next session the following conversation took place:

Therapist: You know, I talked to your foster mom yesterday. She called, did she tell you?

Client: Yeah. She said she would. I don't get it with her sometimes. I guess she gets on my nerves, once in a while, and I wised off with her. Shit. She started to cry. . . . I wasn't that bad.

Therapist: She gets pretty emotional with you, it sounds like. And what is it, you don't know how to handle it?

Client: Well, you know. . . . I been used to a lot of screaming, a whack on the head, and then that's it. But with her, wow, I don't know . . . it's hard to figure . . . she kind of whines, worries you to death, doesn't let up . . . like she's a little drill . . . drilling into your head. . . . I'm not sure where she's coming from.

Therapist: She's got you kind of mixed up, because you've never known anyone like her.

Client: Yeah, that's it. . . . She gets me mixed up. . . . Like she's not mean or anything. I'm beginning to think maybe she even likes me. . . . But, I don't know. . . . She's so damned nervous about it . . . like, like, like maybe she's not sure if I like her. . . . But that's dumb.

Therapist: Is it?

Client [*Long pause*]: Well, maybe not. I really did give her a hard time when they first sent me there. I think I scared her pretty good, the way I was acting. . . . You know, I guess I got to give her credit for hanging in there with me, the way she has.

The following months saw a growing stability in the client's life and in his emotional responsiveness. A major event occurred when, after much hesitation, he went out for spring practice with the school football team and was accepted. His coach and teammates were both enthused and taken aback by his sometimes overly aggressive play. Joey became determined to learn the finer points of the game and to become a "first stringer."

His schedule of school, work, and football practice necessitated a reduction in therapy contact; however, he and Mr. Hollan managed to get together at least once a week. Many of these meetings were purely social. At some sessions, however, there was still work to be accomplished, as for example, when Joey had several nasty confrontations with the football coach. One such incident occurred when the coach struck Joey on the side of his helmet for "lack of hustle" and Joey swung back. He was temporarily dismissed from the team. This prompted some lengthy therapeutic discussions concerning the unfortunate fact of life that not all individuals that are encountered are easygoing and accepting. Joey concluded that indeed distinctions had to be made, that social relations were not all in the same mold, and that there were choices available to him regarding his life. In this instance, because of the importance of sports to him, Joey decided to attempt a reconciliation with the coach, although he knew they would probably continue to dislike one another.

Over the next year, therapy contacts tapered off progressively. There were occasional trips to a ball game and periodic meetings for a coke after practice, and Joey frequently visited the Saturday morning recreational center. Close feelings were maintained and sporadic problems reviewed, but in large measure, Joey was establishing himself as a maturing person outside of therapy.

UNRESOLVED ISSUES AND FUTURE PERSPECTIVES

As with any therapeutic approach, relationship therapy requires the critical eye of scientific study for its sustenance and development. In this regard, it falls far short of other treatment approaches. At the heart of this problem is the virtual absence of what has been termed *outcome research*—that is, scientific evaluation as to the actual effectiveness of this type of treatment. The reasons for this lack are many: some stem from unique developments in the general history of psychotherapy; others are embedded in the special problems encountered when attempting to do research on this form of treatment. To conclude this chapter, a brief review of these issues will hopefully orient the reader to this unresolved area of relationship therapy.

Historical Factors

The early decades of the twentieth century seemed to be a more leisurely time with respect to psychotherapy. In an era dominated by the psychoanalytic movement, most therapists and clients fully expected that treatment would take place over long periods of time in order for resistances to be overcome, to have a deep relationship established, and to allow ample time for self-exploration and analysis. The necessity for frequent and lengthy contact with clients also seemed to be an accepted fact among therapists who worked with troubled or delinquent youth, as, for example, in the well-known Cambridge-Somerville Youth Project of the 1930s and 1940s (Powers and Witmer, 1951), in which therapeutic work was maintained with children and their families from two to eight years.

As we consider the aims and procedures of relationship therapy it is reasonably apparent that it also represents a lengthy endeavor. Sensitively dealing with clients' suspicions and tests, attempting to bring about an emotional breakthrough, and so on, can hardly be done on a rapid, rigid timetable. And yet this concern with time appears as a major stumbling block in the historical developments of the post-World War II era. The many psychological agonies produced by the war, as well as the increased complexity and mobility of life in the postwar years, seemed to dictate the development of more efficient, short-term therapies. Directively helping a client through times of immediate crisis became, perhaps necessarily, the tempo of the times. This trend was later abetted by the ascendency of behavioral techniques of treatment that also were, for the most part, brief and symptom-oriented procedures. In effect, the time-consuming methods of relationship therapy seemed to go into a decline. Naturally in such an era there was not much impetus to do research, especially on an approach that had fallen out of vogue.

During more recent decades the fires have been rekindled somewhat, largely through the efforts of Carl Rogers. His research in defining and studying "therapeutic relationships" and in identifying the personal qualities of therapists that promote growth in clients has led to a mellowing of the strict emphases on efficiency and formal techniques. In addition, Rogers's contention that many nonprofessional and relatively untrained individuals may play effective therapeutic roles opened the door for the paraprofessional movement. This influx of mental health workers has relieved some of the pressures on embattled staffs, thereby permitting the possibility of longer, more intensive and more finely tuned therapies with clients in need of such approaches.

The stage thus seems to be set for the strong reemergence of relationship therapy. As mentioned at the beginning of these chapters, broad cultural forces appear to be operating in today's society that make syndromes of alienation a prominent class of mental health problems. The procedures outlined, representing an amalgam of various theories and clinical practices, are as yet largely untested in a scientific sense. If, indeed, mental health workers are going to meet the needs of a contemporary clientele, then rigorous programs of research will be needed to evaluate and refine these procedures.

Special Research Issues

Conducting outcome research on relationship therapy presents a wide array of problems, many of which are specific to this form of treatment. No ready solutions to all these complexities are available; however, a brief listing may serve to highlight the challenges faced by investigators in this area.

Definition and sequencing of procedures In any well-conducted study of therapy the investigator must be able to specify that the relevant techniques are actually being utilized and, in addition, that the various techniques are being applied at appropriate times in the treatment process. This important general principle of outcome research is especially applicable to relationship therapy, because, as we have seen in this chapter, it is composed of a number of different procedures and tactics whose application depend on the phase of treatment and the emotional-psychological status of the client at the time. Thus, in any research evaluation of this therapy, special care must be devoted to carefully defining each procedure, specifying the sequencing of each, and providing some assurance that the procedures are being invoked at appropriate times. If we contrast this with research that evaluates only a single technique (e.g., an extinction technique to remove an undesirable habit), we can perhaps appreciate the enormous technical problems faced by investigators in this area.

Specification of emotional processes A problem related to those cited in the previous section pertains to the fact that an important component of relation-ship therapy is the emotional response of the therapist to the client. Apart from formal techniques and strategies, the therapist's communication of an honest willingness to enter into a relationship with the client seems to be the essential ingredient. Because of the central role played by such interpersonal factors, research on relationship therapy must include means for their evaluation. The development of rating scales by which independent observers may make such evaluations has already received some attention in the field (see Parloff, Waskow, and Wolfe, 1978).

Personal qualities of the therapist It is probably a fair speculation to state that not all therapists have the emotional-interpersonal qualifications to successfully carry out relationship therapy. Taking this one step further, it is also likely that optimum therapist characteristics may vary considerably depending on the type of alienation problem exhibited by clients. For example, a committed, energetic, reasonably aggressive, and outgoing therapist may achieve the best results with young, alienated delinquents; a more passive, contemplative, but equally committed individual may do better with detached middle-aged clients. Whatever the case may be, in view of the apparent importance of producing a good "interpersonal fit" between therapist and client, research on such compati-bility issues is of great importance in relationship therapy.

Criteria for success Naturally, any research program that evaluates the effec-tiveness of a form of therapy must have some criteria against which to judge success. The alcoholic who gives up liquor after treatment presents a fairly clear outcome. Similarly, the child abuser who no longer harms his or her children meets a well-defined criterion of successful therapy. Comparable standards for the outcome of relationship therapy are probably not possible. Here we seem to be dealing with less defined changes in emotions and internal responsiveness to others and alterations in perceptions and attitudes concerning others. The development of criteria and measurement techniques in these ill-defined areas is perhaps the foremost task facing the researcher.

CHAPTER NINE

INSIGHT THERAPY: CONCEPTS AND OVERVIEW

INTRODUCTION

The woman's face is frozen. Its fragile attractiveness is encased in stiff, mechanical movements. Tailored clothes signal conventional suburban prosperity, and their severe lines continue the motif of her facial expression. Her words are exquisitely precise, and although they speak of anguish, their tone is devoid of emotion.

The image she conveys is one of encasement, of psychological imprisonment; yet slight hints of deeper messages can also be sensed. Something about her manner suggests suspicion and intellectual challenge. Her voice carries remote echoes of Europe—of different times, more exotic roots. Once or twice, her eyes trap the therapist with a look of pleading.

It is the first session of outpatient treatment for a thirty-four-year-old housewife, and the therapist is reacting to the varied and sometimes conflicting impressions that are created. She tells her story in a speech that was obviously rehearsed many times prior to her appointment.

> **Client:** I'm so ashamed and guilty. It's my daughter. She's seven years old. In the second grade. She is terribly nervous. Very tense. No confidence. It's gotten to the point where her second-grade teacher is worried about her, and she called me in for a conference to discuss it. I was dumbstruck because I realized that I was the cause of it. I didn't know it has become apparent to others, but I suddenly knew that the problem had gotten to the point where I have to get therapy. I can't go on harming the child like this.
>
> It's not that I'm a bad mother. I care for my children a great deal. I have two other girls. They're younger, five and three, and I love them all. But with Lisa, that's the seven-year-old, there are frequent times when I lose control of myself. I don't know what comes over me. I rage at her,

yelling, no, scream at her. I rant, belittle, reduce her to tears. I try to stop myself, even while it's happening, but I can't. I become a snarling ogre.

I feel so guilty and ashamed when it's over. It's so inappropriate. These outbursts occur over such trivial things. We'll all be sitting at dinner, for example, and she might accidentally spill her milk, and that starts it. I become engulfed with anger, and lose control. I know that it is ridiculous, but I can't help myself. My husband tries to calm me down and tries to be protective to the girl, but I just continue with my ranting and raving. I'm just ruining the girl's self-confidence, and it's over such silly things.

And it's been getting worse. These outbursts have been happening more frequently . . . much more than last year, or before that. And it only occurs with Lisa, not the others. It's really insane. She's such a lovely child and so well-behaved. What is wrong with me? I'm going to drive the child to an asylum, and over such inconsequential things.

There must be something deeper going on. Things within me that I don't understand. I've got to get a grip on myself before I completely destroy her. I'm so ashamed. Why do I do it? Why?

The plight of this client is typical of many who seek treatment, and the highlights of her therapy will be used throughout our discussion to illustrate insight approaches. The reader is therefore encouraged to follow this case carefully as its various details and facets unfold.

The question "Why?" seems to lie at the heart of insight therapy. Things are going seriously wrong for no apparent reason. Inappropriate behaviors, severe emotional conflicts, grinding unhappiness, and tension may dominate the person's life, and yet the causes are hidden. Clients suffer both the symptoms and the helpless feelings of being unable to understand or do anything about them. In this context, as described in Chapter 4, the aims of insight therapy are twofold: (1) to help clients gain an understanding of the hidden patterns that underlie their distress, and (2) once exposed, to assist the client in changing or resolving these debilitating patterns. Two remarkably different tactics are called for. The first involves procedures that uncover and elucidate the submerged emotional currents and unrecognized behavioral systems in a person's life. Such exploration into the unknown is a delicate process. Areas of intense anxiety or unhappiness may be exposed. Motives and wishes that are surrounded by guilt and revulsion may be encountered. A deep, honest look at one's life may reveal a petty, meaningless existence—barren, loveless, uncreative. This process of self-exploration can therefore be painful, frightening, depressing; yet to become aware, to acquire self-knowledge, is also a liberating experience because now one can do something about malevolent patterns rather than being their unwitting victim.

After an exploration of these unrecognized aspects of a client's personality, therapeutic tactics change to the hard work of bringing about behavioral and emotional change. Old fears may die slowly, and well-ingrained habits do not give up easily, but we saw in the chapter on behavioral approaches that a variety of procedures exist for promoting such change. The replacement of maladaptive patterns with more human and creative ones thus represents the ultimate goal of insight therapy.

It is apparent from this brief introduction that treatment focusing on self-exploration includes aspects of the other therapy strategies covered in this book—relationship, supportive, and behavioral. Thus, as with these other approaches, we will be dealing here with a treatment form that emphasizes a particular dimension, but by no means is exclusively devoted to insight.

CONCEPTUAL BACKGROUND

In one form or another virtually all schools of psychotherapy address the notion that individuals may fail to recognize certain of their own behavioral or emotional reaction patterns or may be unaware of particular aspects of their personality. To be sure, each theory uses distinctive terminology and each makes different assumptions about the processes involved; however, all the theories seem to acknowledge that lack of awareness is an important issue in understanding human maladjustment.

Psychodynamic Viewpoints

Freudian psychoanalytic theory emphasizes the view that during early socialization overwhelming anxiety and guilt may become associated with certain inner drives and emotions (particularly sex and aggression) because of severe and punitive attitudes of parents and the culture generally. Further, in order to escape from these infantile and often intolerable feelings of anxiety, the individual develops psychological defenses that prevent the *experiencing* of the threatening drives and emotions. A variety of mental mechanisms may be catalogued that serve this repressive mission. The individual may develop, for example, habitual thought patterns that are exceptionally flighty, superficial, and externalized. Attention is directed only to the most conventional and peripheral aspects of situations. To probe too deeply, to look after subtleties, to seek complex relations, is dangerous. Safer to be the carefree mental butterfly, flitting from one surface to another, never tasting deeper meanings, always a jump ahead of emotional reactions or the arousal of inner drives. At the other extreme are defenses that rely on a rigid, disciplined intellectual approach to the world. Virtually all one's efforts are devoted to exceptionally precise, rational, unemotional analyses of small details in the environment. Psychic energy is so bound up with such intellectual activity that responsiveness to inner emotional stimuli is forsaken. It is safer to indulge in the narrow, compulsive thought patterns and repetitious rumination about details than run the risk of experiencing frightening emotions.

Such psychological defenses, according to psychoanalytic theory, may become ingrained, habitual and automatic modes of coping with all emotional stimuli and the world generally. In the service of protecting oneself from childhood sources of anxiety, the individual becomes a victim of the defenses themselves—becomes locked in the cold, limiting prison of neurotic thought patterns. Moreover, once these patterns become ingrained and automatic the individual may well fail to appreciate their existence or their negative effects.

We can therefore distinguish two areas of unconscious process in psychoanalytic theory: (1) preventing the experiencing of threatening emotions and drives and (2) a lack of awareness of the defensive mechanisms by which this repression is accomplished.

Theorists following in the psychoanalytic tradition, the so-called neo-Freudians such as Adler, Horney, and Sullivan, also emphasize the role of intolerable anxiety in motivating repression. However, they view the anxiety as stemming from disturbed interpersonal processes, particularly early ones, in the life of neurotic individuals. Childhood fears of rejection, abandonment, overwhelming punishment, and powerlessness threaten the person's security and form the basis for long-term patterns of anxiety. The neurotic individual, according to these theorists, develops specialized ways of relating to other people so as to "cover over" the unbearable anxiety and to provide a measure of day-to-day security. These interpersonal defense mechanisms, as with Freudian defenses, may become habitual and routinized, so that the individual recognizes neither their maladaptive effects on others nor the underlying anxieties that motivate them. Such habitual patterns as aggressive domination over others, slavish dependency, compulsive strivings for one sexual conquest after another, and so forth, are viewed as interpersonal "security operations" that may provide short-term freedom from anxiety but that in the long run will likely produce even more disruption and anxiety. The neurotic person thus becomes a victim of ever-increasing insecurity and is driven to progressively more maladaptive defenses, all with a grim lack of awareness of this gradually spiraling process.

Several other aspects of psychoanalytic theory bear comment. By emphasizing childhood sources of anxiety, these theorists are pointing out the extreme nature of this emotion. They are not referring here to such lesser reactions as the nervousness or tension that an adult might feel at taking an exam or giving a public speech. They are addressing the "life-and-death" kind of terror that might be experienced by a two-, three-, or four-year-old whose whole world is disintegrating when facing parental rage or threat of abandonment. According to these theorists such childhood anxiety patterns still reside within the neurotic adult and continue to threaten personality disintegration many years after their inception.

The intensity of this threat underlies the psychoanalytic notion of *resistance*, that is, the assumption that neurotically repressed individuals will rarely discard defenses spontaneously. To the contrary, it is presumed that such persons require assistance, through the use of special uncovering techniques and therapist pressures, in order to confront anxiety-laden issues in their lives. Further, because of the intensity of emotion involved, psychoanalytic theorists view the insight process as necessarily gradual, having the client confront tolerable doses of anxiety as they are able, without precipitating disorganization, unbearable anguish, or defensive withdrawal from therapy.

Behavioral Viewpoints

A legacy of psychoanalytic views of unconscious processes can be seen, perhaps surprisingly, in certain aspects of the behaviorist school of thought. The entire area of escape and avoidance learning, for example, is fundamentally based on the study of fear and anxiety and an analysis of the means by which these negative emotions are reduced. To be sure, much of the research and theory in this area have investigated simple escape behaviors, such as physically running away from a feared stimulus, and so forth. This line of theory, however, has been extended into the realm of thought processes as well, in the sense that individuals can learn to "not think" about (i.e., mentally avoid) certain inner stimuli that are anxiety provoking. Such cognitive avoidance responses probably come about through a gradual shaping process in which the individual first learns to avoid a feared situation, then acquires a pattern of not speaking about the situation or topic, and ultimately learns to not think or symbolically represent the feared stimulus.

Behaviorists also employ two other concepts that relate to lack of awareness. A person may be undergoing stress, for example, but be unable to discriminate whether the source of stress is internal (e.g., fear-provoking thoughts) or external (threatening environmental stimuli). Despite this failure to detect the origins of stress, the individual responds with fear and defensive behaviors. Similarly, a person may habitually engage in a particular response pattern that leads to very predictable and reliable consequences but may lack awareness of this behavior-outcome relationship. Here again we can see concepts that parallel the psychoanalytic notion that individuals may be unaware of both the sources of anxiety in their lives and the maladaptive effects of their defenses.

Humanistic Viewpoints

Theorists in the humanistic tradition take a broader perspective on unconscious processes than psychoanalytic or behavioral thinkers. Whereas the latter camps focus largely on defensive avoidance of strong anxiety, the humanists address problems in which individuals have lost contact with larger domains of their personalities—notably, the philosophical, spiritual, and emotional realms of living. Philosopher-therapists such as Erich Fromm (1947), Carl Rogers (1951), Victor Frankl (1965), and Rollo May (1961) view the human condition as a continual search for personal freedom and meaning. Important components of this search are the choosing and taking *responsibility* for the direction one takes in life, the capability of deeply *experiencing* one's own personality in all its facets, and the development of an authentic *commitment* to fellow human beings.

Humanists believe that maladjustment occurs when the individual retreats from these conditions, pointing out that there are multiple pressures in our lives to foster this retreat. Strong forces daily encourage us to conform blindly, to adopt unthinking or safe allegiances, to compulsively get on with the job, to gather material goods, to automatically watch out for ourselves first—in short, to give up our individuality and freedom. The pressures toward dehumanization are internal as well, according to these theorists. To exercise personal freedom and choice means departing from the safe haven of routine conformity and obedience to external dictates, a condition that can engender awesome ambiguity and fear.

In clinical terms individuals who succumb to dehumanization pressures seem to suffer some characteristic symptoms that can be only vaguely defined but are nevertheless potent. They speak of the boredom, alienation, superficiality, lack of direction, and a robotlike quality of existence. Their lives are passing by without meaning or spontaneity, without a sense of personal depth or identity. They cannot love.

Although it would not do justice to the depth of humanistic thought, much of the above can be viewed in terms of the client's lack of awareness. The emphasis here is not on the focused repressions or specific, unrecognized interpersonal mechanisms dealt with in psychoanalysis, but rather on the massive denial of broad regions of one's existence. The maladjusted individual not only is unable to experience sexual or aggressive feelings, for example, but is unable to experience any feelings at all. A dehumanized individual may not only display specific areas of interpersonal conflict, but has also lost a basic empathy and commitment to fellow humans.

The notion of insight takes on a comparably broader meaning within humanistic theory. Therapeutic efforts are devoted to promoting greater "experiencing" of oneself in the here and now, rather than uncovering limited areas of anxiety and conflict. In addition, the choices and responsibilities in one's life heretofore unexplored are brought into focus and examined. Finally, personal moral and spiritual issues, which previously may have been submerged in a superficial life-style, find their place in therapeutic discussion.

OVERVIEW OF STAGES IN INSIGHT THERAPY

Many practicing therapists who emphasize insight procedures do not rely on any of the theories mentioned above in an exclusive way. Rather, they seem to approach each client in a pragmatic, eclectic fashion depending on his or her needs (see Goldman and Milman, 1978). In addition, as discussed in Chapter 4, several current-day theorists have suggested that insight alone may not be enough to produce lasting therapeutic change in a client (e.g., Martin, 1977; Phares, 1979). They contend that the active effort to change maladaptive behavioral-emotional patterns, once uncovered, is an important part of treatment. This diversity of theory and practice makes it difficult to present an overview of "standard" procedures in insight-oriented therapy. What follows is my attempt to provide a model of this treatment strategy integrating these diverse viewpoints.

Insight therapy may be seen as progressing through a number of stages, each with its own unique issues. The stages can be viewed as a series of logically sequenced steps in a complex process of self-discovery followed by a lengthy period of behavioral-emotional change. In actual practice these stages may not follow, one upon another, in exactly the series to be described below; however, this rough outline is intended to provide the reader with a broad perspective on this complex form of therapy. An awareness of these stages is important in that different technical problems and treatment procedures, to be covered in the next chapter, are involved in each.

The Self-exploration Phase

Initial contact A large measure of patience and understanding is required of therapists in the opening stage of treatment. Clients enter therapy with perhaps a lifelong history of hiding from their emotions. They may be fearful of and unpracticed at looking within themselves. They do not know what their innermost secrets are, nor do they know how to go about discovering them. It would be unrealistic of the therapist to expect a client to be open and deeply introspective, that is, to be a "good" client, at this early stage of treatment. More reasonable are expectations of a somewhat confused, distraught, and resistant individual who needs guidance and direction from the therapist.

Many clients take the view that their unhappiness and distress are exclusively due to environmental factors. Hence they direct much of the initial discussion to descriptions of their pressure-laden jobs, nagging spouse, money worries, boring home life, and similar sorts of factors. Again, this approach is not surprising in view of the external orientation among most clients who need insight therapy.

Clients may also enter treatment with the attitude that if they provide an honest and complete description of their (external) situation, the therapist will use her or his experience to "diagnose" the problem and then will offer a "prescription" to cure the difficulty. This feeling is obviously a carry-over from experiences in physicians' consulting rooms, and clients do not understand that the "real" (internal) problems have not been uncovered as yet and hence that no quick solutions can be offered.

Individuals also frequently enter therapy with many pent-up frustrations and tensions that have accumulated in their daily lives. Indeed, many of these feelings have probably built up because of clients' maladaptive defenses and their negative effects on others; their present intensity perhaps is what prompted entrance into therapy at this point in time. Such individuals react, in the opening sessions of treatment, with a sense that they have now found someone who will help. An outpouring of emotions occurs. A catharsis of sorts takes place, in which the burden of tensions and problems are transferred to the therapist. The ensuing sense of relief within clients is understandable, but it can also be counterproductive. In the extreme, clients may feel so relieved after several cathartic sessions that they decide not to continue in therapy. In more moderate terms, they may assume that now the problems are in the hands of the therapist and that they can sit back until a solution is offered. What is unrecognized, of course, is that the pent-up tensions were only the end result, the current-day residue as it were, of long-term maladaptive patterns that are yet to be discovered and corrected.

Several therapeutic tasks are apparent in this opening stage. First, the therapist must provide structure and guidance as to the long-range aims in therapy, the procedures to be involved, the client's responsibilities, and points in the process that are likely to be particularly difficult. Second, the attitude that the therapist will in some way magically produce a solution to the client's problems should be contravened. Rather, an attitude of a therapist-client partnership, in which the client carries the major burden of self-exploration, is instilled. Finally, the therapist sets in motion procedures that will help the client to make the transition from an external to an internal locus of exploration—a process that may be both gradual and difficult for many repressed individuals. That these are extremely difficult tasks is reflected in the fact that large numbers of clients (some estimates are as high as 40 percent) drop out of therapy within the first five sessions.

Beginnings of self-exploration Under the guidance of the therapist, clients gradually begin the transition from seeking to "blame" external factors to an assessment of their own behaviors, motives, and emotions. This can be a period of strong anxiety and self-doubt for clients in that habitual and safe ways of perceiving their situation are being discarded. They begin to gain a realization of strong inner turmoil, which may be sensed as menacing. It is ill-defined and somehow alien, and yet the turmoil is experienced as stemming from emotional regions of the personality.

Clients also begin to inspect their own behavior patterns more closely, gradually becoming aware that some of these patterns are self-defeating, inappropriate, irritating to others, or limiting their opportunities for a full, satisfying life. Such self-evaluations are also coupled with a growing recognition that the inappropriate patterns seem to be unplanned and automatic and in some unspecified way are related to the emotional turmoil raging within.

This, then, is the first stage of the self-exploration process—the beginning of a careful, realistic inspection of one's inner life and social-behavioral ways of relating to the world. In this early stage clients obtain only vague glimpses of the strong emotional forces that operate in their personalities. It is difficult for them to place verbal labels on the components of the inner turmoil; hence they have problems in describing their emotions to the therapist. In the same fashion, clients frequently seek to rationalize and "excuse" some of the maladaptive behavior patterns of which they are becoming aware. The anxiety and ambiguity of this phase makes it inherently upsetting, and progress occurs in fits and starts. Periods of openness are followed by episodes of defensiveness and fearfulness. Feelings of anger may erupt toward the therapist, who may be seen as too demanding or unsympathetic. Clients struggle with the conflict of whether the vague hope of a better way of life is worth all of the present upset. Indeed, the beginning of self-exploration can be a very distressing period of treatment.

This stage is complicated by the fact that clients are still getting to know and are evaluating the therapist. It is one thing to divulge factual and environmental information to an impersonal "expert" in the first few sessions, but now the issues are far more serious and sensitive. Clients struggle with the question of whether the therapist is personally capable and worthy enough to share in the exploration of their private, inner world. The dimensions of this evaluation vary from client to client: however, some questions that frequently arise are: (1) Will the therapist really be able to understand this confusing mass of emotions, fears, and fantasies that seems to be emerging? (2) Will the therapist take an evaluative attitude and be condemning or demeaning? (3) Can the therapist be an honest, genuine, and constant helpmate in the difficult self-exploration process, or is he or she merely playing a role? and (4) Is the therapist capable of providing support and guidance during periods of vulnerability and distress?

As is apparent, the tasks facing the therapist are multiple and complex. First, treatment procedures that guide, encourage, and train the client toward continued self-exploration must be maintained. However, the therapist must remain sensitive to periods of excessive anxiety, distress, or discouragement and be prepared to temporarily lighten the pressures for self-exploration in favor of providing emotional support. Second, clients' attempts to resist or sabotage the insight process (to protect themselves from the anxiety) require firm but sympathetic management. Finally, the therapist must stay attuned to the developing relationship with the client. This involves constant assessment of one's own emotional stirrings and reactions to the client's characteristics and overall style of relating, as well as continued sensitivity to the client's perceptions and expectations in the therapeutic relationship.

This early stage of insight also requires discussion at another level of discourse that has important implications for later periods of therapy. We are talking here about a time in therapy when neither client nor therapist knows what is going to emerge in the process of uncovering hidden aspects of the client's life and personality. It is a phase of great ambiguity for both participants. The outlines of a unique individual are slowly taking form, as in the gradual sharpening of a photographic image while being developed. We are here in the blurry, ill-defined stage, when the details of neither the main subject nor the background have yet come into focus.

Since this ambiguity may be prolonged, there is a strong temptation for both therapist and client to prematurely assume that they "know" what the fully developed picture will be. The client, for example, having acquired a vague sense that some terrible and shameful emotions lurk in the recesses of his or her personality, may impulsively conclude that he or she is a despicable or unworthy individual. Or, confronted with strong anxiety, the client may focus on some minor and relatively "safe" problem area and rigidly adhere to the view that this peripheral problem should be the central theme in treatment.

Therapists at times have their own difficulties in managing the ambiguity of this phase. It is tempting to "fill in the picture" through an excessive reliance on theory. If, by way of example, a female client reports early in therapy that she has conflicting feelings toward her romantic partners, therapist A may prematurely conclude, "Aha, unresolved Oedipus complex," on the basis of Freudian theory, whereas therapist B may surmise, "Um hm, confused sexual identity," drawing from social learning theory. Either may be correct, or, as will occasionally happen, both may be totally off the mark. When such inferences are incorrect, at best, valuable time and energy may be lost as the therapist guides the client's exploration down a blind alley. At worst, such incorrect assumptions produce great confusion and anxiety for the client to the point where the entire therapeutic process is subverted.

Early attempts to change As described in the previous section, many clients begin to recognize the inappropriateness of some of their behavior patterns fairly early in therapy. This awareness may prompt several reactions: chagrin at having behaved so ineffectively in the past, guilt for having hurt or upset others, and a resolve to change these maladaptive behaviors. The assumption is made that the solution is clear-cut. All they must do is stop behaving in these unreasonable ways.

Many clients indeed make sincere efforts to alter these patterns during this period of therapy, and they are shocked to discover that they cannot change. Attempts to discard habitual patterns are accompanied by strong anxiety, which literally drives them back to the old, safe behaviors. The inability to change may elicit a sharp sense of discouragement, which frequently takes the form, "What is the sense of trying, I will never change. This is the way I am." Such reactions obviously pose a high risk of leaving therapy prematurely.

In this stage, clients are confronting the fact that habitual behavior patterns are playing a *defensive function* in their personality; that is, they serve to reduce anxiety or are used to manage threatening interpersonal situations. The realization that these patterns play a larger role in the balance of forces in their personality opens new areas of exploration for the client. Recall that in the previous phase clients had a vague sense that their automatic reaction patterns were in some way related to the inner emotional turmoil being experienced. Now, in the face of being unable to change these patterns, interest focuses much more directly on the specific nature of the relationship between behavior and inner, emotional processes.

The therapeutic tasks of this phase are twofold: (1) to help manage clients' sense of discouragement at not being readily able to discard inappropriate behaviors and (2) to enlarge the arena of exploration into the realms of emotional and social sources of anxiety and the defensive strategies that have been used to control that anxiety.

Analysis of psychodynamics We now enter a very complex and difficult period of the insight process. Clients are, in effect, being encouraged and guided into a confrontation with the major areas of agony in their lives. Fears that threaten to overwhelm, murderous rage, gut-wrenching guilt, memories of a whimpering, beaten child, and the devastation of seeing oneself as petty, hollow, and lifeless are just some of the emotions that may now gradually emerge. Clients confront these feelings not only in an analytical, intellectual fashion, but also in a direct, experiential way. The raw power of these emotions, with their awesome threat to the integrity of personality, envelops the client in an immediate, firsthand manner. This is perhaps the period of therapy when the client feels most vulnerable. The raw nerve endings are gradually being exposed.

We can legitimately ask whether this direct experiencing of agonizing emotions is a necessary part of therapy. Is it not enough to identify the problem behaviors and then proceed to help the client to change them? Would it not be sufficient for the client to gain an intellectual understanding of the emotional turmoil, inspecting the ghosts from a safe distance, as it were? Why go through the severe distress and upheaval of deep immersion in these destructive emotions themselves?

These questions can be answered in a variety of ways, depending on the particulars of one's theoretical orientation. A therapist with behavioristic leanings might argue that identification of the problem behaviors, and then changing them, should be sufficient. Cognitive theorists go a step further and suggest that an intellectual understanding of the emotional underpinnings of deviant response patterns is a necessary forerunner to therapeutic change. Psychodynamic theorists, however, extend the process to its ultimate; that is, they take the view that actually experiencing the agonizing emotions (and rationally understanding them) are central components of insight therapy.

The psychodynamic argument runs along the following lines. The underlying emotions are the frightening inner stimuli from which the client has been escaping, sometimes for many years. These are the wellsprings that motivated the development and maintenance of maladaptive psychological defenses. By directly confronting and experiencing these emotions the client is provided with opportunity for several important therapeutic processes: (1) the discovery that he or she will not be overwhelmed or psychologically destroyed by them; (2) a gradual desensitization to the fearful qualities of the emotions; (3) the development of more efficient means of coping with the emotions to replace the maladaptive defenses currently in use; and (4) the emergence of a sense of mastery, as the villainous aspects of one's personality have finally been confronted and conquered.

The therapist is faced with multiple tasks in helping the client through this complex and difficult period. First, of course, is a continuation of the techniques that prompt both the intellectual and experiential forms of insight described above. Second, the therapist must continuously assess the level of distress experienced by the client and provide support and structure as needed. Third, the therapist must assist in providing a broad perspective on the insights that are occurring so that the client can understand them in terms of real-life problems and with regard to tasks still to be faced in treatment. Finally, in order to help combat the dread and loneliness of this phase, the therapist, more than ever before, must continue in a close, empathic relationship with the client.

Review of historical roots A logical question accompanying the exploration of psychodynamics concerns the origins of clients' problems. After having gained insight into threatening emotions, defenses, and areas of anxiety, a natural curiosity spurs the exploration process backward in time. "Why am I this way?" and "Where did all this anxiety and defensiveness come from?" are the types of questions that now emerge. Clients have recently experienced the agonizing emotions, which usually stem from earlier traumas or intolerable family dynamics, and now they seek an understanding of these historical roots. This phase of the insight process may not be essential to effective treatment, but in the context of seeking a full understanding of themselves, many clients find this retrospective analysis an important aspect of therapy.

Clients' tendencies for self-condemnation frequently subside as they gain an understanding of their backgrounds. The deep-seated anxieties and conflicts that were heretofore seen as contemptible may now be perceived as natural outgrowths of tragic or frightening aspects of earlier years. Many clients can now make the distinction between taking personal responsibility for improving their emotional and behavioral patterns and blaming themselves for their condition. In the same light, as a rational understanding of the historical factors emerges, much of the mystery and dread surrounding clients' maladjustment begins to subside. Self-knowledge and logic begin to replace superstition and fear.

Several important therapeutic aims are part of this period. This is frequently a time in therapy when clients gain a broader perspective on their problems—

their current dynamics, the negative effects on present adjustment, and the historical factors that brought them about. It is a time of summary, in which the therapist encourages a wide-ranging, logical review of the self-knowledge gained in earlier phases of the insight process. As such, it is also a period when the client is asked to take a step or two back from the intense emotionality of the previous stage and to engage in a more thoughtful analysis and evaluation.

This is also a period in which the therapist assists in the development of a balanced view of the past. It is often tempting for clients to perceive parents or earlier circumstances as the villains in their lives and consequently to develop a completely cynical and "poor me" attitude toward their present unhappiness. Such a development operates to reduce motivation for changing one's own behavioral-emotional patterns in later phases of treatment. Hence, the historical analysis also emphasizes an understanding of parents, family, and significant others in terms of their strengths, weaknesses, needs, and problems in the earlier times. Clients may come away from such an analysis with a bittersweet feeling about both the positive and negative effects that others have had on their lives, but they may at the same time have stronger motivations to change and correct mistakes of the past.

Negotiating a contract for change After the first half of therapy clients have attained a degree of self-awareness that is remarkably different from that with which they entered therapy. They are in a position to make some critical decisions, based on full knowledge, as to the changes that are desirable and necessary in their lives. In the present stage, these prospective changes are explicitly discussed and evaluated by client and therapist, and an agreement is reached regarding the goals of behavioral-emotional change to be accomplished in the second half of therapy. Although these negotiations may occasionally be difficult and laden with conflict, these decisions must ultimately be made by the client. The therapist's function here is to ensure that the decisions are based on full utilization of the self-knowledge acquired in the first half of therapy.

As part of this *contract for change* the therapist provides careful explanation of the new directions to be taken in treatment, the procedures to be utilized, their likelihood of success, any potential risks, and an estimate of the length of time involved. Taking all this information into account, the client is now ready to embark on the second half of the treatment process.

The Behavioral-Emotional Change Phase

Initiating changes Three parallel processes are set in motion at the outset of the behavioral-emotional change phase of therapy: (1) procedures to help in the elimination of unwanted and inappropriate behavior patterns; (2) techniques to assist in the development of new and effective strategies for meeting needs; and (3) methods designed to extinguish intense anxiety or other debilitating emotions that came to light during the insight phase. As can be noted, these processes emanate largely from behavioral therapy, thus representing a substantial change in direction and viewpoint from that of the insight phase.

In this opening period the mechanics for bringing about these changes are arranged. Instructions regarding procedures, directions for client record keeping, prescriptions pertaining to homework assignments, and a review of behavioral goals are provided. In addition, clients are forewarned about the potential difficulties and anxieties involved in the change process—a caution that strikes home for most clients when they recall their inability to discard maladaptive patterns early in the insight phase of treatment.

Behavioral-emotional changes in the therapy setting It is frequently appropriate to begin the behavioral-emotional change phase by first working to bring about alterations in a "safe" place. The therapist can offer support and encouragement, as well as corrective feedback, as new response styles are attempted, or when old, inappropriate behaviors reassert themselves. Hence, in this stage of treatment the possibilities for more adaptive behaviors can be explored and practiced. Interspersed between periods of practice, client and therapist also assess and discuss refinements that are needed, the possible impact of the new behaviors on other persons in the environment, and specific issues in expanding these patterns into the client's daily routine.

During this period of treatment, as clients actively attempt to discard the old, defensive behaviors, they are again exposed directly to the anxieties and agonies that were confronted during the insight phase. These exposures now represent opportunities to continue a desensitization and mastery process over these distressing emotions. There is a gradual diminution in their intensity, with a concomitant lessening of needs to rely on defensive patterns. Although these early emotional conditionings may not disappear in a dramatic fashion, their progressive decline holds the promise of eventual freedom from them.

Finally, behavioral self-control techniques are introduced during this stage (see Chapter 6). These procedures, through which clients can learn to regulate and modify their own response patterns, become increasingly important as the change phase of therapy proceeds. At this period of time such personal skills as self-monitoring, stimulus control, self-reinforcement, and general problem-solving strategies are taught and practiced in the therapy setting.

Initiating changes outside of therapy As new response patterns become well practiced within the therapy setting and as maladaptive ones become more comfortably suppressed, a gradual transition takes place in the direction of environmental applications. More open ways of relating to others, more efficient ways of solving problems, more assertive means of engaging with the world are ready to be tried. This is frequently a time of tension and nervousness for the client, because the risks of rebuff, social embarrassment, and outright failure lurk in the background. For these reasons, the transition to real-life situations is accomplished gradually and systematically—at first with individuals who are likely to be supportive and understanding of the new behaviors and in settings in which the stresses are relatively minor. Thereafter, as successes and positive reactions accrue, more difficult and problematic situations are approached as part of a general broadening of areas of application.

Throughout this period, self-control skills are continuously practiced and expanded, so that there is a gradually decreasing reliance on the therapist for managing behavioral change. Clients themselves become more proficient in regulating their response patterns, managing times of stress, and rewarding themselves for desired behaviors. We can see, then, as this stage progresses, that newly acquired behaviors are strengthened both by the positive reactions stemming from the environment and self-reinforcements from clients themselves. Along with such positive occurrences is a growing sense of adequacy and mastery.

Permanence and generalizability of changes It is important in devising the program for behavioral-emotional change that attention be paid to bringing about lasting and broadly useful effects. How frustrating it would be for the client to have hard-earned improvements eroded by the passage of time or the gradual reemergence of the old, habitual patterns. Hence, during this stage of treatment the following procedures to increase the chances for enduring changes are invoked: (1) exposing the client to a wide variety of situations in which the new behaviors are required; (2) varying the types of reinforcers utilized; (3) varying the individuals who deliver reinforcement; (4) gradually decreasing the frequency and magnitude of external reinforcements; (5) increasing the emphasis on self-control procedures; and (6) assisting the client in organizing the newly acquired behaviors into broad and flexible strategies for coping with problems, relating to others, and meeting life's demands.

Fade out of the therapist and termination The time required to progress through the stages of insight-oriented therapy seems to be quite variable. In orthodox psychoanalysis, for example, a client may engage in multiple sessions each week for several years. In briefer forms of this approach, which are more usual in outpatient clinics and in present-day private practice, treatment is typically completed in a year or less (Sifneos, 1972). Even with relatively brief therapy, however, the process involves a complex, emotional, and frequently dependent relationship with the therapist. Fearful, intimate, and vulnerable aspects of the client's existence have been shared, and very often strong bonds of trust and friendship have been established. Toward the close of therapy, therefore, a careful disengagement is required in order to protect the client from too sudden a separation, the rearousal of anxiety, and the remorse of losing a confidante. In most instances this disengagement takes place gradually, with a progressive decrease in the frequency of sessions. At the same time,

Table 9.1
Summary of stages in insight therapy

Stage	Therapeutic tasks
The Self-Exploration Phase	
Initial contact	Provide information and structure; orient client toward "internal" exploration; correct mistaken assumptions about therapy
Beginnings of self-exploration	Have client begin to analyze and evaluate habitual behavior patterns and emotional reactions; manage client's anxiety; remain sensitive to client's evaluation of therapist
Early attempts to change	Manage client's discouragement at inability to change; orient client to explore emotional roots of defensive behaviors
Analysis of psychodynamics	Promote intellectual and experiential insight into threatening emotions; continue to explore defensive behaviors; relate insights to current problems; provide support
Review of historical roots	Promote analysis of origins of emotional conflicts and defensive mechanisms; summarize relationship between psychodynamics and current problems
Negotiating a contract for change	Discuss and agree upon behavioral and emotional changes to be attempted
The Behavioral-Emotional Change Phase	
Initiating changes	Instruct client regarding techniques of change
Changes in therapy setting	Assist client in discarding inappropriate defensive behaviors, developing adaptive patterns, and extinguishing anxiety reactions in the therapy relationship; introduce behavioral self-control techniques
Changes outside therapy	Assist client in gradual application of new, adaptive behaviors in environmental settings; help client expand self-control skill
Permanence and generalizability of changes	Prompt client in progressive application of behavioral techniques to prevent extinction of new reaction patterns
Fade out of therapist and termination	Gradually decrease frequency and intensity of therapeutic contact; manage separation from therapy; promote outside relationships and sense of self-determination

alliances with other supportive figures in the environment are encouraged so that an effective transfer of attachments and allegiances can occur as part of the termination process. This gradual tapering of contact reduces the risks of the rearousal of anxiety or symptoms that occasionally occur at the prospect of leaving therapy.

Summary When students begin training in psychotherapy, they frequently make the assumption that insight therapy involves a simple, straightforward uncovering process. Get the client to talk about some conflicts, or reveal some emotions, and therapy is accomplished. It is hoped that the foregoing overview provides an appreciation of the complex and multistage nature of this treatment. Apart from the technical aspects of managing these stages, the reader should also appreciate the very subtle clinical judgments that are part of therapy, particularly regarding: (1) how much distress clients can tolerate; (2) when to provide support; (3) when to exert pressure for more self-exploration; and (4) the timing and sequencing of the various stages. The complexity is multiplied even further when one considers the critical importance of the therapeutic relationship itself in providing a safe and supportive context within which exploration and change can take place.

We can see here, then, elements of virtually all the therapies discussed in previous chapters—supportive, behavioral, and relationship—all occurring in combination with insight techniques to produce a unique therapeutic form. In approaching the material in the next chapter, which deals with the actual techniques of insight therapy, the reader should keep this overview in mind and frequently refer back to Table 9.1 for a summary of these stages.

CHAPTER TEN

INSIGHT THERAPY: TECHNIQUES AND CASE STUDY

TECHNIQUES OF INSIGHT THERAPY

Although insight therapy can be an extremely challenging and fascinating process, a mere description of the techniques used in this treatment would be dull and abstract. Hence, the following sections will include not only a review of insight procedures, but also illustrations of their actual usage in the case example that was introduced in Chapter 9. In this way it is hoped that the reader will gain a more meaningful understanding of the techniques and their relationship to the unfolding therapeutic process.

It is also apparent from the last chapter that the techniques to be used depend on the particular stage of therapy. For this reason, they will be presented here so as to roughly parallel the stages described earlier: (1) initial procedures, (2) techniques of the self-exploration phase, (3) management of the contract for behavioral-emotional change, (4) implementing behavioral-emotional change, and (5) procedures during termination.

Initial Procedures

Recall from the overview in Chapter 9 that three tasks face the therapist in this initial stage of therapy: (1) to provide information and structure for the client as to the therapeutic process; (2) to clarify the client's misapprehensions about the nature of therapy; and (3) to assist the client in making a transition from an "external" to an "internal" locus of exploration. In the following excerpts from the first session with the client who had temper outbursts toward her daughter, note how the therapist handles the first two of these issues.

> **Therapist:** Do you have any ideas about why? Any guesses?
>
> **Client:** You know, it's not that I haven't thought about it a lot. I really dwell on the problem. Really tried to think it through . . . and I come up

with nothing. It's a blank. . . . And I always resolve to control myself, but then, maybe the next day, some little thing triggers it, like her spilling the milk, and my temper explodes.

A friend of mine has received therapy, and she told me it often takes a long time to figure these things out. I'm pretty sure that's what I need. I need someone to analyze my case, and figure out what's going on.

Therapist: I think you're right. It sounds like something needs to be done, and we should talk about some of the possibilities. But, while it's fresh, let me correct one thing. You mentioned needing someone to analyze your case. By that I suspect you mean that I, or some other therapist, should figure out what's happening with you and your daughter.

Client: Well, yes.

Therapist: I'm afraid it doesn't work that way very often, although I can certainly appreciate your wanting to clear this up as directly as possible. Let me give it a somewhat different emphasis. First, as you said a few moments ago, there are probably deeper things going on—within you, and in your relationship with Lisa. And sometimes it's difficult to see and understand some of the deeper processes. But the main burden of discovering and analyzing them would fall on you. Of course, I would help—offering guidance and suggestions—but for the most part you would be doing the digging and . . .

Client: But I've already done that until I'm blue in the face, and, I don't know, . . . I've been unsuccessful. . . . I was hoping that I could describe . . . well . . . you know, tell you, that . . . I don't know. . . . I guess I'm confused right now.

Therapist: Let me describe therapy in a kind of outline form, and then let's see what you think about it. In the beginning we would spend quite a bit of time helping you to learn how to explore the deeper parts of yourself. It's not always easy to do it by yourself, without guidance. Then I would encourage your putting these skills into practice, and we would go through a period where you would work very hard in learning more about yourself—investigating your needs, emotional pressures, things that make you tense, happy, angry, whatever. Once we get a better understanding of these emotional pressures, we'll be in a position to do something about relieving them or perhaps changing some things.

Client: When you say skills, er, what kinds of skills would be involved in learning more about myself that I haven't tried already?

Therapist: Well, there are a variety of procedures. Helping you to become more sensitive to your emotions, looking closely at the relationships in your life, maybe focusing on dreams and fantasies, your attitudes, hopes for the future—in short, having you learn how to focus on all those areas in your life that maybe get lost in the everyday shuffle. And certainly, from what you've told me, we would explore pretty thoroughly your feelings towards Lisa.

Client: I love her very much. I know that sounds defensive. . . . I get what you're saying, though. There's probably a lot that I don't understand about my feelings.

Therapist: While we're on it, I should also tell you that this might take quite a few sessions. It's hard to tell, because people and situations are so different; but it would not be unusual for the business of learning about yourself to take fifteen to thirty meetings. And then, going about changing things that you feel should be changed might take another fifteen to thirty sessions.

Client: Yes, so I gathered. It will take some time, but I'll work at it. I need to get this cleared up. . . . I'm ready. When do we start?

Therapist: We can start now. I think it would be best if we took a few meetings for you to tell me about yourself and what's happening with Lisa. We'll start the business of you exploring yourself, and sharing your thoughts with me as openly as possible. Then we can discuss some of the specifics of how we'll proceed from there. To begin, I think we should plan to have two sessions a week.

Note that in this excerpt the therapist tried to provide an overview of the stages in therapy and at least a rough estimate of the time involved. Issues regarding the client's and therapist's responsibilities in the insight process were dealt with, as well as some of the general areas to be explored. Finally, the therapist initiated the self-exploration process with a general prompt for the client to begin investigating herself, but without dictating the specific topics to be explored. This sort of open-ended entry into the process gives the client wide latitude and may be revealing of her current level of insight and her general approach to problems.

In the next few sessions the therapeutic task shifts toward training and orienting the client to the self-exploration process, while at the same time providing more information and clarification about therapy, as needed. These sessions are extremely important in that the basic work orientation of the client is being established, as well as the interactional style between client and therapist. The specifics of these issues will be described below, but suffice it to say that some of the therapeutic patterns that evolve in the opening five sessions may influence the entire course of treatment.

Training in exploratory procedures takes place at three levels: (1) formal didactic procedures, (2) explicit corrective feedback, and (3) subtle shaping techniques. A fourth factor, which is not a formal training technique, is also important during this opening stage. This pertains to the therapist providing an accepting, empathic atmosphere in the budding therapy relationship so that the client can feel free to work in a relatively safe, nonjudgmental setting. We will review each of these points individually in the following sections, along with examples from the illustrative case.

Didactic procedures A number of formal self-exploration techniques can be utilized and practiced during the opening stages of therapy. The first is instruction in free association, a procedure which aids in the spontaneous and open expression of thoughts, feelings, fantasies, and other mental events. Clients are instructed not to engage in censorship or rehearsal but simply to automatically verbalize mental and emotional contents as they occur. Such an approach tends to reduce inhibitions and superficial defenses that block the expression of sensitive or embarrassing material, and it also sets the general tone for open communication to the therapist. Second, clients are instructed in focusing on and reporting feelings and experiences in the "here and now," a procedure that is related to free association. Recounting events that occurred in the past can obviously be an important aspect of therapy; however, in this initial training period, an orientation towards immediate, inner experience is an important prerequisite for the deeper exploratory work to follow. Third, clients are instructed to minimize chatty or simple accounts of external events, and to focus instead on their interpretations and personal reactions to those events. Fourth, instruction is provided concerning the recording of dreams, fantasies, and daydreams that occur between sessions. Keeping written records prevents the forgetting of such fleeting experiences, and they can be a rich source of personal data useful for therapeutic analysis. Fifth, clients may also be encouraged to keep a daily diary, particularly of significant or upsetting events. Included should be descriptions of the events themselves, emotional reactions, and the circumstances surrounding the event.

All of these procedures are geared toward an "opening up" to inner experience and an analysis of events that trigger personal emotions and reactions. In sum, they serve to sensitize the client to the importance of introspection and self-discovery. The following excerpt from the second session with the case example illustrates some of these instructions.

Client: I'm not sure how to go about this. I mean, you told me to talk about myself. But I've already told you about me. I'm a housewife, a college graduate, mother of three, happily married, we've got a nice house. . . . What should I go into?

Therapist: I know it's hard because I've left things so open for you. It's important though, that I leave it open so you can be free to explore yourself in ways that are most meaningful to you. But let me describe some approaches that will be helpful to you. First, in our sessions, I would like you to be as spontaneous and as open as possible. Just say what comes to mind. Blurt it out. Don't hold back, trying to make it sound correct or plausible. Don't censor thoughts or feelings you think may be silly or embarrassing. Tune in on feelings and reactions that are happening right now, and talk about them with me. . . . This approach won't be easy, because it's not the usual way that people have conversations.

Client: I'll say.

Therapist: But this is one way to help get beneath the surface of things and to begin to look at deeper parts of yourself.

Client: That kind of conversation is very alien to me. I'm a very logical type person. I don't know if I can do it.

Therapist: We'll work on it together. You're right, it's not something that can be done immediately. It does take practice, and as you work at it, I'll try to point out times when it's going well and times when you seem to be straying.

Client: Well, I'll try, but I'm making no promises [*Laughs*].

Explicit feedback Most clients attain an intellectual understanding of the didactic procedures described above but find it difficult to put them into practice. This applies especially to free-association procedures and to descriptions of the ebb and flow of current feelings and thoughts. It is less anxiety provoking to talk about external events and to engage in prerehearsed descriptions of symptoms. Long-term conversational habits as well as psychological defenses prompt an avoidance of unstructured excursions into inner experience. Thus clients need practice in approaching this spontaneous and inner-oriented exploration, and an important component of that practice is the feedback provided by the therapist. As clients at first go through brief periods of this introspective mode, the therapist acknowledges and encourages these successes. By the same token, when the client drifts into an avoidant, defensive approach, the therapist may point this out and encourage a return to the more open style. Even though major insights are unlikely during this early stage of treatment, the feedback progressively guides the client into the arena where self-discovery can take place.

Let us return to the case illustration in the middle of the second session. The client has maintained her rather precise, unemotional, and businesslike approach to therapy.

Client: I feel sort of silly trying to talk this way. I think we should be talking about me and my daughter.

Therapist: That's fine. Talk about what you sense is relevant.

Client: I'm still caught in all this guilt, and, I guess, fear, about what I'm doing to her.

Therapist: Yes, I see. You're doing fine.

Client: But I seem to be stuck. If anything, my outbursts have been getting worse for a number of years now. It's frustrating. . . . You know, a thought just popped into my head. It doesn't fit in anyplace, but since you want me to describe such random thoughts, here it is. Lisa is my husband's favorite among the children. I don't see where that has anything to do with the situation, but there it is. As I think I told you earlier, my husband, Herb, is very understanding during my little episodes. And he's generally a very easygoing person. . . . He works as the office manager in the _____ Company, which I'm sure you know is one of the biggest firms in the city. I think they have something like five hundred employees in the home office alone, and I saw in yesterday's paper that they may even be taking over the _____ Company. . . . Well, where was I? I, er, how should I say it, I can't seem to get the knack of what I'm supposed to do.

Therapist: You were going along fine, but then maybe you began to, I'm not sure, but, back off a little? Did you sense that?

Client: Yes, I guess I did. It's really not important how many employees his company has. Do I do that a lot? I'll have to watch that.

Subtle shaping techniques Deep and honest self-exploration seems to take place in some contexts more than others. It probably does not occur very often when someone else (i.e., the therapist) is dictating what the client should be feeling. It is not likely to occur in passive responses to a series of questions through which the therapist is trying to guide the conversation. Self-exploration appears to be a far more active and complex process in which the client is both immersed in the flow of memories, current feelings, needs, and inner experience and can also step back, so to speak, and logically analyze and evaluate these experiences. In its ultimate form, self-discovery seems to involve a very private process of digging deep within oneself, being totally open to inner stimuli, logically appraising one's own reactions and behaviors, and gaining a broad and valid perspective on one's way of life. It is this overall orientation that the therapist is attempting to foster within the client during these early stages of the insight process. The didactic training and feedback techniques described above help to instill this exploratory frame of mind. It can also be fostered at a more basic level, that is, in the moment-by-moment verbal and emotional exchanges that take place between therapist and client.

At a structural level we can analyze the client-therapist interaction as follows. Let us say that the client makes a fairly complex statement that is composed of (1) a recounting of what someone else said to her yesterday, (2) a description of the setting in which this speech occurred, and (3) her emotional reaction to the other person. Upon hearing this incident, the therapist, if she or he is going to respond at all, has a choice of which component of the client's communication to comment upon. If the therapist directs attention to the other's statement ("I wonder why she said that") she or he is, in effect, guiding the client to talk about something external (the possible motives of someone else). Similarly, should the therapist respond to some issue pertaining to the setting, the client's attention is drawn to external factors. However, by responding to the third component (the client's emotional reaction) the therapist is communicating the message that *this* is the relevant territory for the insight process.

Such points occur with great frequency in each therapy session and hence provide many opportunities to shape and guide the client toward an internal and introspective frame of reference. One particularly effective interview technique that accomplishes this aim is *reflection of feelings*. Originally popularized by Carl Rogers, this technique is widely used by insight therapists of diverse theoretical orientations. In essence, the therapist attends very closely to the emotions being communicated in each of the client's statements and then attempts to state (reflect) those feelings to the client in an empathic, nonjudgmental fashion. The therapist is thereby communicating to the client several ends: (1) that his or her emotions are especially important issues; (2) that the therapist understands and accepts these feelings; and (3) that further communication of these inner experiences are (implicitly) expected. An important feature of this technique is its unobtrusiveness; that is, it tends not to interrupt the smooth flow of a client's exploration of inner processes.

Toward the latter part of the second session with the case illustration is an excerpt involving the therapist's shaping procedures, which include, among other responses, reflections of feelings.

Client: My husband surprised me last week when I told him I was going to seek therapy. He's usually so easygoing that he'll go along with whatever I want to do. But when I told him about therapy, he was taken aback. He said that he would not try to talk me out of it but that he did not feel therapy was necessary and that he would not be a part of it. I suppose he feels it's a problem we should work out between ourselves. His firmness on the point was quite surprising.

Therapist: Describe your reactions some more.

Client: Well, it's just that it came as a surprise. Uncharacteristic of him, you might say. . . . Sometimes I wish he would be more firm with me generally . . . or at least control me when I'm having an outburst towards Lisa. But he just seems incapable of it . . . or maybe these temper tantrums of mine catch us all unawares. They happen so fast nobody can control them. . . . It's me who has got to control myself.

Therapist: Right now your feelings about it maybe go in several directions. "Why doesn't he control me when I act that way? But, they happen so quickly, he can't be blamed . . ."

Client: No! It's clearly illogical to blame him. It's my responsibility. I'm the one doing it to Lisa. He can't be expected to get inside my head and prevent these outbursts before they occur.

Therapist: And if I sense your feelings right now, it's kind of, indignation, saying, "Hey, wait a minute, Herb can't be blamed for these temper outbursts."

Client: That's right. I'm the one who is responsible [*Pause*]. I don't know, when I talk about it like this, or even think about it by myself, I feel kind of, I don't know what you'd call it . . . unresolved, or something. I get the feeling that there are other things going on, underneath. It's disturbing. I get upset with myself when I can't figure things out logically. . . . What do you think? I see that our time is just about up.

Therapist: I'm very pleased with the way it's going. You're working hard—analyzing, exploring. You sense some unresolved things within you, for which there are no ready answers. But that's to be expected. That's part of therapy. They will become clearer as we continue to work at it.

The use of didactic training procedures, corrective feedback, and subtle shaping techniques seem to be producing a gradual but progressive "opening up" to inner experiences within the client. She can sense some underlying issues and anxieties within herself that seem to represent both a mystery and a challenge. During the first four sessions, however, her mode of approach to therapy continues to be predominantly unemotional and precisely logical. Her occasional forays into feelings and self-analysis result in heightened anxiety, which prompts a hasty retreat to a rigidly intellectual style. Also, throughout these sessions her means of relating to the therapist is extremely formal and tense. She appears to be working very hard to follow instructions and to enter an "exploratory frame of mind." It's as if she were being an exceedingly good student who is working so hard at the assigned tasks that there is rarely any opportunity for interpersonal spontaneity. In sum, she has gained an intellectual understanding of the approach to be taken in the insight process and she has begun an orientation toward self-exploration, but a great deal of work has yet to be done. The time is ripe in therapy for an expansion of techniques that encourage insight and self-discovery.

Techniques of the Self-Exploration Phase

The "turning inward" by the client accomplished during the beginning sessions is followed by a progressive elaboration of treatment procedures designed to promote self-exploration. Thus is entered a period of therapy in which anxieties and resistances need to be overcome, threatening emotions are confronted, and eventually, a broad-ranging self-evaluation takes place. A journey into the unknown is begun in earnest.

Three classes of therapy techniques are available during this phase, and they are used concurrently during this relatively lengthy period. These techniques are:

1. Interview techniques that promote intellectual analysis, including (a) nondirective leads, (b) open-ended questions, (c) requests for logical analysis, (d) elucidation of inconsistencies, (e) dream analysis, (f) summary of repetitive patterns, and (g) interpretations of motives and feelings.

2. Interview techniques that promote direct experiencing, including (a) free association, (b) reflection of feeling, (c) guided fantasy, (d) role playing, and (e) confronting resistance and defenses.

3. Relationship techniques that promote insight, including (a) the anonymity of the therapist, (b) management of early signs of transference, (c) control of the intensity of transference, and (d) interpretation of the client-therapist relationship.

We can see the relation of these classes of procedures to the overall therapy process in Fig. 10.1. Note that after the initial stage of therapy, which roughly encompasses the first five sessions, the self-exploration procedures all come into play for the remainder of the insight phase of treatment. After this phase, in which clients have analyzed and evaluated their inner dynamics, they are prepared to engage in a period of negotiation and decision as to what personal changes are to be accomplished; thereafter, treatment enters the relatively lengthy period of behavioral-emotional change.

On the following pages, each of the insight procedures will be described, along with excerpts from the case study to illustrate their application. Even

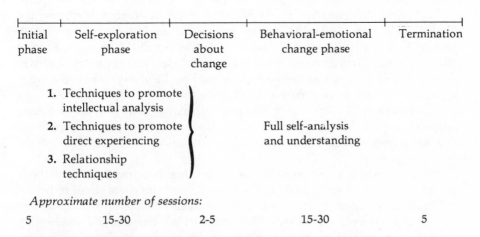

Figure 10.1 Relationship of self-exploration techniques to overall therapy process.

though the techniques are described individually, it should be kept in mind that they are most often used in various combinations throughout the self-exploration phase, depending on the needs of the moment.

Techniques promoting intellectual analysis *Nondirective leads* and *open-ended questions* represent two of the more frequently used "bread-and-butter" interview techniques. They are relatively mild, nonintrusive therapist responses that serve as prompts to the client to continue exploring and communicating. Nondirective leads usually consist of brief verbal statements urging further analysis of the ongoing topic and can be illustrated by such comments as "Yes, please go on," "Try to look into that some more," or "Tell me what you're thinking." Open-ended questions convey the same sort of encouragement, with perhaps slightly greater demand for response. Examples here are, "What does that mean to you?" and "What would you like to talk about today?" Both techniques are relatively nondirective as to topic and permit a wide range of choice as to how clients will react to these prompts.

Requests for logical analysis, as the term implies, are requests for the client to engage in a rational consideration of a topic or a set of experiences that has recently been discussed. Depending on the content, this may involve an analysis of motives, evaluation of the effects of one's behaviors on others, a review of a particular, recurrent pattern, and so forth. Several examples would be: "You mentioned how very nervous you get when we discuss school. Why do you think that occurs?"; "Let's figure that one out some more. How would you explain it?"; and "Is it possible that there are some other factors that we haven't considered yet?"

Elucidating inconsistencies is a more confrontive technique than those cited above. Here the therapist may ask clients to consider two (or more) seemingly contradictory aspects of their behavior. Such inconsistencies may reflect conflicts or vacillations in interpersonal affairs or may represent contending emotional patterns. By highlighting these discrepant reactions, the therapist encourages and stimulates analysis of unconscious or dimly perceived conflicts in a relatively directive fashion. Illustrations of this procedure are as follows: "Yesterday you mentioned that your brother was the greatest guy in the world, and yet you just finished telling me how he always takes advantage of you and the rest of your family. I'm having trouble fitting these two images of him together." "You're very insistent in saying that you are a tough, independent person who doesn't need anybody. Yet I couldn't help noticing your sad expression and misty eyes when you said that. Is there something more going on here?"

Dream analysis is, of course, one of the time-honored insight methods stemming from the psychoanalytic tradition. Clients are encouraged to record and then report dreams, fantasies, and daydreams in therapy. Since dream content and symbols are so individualistic and are frequently prompted by everyday occurrences in the lives of clients, therapists usually adopt a nondirective approach with such material. That is, clients are encouraged to actively interpret their own dreams, with the therapist playing a relatively passive role. Adjunct techniques used here are to prompt free associations to the dream content, request clients to logically analyze the symbols, mood, or emotional currents in the dream, and to point out inconsistencies in the dream material. Various therapist responses in this realm are: "What does the dream mean to you?"; "Tell me everything that pops into mind as you think about the dream"; and "As you think about the mood in your dream, how does that relate to the way you've been feeling lately?"

Summarizing repetitive patterns is a technique that has the client inspect and evaluate behavioral and emotional responses that seem to recur with some frequency in his or her life. As such it encourages taking a broader perspective on the repetitive problems that may characterize the client's maladjustment, rather than merely focusing on individual events. Because of this summarizing quality, the technique tends to be used more frequently during the middle and later portions of the insight phase. Two examples of actual therapist responses in this area are: "It seems to me that whenever someone gets close to you, you react in the same way. Is there a pattern there? What do you think?" and "Okay, you just finished telling me how badly you reacted when your boss criticized you. Wasn't that the same reaction you described last week when you were talking about that tough teacher you had in high school?"

Interpretation of motives and feelings is perhaps the most directive and confrontive of the insight techniques. Here the therapist attempts to point out emotional and motivational patterns of which the client is unaware. It is considered a relatively risky procedure for several reasons: the confrontation with the unrecognized material may be too anxiety provoking for the client; the interpretation may be rejected by the client and thus result in a degree of disharmony in the therapeutic relationship; or the interpretation may actually be incorrect, leading to confusion and misdirection in the treatment process. For these reasons, this technique is used relatively infrequently and with considerable caution. When utilized, it is usually under conditions in which the client is open and responsive to new insights and the "evidence" upon which the interpretation is based is reasonably clear and apparent to both participants. Examples are as follows: "You've been telling me that you're always quitting jobs because they're so boring and meaningless, but aren't there some strong elements of fear also mixed in here?" "I really think you're rationalizing. You do all these marvelous things for your son, because, as you say, you love him so much. Then why do I get this sense that you're also very angry with him?"

The techniques described in this section, for the most part, lead to logical analyses of client behaviors and emotions. They represent therapist activities that orient the client toward an intellectual understanding of his or her problems. As indicated earlier, they are used in conjunction with techniques stemming from the two other classes of insight procedures (experiential and relationship) throughout the self-exploration phase of treatment. It is virtually impossible to describe the exact ways in which these various techniques are combined and sequenced in actual practice, since these issues depend on the unique quality of each client's management of the insight process. As a general rule, however, the three classes of techniques may be utilized in a fairly balanced manner during self-exploration. That is, clients are encouraged to directly experience underlying emotions, needs, and reaction patterns, to "see" their operation in the therapeutic relationship, and ultimately, to rationally analyze and understand them.

Before proceeding to a description of the experiential and relationship techniques for promoting insight, excerpts from the illustrative case will be presented. Note in these excerpts that not all of the therapist's activities represent techniques that promote intellectual analysis. Some involve providing support and structure for the client. Others are illustrative of insight techniques to be described in subsequent sections. Nevertheless, these excerpts are representative of the course of the self-exploration process in its early stages.

As we get into deeper and more emotional material with this client it will be instructive to include several commentaries on the therapist's personal reactions during the treatment process. These are included to convey not only the therapist's emotional involvement but also the factors that went into various therapeutic judgments and decisions during the self-exploration phase.

Fourth session

Client: Before we get started today I want to ask your opinion on something. I was thinking pretty hard on how to approach this whole business, and I believe it's important that I should start by telling you my background—the story of my life, so to speak. Maybe as you hear it you can pick up some things that may be helpful. What do you think?

Therapist: You sound as if you think this could be important, and I'd like you to feel free to explore what seems relevant to you.

Client: Okay, let me try it. I'll go back to the beginning. [*The client proceeds with a very bland, unemotional account of her history. Throughout this fairly lengthy narrative her very precise, intellectual, and emotionless approach does not change.*]

I was born in Belgium. My parents were Jewish, pretty orthodox, and they were both professional people. Doctors. They were both on the staff at _____ Hospital. I had one younger sister, two years younger than me. You know, the one who is now living in Arizona. We were a very close-knit family. I can remember my parents in those early years as being absolutely wonderful. The house was always filled with affection. They gave us a great deal of time. Everyone was close to one another. . . . It's hard to describe. How should I say it? Those early years just seemed brimming with affection [*Pause*].

I was young, five or six, when the war broke out. I don't think I even noticed it really, to tell the truth. Oh, I suppose I must have noticed a general increase in tension. My parents had to work long hours, and so forth, but I think they were so protective, and at ease with us girls, that we didn't realize what was going on.

A short time after the Germans occupied, it happened. I remember I was standing at the front window. I was six. A covered truck stopped in front of our house, and men in uniform jumped out. I really didn't know what was happening, but my parents were wild. In a matter of seconds my parents had my sister and I at the back door, and they sent us across the alley to our neighbor's house. It all happened so fast. The next thing I knew my sister and I were looking out the neighbor's window, and the soldiers were dragging my parents to the truck. Naturally, we didn't understand about concentration camps as children, but I think I somehow realized—perhaps from the reactions of our neighbors—that we would never see our parents again.

[*Therapist commentary:* As I listened to this account I was plunged into a deep, fearful despair. All the unspeakable agonies of the holocaust enveloped me. Even more, the image of a six-year-old child, seeing her parents being dragged off to their deaths, gripped me with grief and anxiety. How terror-stricken she must have been at the time. Absolute, stark, childlike terror.

Then why was I not seeing signs of that terror now, however remote, as she described this incident? She was recounting the story in a thoroughly businesslike, unemotional way. Not a flicker of anxiety or grief was in evidence. I became confused. How could I be responding to all this with devastating inner reactions when she was merely telling it in simple narrative form? What was going on with her?

One possible answer suggested itself almost immediately. The terror of the incident must have been so shattering to her childhood personality that she long ago learned to repress and hide from those emotions. She can recall the incident itself, but the horrors associated with it seemingly are not being experienced.

Whatever the reason for her apparent lack of feelings, it seemed inappropriate for me to interject my overwhelming reactions at this point. I decided to simply continue listening to her story.]

Client: It didn't end there. The Gestapo knew about us. They were searching . . .

Therapist: Yes, I understand. Go on.

Client: Well, my memory is blurred on the next period of time. Maybe several months. We were moved from place to place. Smuggled, as it were, from neighbor, to friend, to relative. It may not be accurate, but I felt that we were just a step ahead of being dragged off ourselves.

Therapist: It must have been frightening for you.

Client: Yes, I suppose so. Somehow we were brought to England. I vaguely remember other refugee children for a brief time. And then my sister and I were adopted by an elderly couple. We went to live with them in the country. It was a beautiful, elegant place. They were wealthy—very upper class. They were old and lonely. We became the center of their lives. They showered us with love and support. They must have known that we needed it. And I suppose, in their loneliness, they needed us as well.

Therapist: Sounds as if it was a very important time for you both. For helping to put your life back together.

Client: I was six years old, and I settled into their way of life very quickly. We received all the privileges of the English upper class, even though a war was going on. Clothes, private tutors, many advantages, and most of all, the couple's constant love and attention. It didn't take long before I started to view them as my real parents. I was young. I needed them. . . . My sister and I lived with them for the next nine years, and I loved them very much.

Therapist: What happened then?

Client: One day, quite unexpectedly, we got a letter from the United States. It was from my parents. . . . They had survived. Somehow they had survived the camps. They had looked for us all over Europe after the war, but it took all that time. Now they wanted my sister and me to pack immediately, leave our foster parents, and join them. . . . I was really torn. I wanted to go to my parents, but I was crushed by the thought of leaving the old couple. Within a matter of days we left for the United States. I never saw those lovely old people again.

Therapist: All this must have had some strong effects on you. What do you think they might be?

Client: Well, for one, I'm a very, very tense person . . .

Techniques promoting direct experiencing Before continuing with the case presentation, let us review insight techniques that are aimed primarily at focusing the client on immediate inner experiences. Recall that these procedures are used concurrently with other insight techniques during the self-exploration phase.

We have already encountered two of the most important techniques in this area in the discussion of the opening phase of therapy: *free association* and *reflection of feelings*. Both are designed to foster sensitivity to moment-by-moment internal stimuli and the spontaneous, uncensored communication of these experiences. Relative to the other procedures to be described in this section, these two are by far the most frequently used.

On occasion, the techniques of *guided fantasy* and *role playing* are used to focus attention on the feelings associated with specific incidents or interpersonal events. In each technique the therapist verbally describes a situation to the client and requests that the client remain sensitive to the emotions that are elicited. These feelings may then be analyzed in subsequent discussion. An example of guided fantasy, drawn from our case illustration, is as follows:

Therapist: I want you to picture in your mind that time when you were packing—getting ready to leave the elderly couple. . . . There you are putting clothes in the suitcase. . . . Tune in your feelings. . . . Describe them.

Client: It's funny, because I know that I'm terribly frightened, but there is a sort of shell around the feelings. It won't let the feelings burst forth . . .

An example of role playing, dealing with this same episode in the client's life, is as follows:

Therapist: Imagine yourself during that same time, talking to your sister. You had both just heard that your parents were alive, and you were to go to the United States. . . . Get in the mood. You're sixteen years old. The two of you are alone. Tell me what you're saying and feeling.

Client: I'm telling her I don't want to go. No! I can't go. It's too much to ask. It's unfair. She's crying. . . . How can I say it's unfair? My God, they're alive [*Pause*]. What's the matter with me? [*Pause*]. I can't do this. It's too silly. . . . I want to return to telling you the rest of my background.

Techniques that promote direct experiencing are probably most prone to elicit resistance and defensiveness. This is understandable, since direct exposure to emotions and needs is perhaps the most threatening aspect of the insight process. It is appropriate, therefore, to discuss the management of defensiveness in the present section. A number of options are open to the therapist on this issue, and their use is determined largely by the degree of distress being experienced by the client.

Under most circumstances when clients avoid or withdraw from certain topics or emotions, the therapist will increase levels of personal support and reassurance. This is done under the assumption that an anxiety system has been touched upon and hence the client may be better able to confront the threatening material when external supports are provided.

In most cases therapists also point out to the client that avoidance or "backing off" seems to be occurring. This sort of feedback helps clients become aware of the momentary emotional dynamics in the situation and also serves to make them more sensitive to their defensive tactics in the future.

The more critical choices regarding the management of resistance occur with respect to how much pressure the therapist will exert to have the client return to the threatening material. Obviously, at one extreme, the therapist may respond passively and merely acknowledge and accept the client's defensiveness. This option would be chosen when, in the therapist's judgment, excessive distress would be generated by further confrontation with the difficult material. Another option, perhaps the one most frequently used, is the application of mild exhortations to return to the threatening issues, along with encouragement to tolerate the distress that is evoked. This therapeutic tactic may be accompanied by continued use of insight techniques that prompt direct experiencing (e.g., reflection of feeling).

Continuing with the case example, the following illustrates a relatively mild response to the client's defensiveness when she was role playing the conversation with her sister:

Client: I can't do this. It's too silly. . . . I want to return to telling you the rest of my background.

Therapist: You seem to have touched on something disturbing just now, and want to get back to more straightforward material.

Client: Well, maybe. . . . I really can't tell if I'm just not in the mood for that kind of imaginary conversation, or if it triggered some darker issues I'm not ready to face.

Therapist: I realize it can seem confusing and vague and sometimes upsetting. That's part of therapy, however. It can be worth taking some risks in order to get at the difficult issues.

Client: You're right, I know. Let me see if I can get back in the mood. . . . I really didn't want to go, but I felt obligated to my parents, and . . .

[*Therapist commentary:* In the case example, the various techniques for promoting intellectual analysis and direct experiencing were continued through subsequent sessions. However, because of the client's predominantly unemotional, businesslike approach throughout the early period of treatment, a decision to rely more heavily on direct experiencing procedures was made.]

Seventh session

Client: Well, I told you last time how much I disliked the United States when I first came here. I didn't have any friends. School was boring, although I was doing very well academically. . . . I just didn't fit in. . . . That went on for two years, and I was miserable. . . . I corresponded with my foster parents, and their letters were bright spots, but basically I was very lonely.

Therapist: Even as you talk about it now, I guess I can sense the gloomy feelings.

Client: When I was eighteen, things took a dramatic turn for the better. I met this boy, man, I should say, who was in law school. We started seeing each other . . . and we both fell head-over-heels in love with each other. It was amazing. We were on the same wavelength on everything. We saw each other all the time. . . . We had what you might call perfect communication. We could be together and not say a word, and yet we both knew what was going on in the other. I just let myself go completely in that relationship. It was complete and mutual in every respect [*Sad expression on her face*]. I loved him so much, he could have used me for a doormat and I would still have been supremely happy.

Therapist: Sounds as if you . . .

Client: And what's more, the relationship was getting stronger and stronger. I didn't think it was possible, but it was. . . . We had been going together for seven or eight months, and then, out of the blue, he said it was all over. I thought he was joking. No signs, no warning. Just finished. . . . Oh, I don't know, he said we were too serious, you know. He wasn't ready to settle down, that sort of thing. It, it was, was all over. . . . I really went off the deep end. It was too much for me. Everything within me shut down. I become deeply depressed . . . and stayed that way, it seems, for a long time. Two months, three, I don't know. But then I slowly started to come out of it, and some new emotions took over . . . I came out of it very angry — at him, at men in general, I guess, at the whole world. And I also remember, very vividly, that I made a solemn promise to myself never to again let my feelings go out to anyone. I couldn't tolerate that sort of thing happening to me again. I didn't think I could survive another loss like that [*Starts to weep*].

Therapist: The hurt is just too much. It touches you too deeply.

[*Therapist commentary:* I had been working very hard during these early sessions to develop a formulation of the major forces operating in the client's personality. There were many factors, many possible interpretations, but the one that began to take shape most insistently in my own mind, involved the central theme of *separation*. This woman had undergone three devastating losses of loved ones in her life: her parents, her foster parents, and her first romantic partner. Moreover, all three losses occurred under special circumstances. They were sudden, unexpected, and lire altering. To be sure, the separation from her parents must have been the most shattering and overwhelming, producing childhood terrors so strong they had to be repressed. Each subsequent loss produced agonies of their own, but also must have rearoused the horrors of the original separation. The repeated cruelties of fate left her, in her own mind, a marked woman.

One other factor assumes importance in this interpretation. Each of the sudden, unexpected separations occurred when the relationships involved were at a height of affection and openness. The emotional conditioning that took place resulted in the feeling that when you are close, open, and affectionate with someone, this sets the stage for loss and abandonment. Fate will now strike. Is it any wonder that she vowed, when she was eighteen, never to open her feelings to anyone ever again?]

Eighth session

Client: I'm not sure how to explain it, but I can feel some changes taking place within me. Right now I'm calmer than I've been in a long time. I've become much better with Lisa. I haven't had an outburst in over a week, and not many before that. . . . But at the same time I feel some deeper things, I just get vague, what should I call them, premonitions, of darker issues that I have to deal with [*Laughs*]. The curious workings of the feminine mind.

Therapist: Some deeper stirrings are there, and they're hard to identify. Can you get in the mood to work on it? See if we can get closer to them?

Client: No. Not now. I'm kind of enjoying the relaxation, and my improvement with Lisa.

Therapist: Okay. What should we work on today?

Client: Well, I wanted to tell you about graduate school. . . . When I finished college, I was accepted in the graduate program at _____, so I left home, and [*Laughs*] struck out on my own. It was exciting and I was doing very well. During the first year I met Herb, my husband. He was just starting out with his firm. Very hardworking, but with me, terribly attentive. He was always there when I wanted to see him. No pressures, no hassles. Just a nice, retiring, very attentive person. . . . The relationship stayed that way for a year, and we decided to get married. I was to continue in school, while he made his way in business.

Therapist: Seemed like a comfortable, relaxed arrangment?

Client: Yes it was. You know how busy graduate school is. And he was good about it. After the children started coming he took on a lot of the responsibility for the household and their care, while I was at the library, or whatever . . .

[*Therapist commentary:* During the eighth and ninth sessions the client seemed to be more responsive to inner stimuli, and she worked hard to communicate the vague feelings and ideas that were emerging. The many crosscurrents seemed to come together in the tenth session when, for the first time, she felt she had gained some perspective on her problems.]

Tenth session

   Client: I had a dream last night. It was very short, but also very vivid. I think it could be important. . . . Here's the way it went. In the dream, my husband and I were giving a cocktail party for an out-of-town guest, and the party was taking place in our living room. All the people at the party were hovering around the guest of honor, being attentive, making small talk. My husband was in the group, and in the dream I walked into the living room. I fully expected Herb to kind of turn, acknowledge that I had arrived, and invite me into the group. But he ignored me. Just at that point, still in the dream, Lisa called from her bedroom and asked me for a glass of water. A perfectly normal request. But in the dream, I flew into a rage and had a violent temper tantrum towards Lisa. I woke up still feeling that rage, and then a terrible guilt came over me.

   Therapist: What do you think it means?

   Client: Well, I've already interpreted it. I stayed up all night thinking about it. And my interpretation, although not very pleasant, really makes sense to me.

   Therapist: Yes?

   Client [*Very serious and determined*]: You know, the real problems in my life are not between me and Lisa. They're between Herb and me. I've been hiding from that fact for months, years even, but there it is. Whatever these problems are with me and Herb, I've been taking them out on Lisa. Sort·of diverting my anger and frustration onto her—his favorite, remember? I'm afraid I've led us both down a blind alley in therapy. . . . I need to start exploring my marriage . . . but I sense that it will be a hard thing to do.

   For the next four sessions the client, with great difficulty and considerable anxiety, began to explore her marital relationship. A number of important themes gradually emerged, which are summarized below and are then followed by excerpts that convey the emotional quality of each.

   1. After ten years of marriage, she feels totally "shriveled up" and unfulfilled emotionally. The underlying feelings of anger and frustration have been growing for the last five years.

   2. She blames her husband *exclusively* for her condition. She views him as having been a chronically passive and unromantic person whose lack of assertiveness and responsivity produced an emotional void in all realms of their relationship. She now feels strong anger towards him; however, this is not expressed openly.

   3. Despite her underlying anger and frustration, she also can recall suffering throughout her marriage (and now as well) from a pervasive anxiety that somehow she might lose her husband. At times, this chronic anxiety would rapidly escalate to near panic levels, during which she would experience frenzied worries that the loss was imminent. She described how inappropriate these fears were, because Herb continued to be a remarkably attentive and constant companion throughout their marriage. Nevertheless, the intense fears remained that some sudden, unexpected disaster would occur that would result in his being taken away.

[*Therapist commentary:* Throughout these sessions I felt that an important door had been opened and that extremely important material was now emerging. I was also struck by the fact that her rigidly intellectual approach to therapy had given way to considerable expressiveness and a greater openness to her emotions.

Perhaps most striking to me was the observation that, despite her deeper explorations, she could not see her own role in the marital unhappiness. She rigidly maintained that all the blame fell on her husband. The fact that she had "walled off" her own emotions after the disastrous separation from the law student and that she had in many ways structured the marriage to be a convenient, unemotional arrangement went unrecognized during this period of treatment.

Moreover, the deeper dynamics of her fears about separation, and their childhood roots, were still far removed from therapeutic discussion. My earlier, tentative interpretation was becoming more defined: that is, that after the three major interpersonal losses in her life, she had developed a very strong defense of rigidly withholding her feelings of affection and closeness in any new relationship (including the marriage). Should she let these feelings emerge, she would run the double risks of (1) being terribly hurt once again if a separation occurred, and perhaps even more shattering, (2) rearousing the childlike terrors connected with the loss of her parents—terrors that have been lurking in the background for most of her life.]

Fourteenth session

Client: There were times when I would almost go crazy with fear. I became absolutely convinced that in some way I would lose Herb. It was totally ridiculous, but I would be paralyzed by the fear itself. . . . Look at me, I'm a nervous wreck just talking about it. . . . I want to run away from it . . .

Therapist: It was just that overwhelming fear that something undefined would happen to make you lose him.

Client: Yes, I've lived that way through all of my marriage . . . fearful all the time.

Therapist: Where do you think that comes from?

Client: I really don't know . . . maybe because he was such an unloving person. You know how frustrating that is. . . . I don't know. He just can't seem to give me enough reassurance. . . . I can't tell what it is. . . . I don't feel like I'm on the right track . . .

Relationship techniques promoting insight The third of the major classes of insight procedures involves the relationship that the client gradually develops with the therapist. Under certain specialized circumstances the behavioral-emotional aspects of this relationship can serve as important vehicles for self-exploration. We are discussing here outgrowths of the psychoanalytic notion of *transference*.

In essence, this concept suggests that individuals tend to repeat the behavioral-emotional patterns developed in their early, formative (parental) relationships in their later social encounters. Thus the feelings, expectations, defenses, and fears that were part of the child-parent relations become important emotional cornerstones of adolescent and adult interpersonal patterns. As the therapeutic relationship develops beyond the initial amenities, and these more unique and deeper aspects of the client's personality become involved, a sort of window into the past is opened. Here then is a relationship in the "here and now" that can reflect both the positive elements and the tragedies of the past. As such, the therapeutic relationship itself can be a profitable area for inspection and analysis. As clients come to understand their contributions to the therapy relationship, they can gain firsthand insight into how their emotional history is affecting current interpersonal affairs.

This "transferred" relationship seems to emerge more clearly and intensely under certain conditions. First, transference is enhanced when the therapist remains relatively *anonymous*; that is, although the therapist interacts with the client in a generally encouraging, supportive fashion, he or she does not typically reveal many personal details. This relative anonymity allows ample room for clients to "fill in the blanks" with their own assumptions, hypotheses, and projections about the therapist's personality. The concept of transference proposes that these assumptions are drawn from the client's own history and emotional needs, and as they emerge, the client begins to relate to the therapist *as if* the assumptions were true.

Transference also seems to develop more quickly and intensely when therapy sessions are relatively frequent. With two or more meetings per week the client's general emotional involvement with therapy is heightened, and this in turn seems to promote the emergence of transference. In addition, the process is intensified when considerable portions of therapy focus on childhood relations with parents, as opposed to an analysis of contemporary interpersonal affairs. Evidently the attention devoted to childhood needs, emotions, and modes of relating, creates a frame of reference that rekindles these patterns in the therapeutic relationship.

Apart from the theoretical bases of transference, the important issue to be borne in mind is that the client's mode of relating to the therapist represents immediate, ongoing behavior that can serve as important data for the insight process. As the client relates in maladaptive ways, develops unusual emotional reactions, or expresses unresolved conflicts and needs right in the therapy relationship, these become fruitful areas for inspection and analysis. For example, through this vehicle, clients may gain their first understanding of the negative effects on others of their behavior patterns. Or they may become aware of how unrealistic some of their emotional demands are. The immediacy of these insights, the fact that they are happening "right before their eyes" in therapy, makes this a potentially dramatic form of self-exploration.

Returning to our case example, recall that the client has been exploring her marriage with deep emotions for a number of sessions. The fifteenth and sixteenth meetings are especially important. In the fifteenth session the client reports feelings of strong anxiety and depression and a vague sense that she is getting close to some very threatening material. She even considers leaving therapy at this point, but recognizes that this would represent an avoidance of significant issues. In the sixteenth session she reports having confronted this threatening material during the previous few days, and now, in a highly emotional state, she talks about the confrontation. This pivotal session involves a convergence of transference, experiential and intellectual procedures of insight.

Therapist: Having a hard time getting started today?

Client: No. I know what I want to say. It's just so hard to say it. . . . I've been waiting to tell you for several days, but now that it's upon me, I don't know how to start [*Crying, wringing hands, very upset*]. I'm so frightened and guilty, I feel like I'm coming apart.

Therapist: Try to talk about it.

Client: Well, you remember that I was depressed and tense at the last session. I tried to shake it, but I couldn't. . . . Herb noticed that something was wrong, and suggested that we go to a play at the theater that night. . . . So we went [*Crying*] . . . and I just had a feeling that you would be there. . . . So I looked around, during the intermissions, but of course you weren't there [*Very agitated*]. And then I realized what was the matter with me. . . . I'm in love with you . . . Need you very badly . . . completely dependent [*Weeping anxiously*]. And I'm overwhelmed by fright. I feel completely helpless. I know that disaster will strike, and I'll be left completely alone [*Childlike terror in her voice*]. It's too much for me to bear. I feel like my whole personality is crumbling . . .

Therapist: These feelings have really touched on something deep and agonizing within you.

Client [*Almost screaming*]: I feel like an infant. So helpless, vulnerable. . . . I just know that I'll be left alone again. . . . These feelings . . . of closeness and affection for you . . . I feel completely at their mercy . . . I'm at the mercy of the fear . . . I just can't function . . . it's as if the feelings are tormenting me, saying . . . you let down your defenses, thought you could jig around. Okay, now cope with us . . . I can't stand it. I have to resolve these feelings or I'll crumble [*Continues in this way for several minutes, becoming more and more frightened*].

[*Therapist commentary:* As the client says, she has let down her defenses and allowed her needs for affection and closeness to be felt and expressed. These are the very emotions that in the past have been associated with life-shattering separations from loved ones: the law student, her foster parents, and primarily, as a six-year-old, from her parents. By allowing these needs to burst forth in the transference relationship, she is also rearousing all the overwhelming terrors of her parental loss, and it seems that it is these childhood terrors that she is reexperiencing in this therapy session.

Her obvious and intense suffering during the first half of this session tore at me. I wanted her to gain some relief, but at the same time I wanted her to gain some perspective on her terrors, so that she could see how they affected her emotional life and her marriage. I also wanted her to gain an understanding of where these horrible feelings came from and thereby learn that she did not have to continue to be dominated by tragedies and fears of the past. In essence, she needed to learn that it could be safe to feel open and affectionate toward others—particularly her husband and children—without having to be frightened of sudden, unexpected disaster.]

Therapist: I can't help feeling that your emotions right now are touching on deep things in your past.

Client [*Long pause; weeping subsides*] I haven't really looked at it that way. I'm just so caught up in my feelings right now [*Pause*]. I had the same intensity of feelings toward the first boy I was in love with—the law student. . . . And I suffered so much afterwards—I nearly died—that I made a promise to myself never to feel that way toward anyone again. . . . That was so many years ago, I thought I had gotten over it.

Therapist: But now you're . . .

Client: Now I'm wondering if I really did get over it. . . . I knew when I started going with Herb that it wasn't the same. I didn't have the same intensity or depth of feeling with him. . . . I thought it was more mature . . . that affection would grow . . . but, but [*Starts weeping uncontrollably*] as I look back at ten years of marriage now, I know I never once let myself go . . . never once gave my feelings to him. . . . Oh, my God! What a waste! . . . Ten years of marriage down the drain. . . . And it wasn't Herb's fault—the poor, sweet, tolerant guy—it was mine. I was too scared to give him the feelings that rightfully belong to him. . . .

It was safer, the way I made it happen. . . . Oh, my God! Herb, what have I done to you . . . and the children?

Therapist: Those fears, and the hurt, must have really been profound.

Client [*Getting very agitated again*]: Well, I couldn't risk letting my feelings go. After the breakup, when I was eighteen, I knew I'd be destroyed if I let myself love someone again, and, and . . . if they left me again [*Crying*].

Therapist: Being left *again* . . .

Client [*Crying suddenly stops. The same frozen expression as in the first session of therapy comes over her face. And then it melts into a look of absolute anguish and terror. She wails desperately*]: Mamma! Mamma, ahhh, eeeah! Pappa! No. Come back. . . . Mamma, *ahhh, argh* [*Convulses in tears for long period*]. Those bastards. Those filthy, Nazi bastards! . . . They took them away. Left me alone [*Shivering*]. Why me? I could have gone with them. Holy God, why did they leave me? [*Long pause*]. Is it any wonder I can't love anyone—can't let my feelings go? . . . I can feel it freezing over now. . . . Oh, Mamma, Poppi . . . Herb.

Therapist: You've faced it. The agony at the bottom of the pit.

Client [*Exhausted, withdrawn*]: Yes. That's it. . . . What filth. Excrement [*Long pause*]. How can people do that to fellow human beings? I'll never fathom it. Never get over it [*Pause*]. You know, I can see myself, in my mind's eye . . . the little girl in the window [*Embittered, distant*] . . . the filth of the world burying any tenderness and love she might have been capable of.

Therapist: But . . .

Client: No, it's okay. Don't say anything. I'll be all right [*Bitterly*] . . . Just sit with me for a while and let me pull myself together [*More emphatically*]. . . . I'm going to be all right . . . I need to talk to Herb . . .

End of the self-exploration phase The end of the self-exploration phase of treatment is usually a time of review and summary. As the intense emotions of the earlier sessions subside, the major insights are analyzed in a more careful and rational manner, with particular emphasis on their implications for current adjustment. This work is an important forerunner to the next phase of therapy: that of negotiating and deciding on the behavioral-emotional changes to be worked on during the second half of treatment.

Table 10.1 summarizes the many techniques used during the self-exploration phase, along with a review of their applications to the case example.

Procedures in Negotiating a Contract for Change

A relatively brief phase of therapy of negotiating a contract for change occurs as a natural outgrowth of the self-exploration period. Clients at this point have

Table 10.1
Summary of principal self-exploration techniques

Techniques prompting intellectual analysis	Techniques promoting direct experiencing	Relationship techniques
Nondirective leads	Free association	Anonymity of therapist
Open-ended questions	Reflection of feelings	
Requests for logical analysis	Guided fantasy	Frequent sessions
Elucidation of inconsistencies	Role playing	Focusing on childhood relations
Dream analysis	Confronting resistance and defenses	
Summary of patterns		Interpretation of client-therapist relationship
Interpretation of motives and feelings		

Contributions to "Insight" with the Case Example

Recognition of client's role in marital problems	Facing feelings of neglect and frustration in marriage	Recognizing that intimate feelings had been withheld in marriage
Understanding effects of earlier separations	Experiencing intense fears of separation	Permitting feelings of closeness to be experienced, with accompanying anxiety

achieved an understanding of their maladaptive behavior patterns, the emotional forces associated with these patterns, and their historical roots. Toward the end of the self-exploration phase, clients have also gone through a period of reviewing and organizing their insights within the broad perspectives of their current life. They are now in a position to make decisions about desirable and feasible changes in their mode of adjustment.

During this phase, which may take roughly from two to five sessions, a number of steps usually occur in sequence: (1) explicit identification of the maladaptive patterns; (2) mutual assessment of the potential for changing each pattern; (3) decisions regarding the priorities in changing maladaptive patterns; (4) discussion and decisions about new patterns to be acquired; and (5) the development and review of strategies to bring about changes.

In order to illustrate portions of this negotiation of treatment, let us return to excerpts from several sessions with our case example.

Eighteenth session

Client: I feel as if a monstrous weight has been taken off my back. It's not going to be easy, but I can see where I need change.

Therapist: Let's talk about it . . . where you see yourself needing to change things.

Client: Well, I guess it's fairly clear, from all we've gone over. I've got to be able to let myself go with Herb. Express affection—let my feelings go out to him. . . . But you know, just talking about it . . . I can feel the waves of anxiety coming over me . . . and it's not just nervousness, or anything like that. I really get paralyzed with it. . . . God, it must be deeply ingrained in me.

Therapist: You went through some very shattering experiences.

Client: But I've got to do it. . . . If I'm going to be a full human being, I've got to let myself feel . . . and express my feelings. . . . I've got to fight the fear . . . overcome it. . . . But it's almost ridiculous when you think about it. When I allow myself to feel love and closeness with Herb, I'm also in near panic that I will lose him.

Therapist: I agree with you. It's important for you to learn to be open . . . to be able to feel and express your affection . . . and to learn to overcome the fear. These seem to be high priorities in the things we need to work on.

Client: What other things are there?

Therapist: I'm not sure, but I think we should talk some more about it . . . and maybe look more closely at some of the complexities. . . . For example, how do you think Herb will react if you now change your style of relating to him? After all, it's been over ten years.

Client [*Long pause*]: You know, I'm not sure. I do know that he's been deprived—cheated in a way—by my having withheld my emotions from him. . . . But he also seems to be comfortable the way things are—except for the problems with Lisa—and maybe he is in a comfortable emotional rut.

Therapist: Do you see any possible problems there?

Client [*Pause*]: Yes, I do. Whew! I know one thing. . . . If I go through the terrible fears involved in opening up to him, and he doesn't respond in kind, I won't be able to do it. . . . I would really be crushed . . . and very angry, I guess.

Therapist: So there are at least three things we'll need to keep in mind and work on. . . . Proceeding in such a way that Herb can kind of keep up with your changes. . . . Helping you to keep trying even though you might face some temporary disappointments. . . . And that last one, working on how best to cope with anger and frustration when they crop up.

Nineteenth session

Client: What about this fear? Am I ever going to get over it? All day yesterday I was getting myself psyched up, as they say. I wanted to be close and attentive with Herb when he came home, but by late in the afternoon I had frozen over again. The anxiety, the images and thoughts of my parents, and the fear that Herb might leave, all got mixed up together . . . and I just withdrew into myself.

Therapist: I know how upsetting it can be. You try hard, but then the fear closes in. . . . But I'm very optimistic about your being able to master it. I don't think it will go away immediately, but there are some approaches we can take that will bring about a reduction in its intensity. Also, as we work on your becoming more open with Herb and the children, and as you get good reactions back from them, that will help greatly in reducing the fear.

Client: I guess that I share your optimism. . . . I'm not saying that just to be agreeable. . . . But as we've talked about my being separated from my parents, over the last few sessions, the fright hasn't been as bad as it was. Maybe by grappling with it over and over, I'll get used to it . . . or it won't have such power over me.

Therapist: Yes. I think that will be an important part of mastering it.

Client: And you know, I don't want to get us all upset again, but I have continued to feel very open and close to you, and I obviously don't feel so distraught by those feelings.

Therapist: That's good.

Client [*Laughs*]: But the heavy artillery comes in my relationship with Herb—but even there I guess I can see the fear gradually going away in time.

[*Therapist commentary:* After four sessions of the negotiation phase, we agreed that the following issues needed to be worked on in the change phase of treatment: (1) increases in her emotional feelings of openness and expressiveness with her husband and children; (2) improvement in her abilities to communicate her feelings; (3) a decrease in the intensity of her fears of separation; (4) learning skills by which to cope with frustrations or anger-provoking situations at home. It was also decided that we would slow down the pace of therapy to one meeting per week, to allow time for these changes to develop.]

Techniques of the Behavioral-Emotional Change Phase

The procedures available to assist the client in discarding maladaptive reaction patterns and in developing new adjustive ones come largely from behavioral approaches to treatment. Since the techniques involved in behavioral treatments have already been covered in Chapter 6, they will not be repeated in detail in this section. Rather, a brief review of how these procedures were used with the case example will hopefully illustrate their applicability. Figure 10.2 provides a perspective on the relationship of the behavioral-emotional change phase to the entire treatment process and a summary of the change techniques.

Beginning the change phase with the case example As a first step in this phase of treatment the client was instructed in keeping daily records on her behaviors and feelings in four areas: emotional openness, communicating feelings, fears of separation, and the management of angry feelings. Procedures for keeping a log in which to enter these self-monitored data were reviewed in detail and it was agreed that entries should be made every day.

During the beginning sessions of the change phase, treatment plans were discussed and reviewed with the client. It was decided that the four problem areas would be worked on concurrently during this period of therapy. Further, it was agreed that in the initial stages emphasis would be placed on acquiring the necessary skills and practice in therapy itself, to be followed by her applying these skills outside of treatment as soon as was feasible. The treatment strategy for each of the problem areas was tentatively planned as follows.

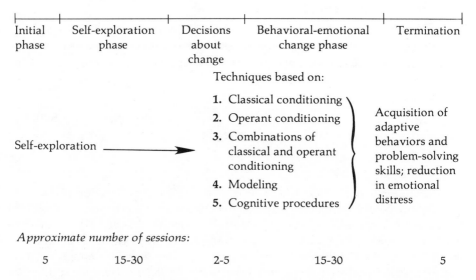

| Initial phase | Self-exploration phase | Decisions about change | Behavioral-emotional change phase | Termination |

Techniques based on:

1. Classical conditioning
2. Operant conditioning
3. Combinations of classical and operant conditioning
4. Modeling
5. Cognitive procedures

Acquisition of adaptive behaviors and problem-solving skills; reduction in emotional distress

Self-exploration ⟶

Approximate number of sessions:

| 5 | 15-30 | 2-5 | 15-30 | 5 |

Figure 10.2 Relationship of behavioral-emotional change techniques to overall therapy process.

On the issue of emotional openness, therapy would begin with discussions and analysis of the environmental and interpersonal circumstances that seem to accompany both periods of openness and times when she feels "walled off." Once identified, the client could then utilize the technique of *stimulus control* to arrange her daily routine to increase those circumstances that foster open and spontaneous feelings. In addition, an analysis would be made of the trains of thought that seem to lead to periods of emotional blunting versus those that precede periods of openness. Here again, once the negative patterns are identified the cognitive-behavioral techniques of *thought stopping* and *coverant control* would be invoked to acquire skills in interrupting ruminations that lead to being emotionally closed. (These techniques, covered in Chapter 6, refer to guided practice in which at first the therapist vigorously directs the client to stop engaging in maladaptive trains of thought, followed by improved client skills in ceasing such obsessive patterns.) Finally, it was planned that the client would practice *self-monitoring* and *self-reinforcement* skills to increase those trains of thought that lead to feelings of openness and emotional responsivity.

With regard to the second problem area, that of communicating feelings, a program that involved modeling, rehearsal, corrective feedback, and reinforcement was planned. Subsumed under the general label of *participant modeling* (see Chatper 6), these procedures involve therapist displays of how various emotions might be appropriately communicated to others, followed by client practice and refinement of the expressive behaviors. However, it was assumed in this area that since the client had an extensive history of emotional involvements and expressiveness (with the law student, foster parents, etc.) the modeling component of this program might be minimal. Greater emphasis would be placed on the reawakening of expressive patterns that are already a part of her personality makeup, coupled with their practice and refinement.

It was also assumed that, as she increased her communcation skills with husband, family, and others, naturally occurring reinforcements would strengthen this mode of relating to people.

With regard to lessening her general fears of separation, procedures akin to *counterconditioning* and *desensitization* were planned (see Chapter 6). Here, at a pace judged to be tolerable by the client, she would be exposed to increasingly intense discussions of the separations that occurred in her own life, and to anticipations of separation from her husband (however unlikely). These graduated exposures to fearful stimuli would be carried out in a context of her practicing to remain calm and gaining mastery over these fearful remnants of her past. As earlier, it was also assumed that as her emotional relationship with Herb improved, naturally occurring signs of his steadfastness would reduce her specific anxieties about losing him.

Last in the treatment plan were procedures pertaining to the management of frustration and anger. Here it was decided that a program of learning general *coping and problem-solving skills* would be instituted, with particular emphasis on how to deal with anger-provoking situations. This would begin with an analysis of those events in the client's life that usually provoked anger (for example, Herb being unromantic or emotionally bland). This would be followed by consideration of the alternative ways in which these events could be handled by the client (e.g., a temper tantrum; sullen, angry withdrawal; direct confrontation; playful seductiveness; intimate, supportive discussion).

Implementing the treatment plans The procedures outlined above were carried out over the next twelve sessions of therapy. A weekly review of her self-monitored data indicated that satisfactory progress was being made on three of the four problem areas. On the issue of emotional openness, however, the records revealed (and the client reported in therapy) that her progress was very uneven. There were times when she felt exceptionally emotional and affectionate with her husband, for example, only to become despondent as she sensed her fear rising and the defensive shell hardening. This pattern of withdrawing from emotions showed some tendency to decline as treatment progressed, but it was agreed that a considerable period of time would be required after therapy was formally terminated before this problem would be brought under control.

The following are excerpts from therapy sessions during the change phase that illustrate some of the procedures outlined above.

Twenty-third session

Therapist: We were going to work again on the fears for part of today's session.

Client: Yes, I remember. I'm ready . . . I really don't look forward to it. It's distressing, but it seems to be helping.

Therapist: Okay. Get in a fantasy mood. . . . Close your eyes, and listen to me. . . . As before, I'll describe some scenes, and I want you to let your fantasies go as I talk. I'll describe a scene that's a little stronger than last time. Okay? . . . You're in your car driving Herb to the airport. You've both been feeling close to each other, but now he is going on a three-day business trip. . . . Neither of you is saying much as you drive. . . . Get in touch with what you're feeling and thinking in this scene.

Client: I can feel some fright, but it's not too bad.

Therapist: What else?

Client: The same old stuff . . . in this case, thoughts that his plane will crash . . . and I won't see him again . . . and then what would become of me? [*Pause*]. But then another part of me says, "Stop this nonsense. It's just a simple business trip. . . . Don't be such a baby. Get with it. There's lots of things you have to get done today, and you don't have time to mope around."

Therapist: You can talk yourself out of the fears somewhat . . . sort of get control over them.

Client: Yes, maybe a little bit.

Twenty-fifth session

Therapist: Let's talk about the times you've gotten angry this week.

Client: It's interesting that you should bring that up. I was going to talk to you about that. Last Saturday was a horror. . . . It was raining, the girls were very obnoxious . . . fighting, bickering . . . all cooped up in the house. . . . Herb was no better. He was grouching around, not talking to anybody. . . . I could feel it building up within myself. First it was a general tension. Then thoughts that somehow this was all my fault. And then came the anger. . . . I knew it was one of those times when I might explode.

Therapist: Did you try some of the things we had practiced?

Client: Yes, but I don't know how successfully.

Therapist: Tell me how you went about it.

Client: Well, first I tried the analysis. It was not hard to figure out. We were all bored, confined. The kids' noise was getting on my nerves. I suppose that same was happening to Herb.

Therapist: Yes. Anything else that was making you tense?

Client: Well, I don't know [*Pause*]. Yes, I guess so. . . . It was Herb's attitude. Withdrawn, tense, as if it was my responsibility to make everything right [*Pause*]. I guess what got me most was his being withdrawn.

Therapist: I see. What did you think about on how . . . er . . . how to handle the situation?

Client: I knew I didn't want to have a tantrum toward the children. . . . I guess I also knew I shouldn't just stay in my own funk. That would just perpetuate everything. . . . I thought maybe I could get the girls playing some quiet game . . . and I, I, er, wanted to come and talk to you . . . but I figured I really should be talking to Herb. . . . But that is hard for me anyway. And especially when we were feeling the way we were.

Therapist: So far, you seemed to be putting our exercises into practice very well. . . . How did you finally handle it?

Client: It'll sound silly, but I got everyone involved in a big game of Monopoly. Even Herb played. . . . With the little ones playing it was really a mess, but we all relaxed and had a few laughs. . . . Later in the afternoon I tried to talk to Herb about my feelings, and what I'm trying to accomplish in therapy. . . . It's not so easy because I'm never sure what he's thinking . . . I suspect he still has reservations about my coming to therapy . . . but at least I tried.

Twenty-eighth session

Client: I have to tell you something that happened after our last meeting [*Laughs*]. I hope you don't think me a schoolgirl when I tell you.

Therapist: That might not be so bad, but go on.

Client: Well, remember we had been talking about my loosening up with Herb. Not being so tense, letting him know my feelings, and things like that. . . . Well, I was feeling very vulnerable and scared on the way home, but I really wanted to try to be different. When I got there, he was home for lunch, and he was very tense himself. . . . Things hadn't gone well at the office and he was just sitting there staring at the newspaper, withdrawn and uncommunicative.

Therapist: Sounds like one of those situations we discussed that makes you worried and frustrated.

Client: Yes, it was, but I decided to try something different. It sounds so trite when I say it, but I can't ever remember doing this with him [*Pause*]. . . . Well, I got my courage up and went over to him, and put my arms around him . . . mussed up his hair . . . and told him to try to relax.

Therapist: Super.

Client: Well, I don't know. I really think he was surprised . . . maybe even stunned, because that was so uncharacteristic of me. . . . He put down the paper, and gave me this very long look. . . . I didn't know what to expect. . . . He pulled me down on to his lap, and well, he loved me up a little bit . . . and that surprised me. . . . I don't know how to say it . . . his tenderness . . . his [*Laughs*] friskiness . . . I got all caught up in it too. . . . One thing led to another . . . and you know . . . we went into the bedroom. [*Serious*] I think it's the first time I really let myself go with Herb . . . we both knew it . . . I felt very profound. It was an extraordinary experience. . . . It all ended up in what I guess you would call a massive reinforcement.

Therapist [*Laughs*]: It's beginning to work just fine for you, isn't it?

Client: Yes, at least partially.

Therapist: How do you mean?

Client: Because later that evening, the old fears swept over me . . . crazy mixed-up fears. . . . I knew where they were coming from, but they are still hard to deal with . . .

[*Therapist commentary:* I guess that I am feeling pretty pleased with myself about this case. Here is a woman who was emotionally stifled by her own fears and tragic background. She is now working hard to overcome these destructive patterns, and is meeting with success. Naturally, the road ahead of her has its pitfalls and obstructions; but at the same time she seems to be developing ways to cope with them.

There were many other issues that could have been considered in her case—the deeper dynamics of her aggression, guilt feelings about her having survived the holocaust, the complexities of her relationships with her daughters—but as the therapy developed it appeared that her deep fear of separation was the central dynamic in her problems.

During the thirtieth session she casually asked about how much longer therapy would continue. I felt some pangs of separation anxiety, but I was also far more concerned about her reactions to the end of therapy. I was pleased and, I suppose, relieved to hear her say that she was now on the "right road" and that she and Herb could work together in dealing with the problems. She was still concerned about her periods of being "emotionally closed"; however, she felt she understood the problem and how to eventually overcome it.

Despite her optimism, she expressed some fears of leaving therapy. She felt, nonetheless, that it was time to think about the end and that she needed to prepare for it. We agreed to have two more regular sessions in which we would continue to work on refinements in her new coping skills and then to have three additional meetings that would be progressively more spaced to allow for a gradual disengagement.]

Procedures of the Termination Phase

A number of important factors are involved in bringing about an effective ending to therapy. Many of these are rather obvious and have been discussed earlier; hence a fairly brief summary should suffice.

Needless to say, ample warning is needed with regard to termination. Indeed, in many instances, clients are given a rough estimate of the number of sessions involved right from the start of therapy, and this estimate can be made somewhat more precise during the negotiation phase midway through treatment. More explicit discussion and plans for termination should take place towards the end of the change phase.

The gradual "fading out" of the therapist during termination takes place on several dimensions. Most obvious here is the progressive reduction in the frequency of sessions, a process that encourages more independent and self-reliant functioning by the client. Second, throughout the last half of therapy there is a trend toward having clients successfully apply new coping skills in their daily lives, a process that again decreases reliance on the therapist for direct advice and guidance. Finally, as clients begin to develop or reestablish bonds with significant individuals in their lives, a naturally occurring shift in the focus of their emotions takes place away from therapy. Again, this is a trend that the therapist fosters throughout the latter portions of treatment.

At a more subtle level, there are several possible emotional dynamics that may complicate termination and hence that should be carefully monitored. Some clients, fearful of the prospect of facing the future alone, may exhibit a temporary return of symptoms. Mild interpretation coupled with support and encouragement in most instances helps clients over this last-minute loss of nerve. More difficult to deal with are occasional lapses of judgment by therapists during the termination process in which they underestimate clients' capabilities for independent living. Perhaps to pamper their own egos, therapists at times feel that their clients still need them, and hence they unconsciously prolong treatment. Careful assessment of both the client's status *and* the therapist's emotional needs are thus required throughout this process.

UNRESOLVED ISSUES AND FUTURE DIRECTIONS

From this writer's perspective, three major issues still have to be investigated with regard to insight therapy. For want of better terminology let us call these issues (1) specifying the techniques that promote insight; (2) the role of the therapist's personality; and (3) the need for adequate theory.

On the first of these issues, that pertaining to treatment techniques, we find considerable vagueness and ambiguity in the field. This applies particularly to specification of techniques to be used during the self-exploration phase of therapy. Practicing clinicians are faced with a wide array of general procedures that are recommended by textbooks and supervisors for the promotion of clients' insight; however, there are several problems with these textbook expositions. First, very few of the recommended techniques are based on scientific research. Rather, they stem from very general theory, opinion, or the relatively limited clinical experience of the author or supervisor. Second, these techniques are often presented in a compartmentalized fashion, so that each may be understood individually but with little appreciation of how they may be most effectively combined and sequenced. Finally, the role of clinical evaluation and judgment in the selection of appropriate techniques during the insight process is almost totally unexplored. Taken together, these deficits in our knowledge indicate that the therapeutic procedures for promoting insight are still far removed from science. Because the insight process is so complex and subtle, developing a rigorous, scientific basis for this phase of treatment represents a major challenge to future investigators.

The second issue deals with the role of the therapist's personality in producing positive treatment outcomes. Although considerable research has been conducted on this question, recent reviews of this work suggest that the surface has barely been scratched. For example, Parloff, Waskow, and Wolfe (1978) conclude in their thorough summary of this area that the research has suffered from such general and simplistic concepts that it may be facing "terminal vagueness." Despite these pessimistic findings, practicing clinicians and researchers alike seem to share the strongly held belief that therapists' personality characteristics do make a difference. It is quite easy, for example, to conceive of a therapist who is technically competent, says and does all the right things, and goes "by the book," yet has clients who essentially refuse to confide or explore with him or her. On the other side of the coin, some inexperienced clinicians who are unsure or unpracticed in the actual techniques of therapy are very successful in having their clients highly motivated in analyzing emotions, talking about delicate topics, and so forth. Identifying such characteristics in future investigations will hopefully pave the way for more effective selection and training of therapists.

The last issue deals with the vague and at times confusing array of theories that underlie insight therapy. Many of these theoretical underpinnings have dictated the actual techniques utilized in therapy. For example, a number of procedures stemming from the psychoanalytic tradition are aimed at uncovering childhood traumas and conflicts, yet there is really no adequate theory of how childhood events influence adult maladjustments. Similarly, recent research has suggested that many of the basic cognitive-behavioral principles upon which some treatment techniques are based may not be the relevant ingredients that are producing client improvement (see Marks, 1978; Mahoney and Arnkoff, 1978). In sum, it appears that the area of insight therapy is suffering some serious conceptual problems. As the diverse traditions of psychodynamic, humanistic, and cognitive-behavioral psychology converge on this important area of treatment, considerable evaluation, refinement, and integration of theories will be required.

PART FOUR

ADVANCING THE FIELD

CHAPTER ELEVEN

EVALUATING PSYCHOTHERAPY

INTRODUCTION

Psychotherapists, like most people, want to feel that they are right. They devote years to being trained. Much effort and emotion goes into treating their clients. They receive good pay for their services. It is easy to say to oneself, "Of course the therapy that I'm administering is effective."

There is, however, a major flaw in this line of thinking. In many other forms of work, individuals receive fairly clear feedback on the adequacy of their performance. A carpenter who builds a house with a faulty design or slipshod methods learns rather quickly that something is wrong as the structure gracelessly creaks to the ground. The businessman who has made a faulty investment decision discovers the error when the steely eyed accountant announces bankruptcy. This is not the case, however, in the practice of psychotherapy, where bringing about improvement in clients' mental health is the business at hand. Deciding whether improvement has occurred is frequently a subtle, subjective matter in which judgments may be biased by therapist and client alike. Often, even the criteria of what constitutes improvement are vague, as, for example, when the goals of treatment are such global things as increased self-esteem or improved coping skills. For these reasons special care is required in the evaluation of therapy. Such assessment is obviously important, not only to protect clients, but also to bring about continual improvement and refinement of treatment practices.

Exaggerated claims about the effectiveness of therapy also are an outgrowth of an unfortunate tendency in the field for many clinicians to form strong, emotional allegiances to a particular "school" of therapy. Becoming a "Freudian," a "behaviorist," or what have you often produces a dogmatic attitude that one's own approach to therapy is obviously correct, while other schools are suspect. Not only do these ideological commitments produce artificial professional barriers among clinicians, they also tend to reduce the rigorous and unbiased evaluation of one's own theory and practice.

We can see, then, several factors, both personal and ideological, that pose a threat to the profession. Individual clinicians may become too comfortable in the well-established daily routines of their therapy practice. They may fail to recognize that the field of psychotherapy is relatively young and that it is still evolving. The development of more effective treatments requires a systematic application of scientific methods, first, in testing current practices and second, in devising and evaluating new therapeutic approaches.

The intent of this chapter is to survey the major issues in the area of psychotherapy research. First we will review a number of historical trends and then we will discuss the measurement problems that are inherent in this research. This will be followed by a section on the design of experiments in this area, along with a summary of the current status of research findings. The chapter will conclude with consideration of future directions of research.

HISTORICAL OVERVIEW

Prior to the 1950s most therapists seemed to live in a protected fantasy world, satisfied that they were performing effective therapy. They did not pay particular attention to the relatively few research studies which were done. They assumed that progress would come about, as it always had, through the intuitive insights of a few prominent theorists in their particular school of therapy. Although this is overstating the case, it appears that most clinicians at the time fit the mold of the "too comfortable" therapist described earlier.

Imagine the shock when, in 1952 and again in 1961, Hans Eysenck published two very influential reviews of the therapy research literature that led to the conclusion that there was no evidence to indicate that psychotherapy worked. Eysenck based this conclusion on a survey of twenty-four studies (involving some eight thousand cases) that evaluated the effectiveness of dynamically oriented therapy (the principal therapy of the day) in treating neurotic clients. These data seemed to show that about two-thirds of clients receiving therapy improved within two years and that about the same percentage of *untreated* clients improve within the same time span. This failure of the treated neurotic clients to show a better improvement rate than the untreated clients was the pivotal issue leading to Eysenck's negative conclusions. His argument, in effect, said that if psychotherapy cannot beat the "spontaneous recovery rate" of untreated neurotics, then we have no evidence for its effectiveness.

The response of the field was electric. It was as if a slumbering giant had been taken by the throat and been shaken very violently. A tremendous outpouring of criticism, invective, and research occurred. If nothing else, Eysenck's work mobilized clinicians to counter his challenge to the profession.

Many of the published papers in the years that followed were aimed at careful evaluation of the earlier research upon which Eysenck had based his conclusions. Most of Eysenck's studies were found to be scientifically unsound. Their faults seemed to lie in three major areas: (1) problems with the ways in which improvement was defined and measured; (2) inadequate research design (lack of appropriate control groups, etc.); and (3) failure to take into account variations in client and therapist characteristics. The discussions and controversies on these issues that ensued for the next decade (cf. Bergin and Strupp, 1970, and Rachman, 1971) were both heated and instructive. The net result was a dramatic improvement in the quality of psychotherapy research during the 1970s and an increase in the precision with which research questions themselves were formulated.

Much of the material to be covered in the remainder of this chapter will take a closer look at the specific problems encountered in carrying out successful research. In an area as complex as psychotherapy there are, as can be imagined, numerous pitfalls, and the progressive improvement in the quality of research will challenge readers to make their own future contributions to this continually developing area.

Evolution of Research Questions

The research question addressed by Eysenck's reviews was quite simply, "Does psychotherapy work?" On the surface, this issue appeared to be very basic, and Eysenck's negative conclusions prompted at least another decade of research aimed at investigating this same general problem. Although the later, better done studies found more promising results (see below), researchers also began to discover that the question being asked was too global. Critics of this approach commented that the *type of therapy* was an important issue that had to be taken into account.

There followed a rash of studies that asked, "Do the various schools of psychotherapy differ in their effectiveness?" Typical of such research was a project by DiLoreto (1971) in which three therapy approaches (behavioral therapy, Ellis's rational-emotive therapy, and Rogers's client-centered therapy) were compared as to their effectiveness in treating general anxiety problems. The many studies of this type have also had their critics, however, although most agree that the research question itself is a decided improvement over the earlier one. Several problems with studies that attempt to compare "schools of therapy" are as follows:

1. Although the therapists who participate in such studies may identify themselves as utilizing a particular approach, there is no guarantee that they actually follow the procedures of that school in an exact and exclusive way.

2. The research therapists may differ in their level of training and experience and in their personality characteristics—factors that could influence the effectiveness of their treatments quite apart from the overall therapy approach they are using.

3. Certain therapy approaches may be effective only with particular types of problems, and hence characteristics of the client also have to be taken into account.

These criticisms led Kiesler (1971), in his important review of experimental designs, to recommend even greater specificity in the formulation of research issues. He suggests that researchers ask such questions as, "Do specific types of procedures, administered by therapists with designated characteristics, lead to improvement among specific types of clients?" As can be noted in this proposal, the level of precision and the multiplicity of factors that are required to answer such questions are enormous. And yet, if the field could develop a large body of data answering these issues, we would be well on the way toward evolving a science of psychotherapy.

Gottman and Markman (1978) place a somewhat different emphasis on the specificity problem in their formulation of a productive approach to research. They suggest that the focus of attention should be on *intervention programs* that contain carefully designated and specific treatment procedures. Within this framework they indicate that several interlocking questions can be asked of research: (1) What should be the content (specific procedures) of the program? (2) How can that content be most effectively delivered to clients? (3) What types of clients make what kind of improvement with the program? A major advantage to this approach, they argue, is that it lends itself to a systematic series of small, manageable studies, as opposed to the large, multi-factor, "grand design" study urged by Kiesler.

We can see, then, in the evolution of research questions, that things are far from settled in the field. Investigators differ even on the basic ways in which experimental issues are formulated. What does seem clear, however, is a definite trend toward increased sophistication in specifying the therapy techniques being studied and in identifying the target populations for whom they are intended. As we will see in the next section, researchers are also devoting considerable energies in trying to develop more meaningful measures of improvement—a task fundamental to the whole research effort.

MEASUREMENT AND DESIGN ISSUES

The Measurement of Improvement

Any scientific endeavor must include the capability to accurately and reliably measure the phenomenon under investigation. This is especially true in the area of therapy research in which the changes that take place are both complex and subtle. As mentioned earlier, the very complexity of the process allows ample room for biased and self-serving judgments; hence there is a need for special care in devising measures of improvement.

Over the years, a variety of different approaches to measuring therapy outcomes have been adopted. Investigators prior to 1960, for the most part, utilized global measures of psychological adjustment to evaluate the effects of treatment. These general indices of improvement, such as improved "ego strength" or "impulse control," were based on therapists' judgments or ratings of the changes that occurred in their own clients. Some studies also used projective tests, such as the Rorschach (ink blot) test to derive similar overall measures of mental health. Both of these methods have been seriously criticized by recent investigators in virtually all schools of therapy (see Bergin and Lambert, 1978). Therapists' global ratings of improvement lack credibility because the person making the judgments (the therapist) is hardly an uninvolved, dispassionate observer. After having provided many hours of "expert" therapy, and having accepted fees for services rendered, it would be difficult to envision the therapist making a completely unbiased rating of client improvement. Projective tests have other types of problems when used as outcome measures, notably an ill-defined conceptual basis for interpreting scores and poor consistency; that is, clients' responses on the test are influenced by situational factors or transient moods.

With the rise of behavioral therapies during the 1960s and 1970s a sharp swing away from global measures occurred. Researchers in this mold were far more concerned with precise measurement of specific, symptomatic behaviors being treated. These early behavioral studies unfortunately let the pendulum swing too far in the direction of specificity. Their focus on single "target" behaviors and their reliance upon simply counting the occurrence of these responses failed to capture the complexity of maladjusted patterns (Ross, 1978). Present-day behavioral researchers emphasize the interrelationships among response systems, as well as the importance of measuring the cognitive processes that accompany them. Illustrative of the too-narrow approach is the early behavioral investigator who, let us say, used aversive procedures in an attempt to reduce the frequency of disruptive behaviors among five-year-olds in a nursery school. Such a project might employ several "observers" to make a frequency count of disruptive acts in class throughout a six-week treatment period. Let us assume that the tally of such behaviors actually did decrease by the end of therapy. By using only that single measure it would appear that the treatment was successful. However, were a wider battery of measures utilized we might also find that (1) the children's aggressive behaviors increased dramatically in the schoolyard and at home; (2) a proportion of the children started wetting the bed with increasing frequency; and (3) their level of social anxiety escalated substantially. Given these other (unmeasured) changes, could we really say that the treatment was effective?

One of the critically important features of the scientific method is that it is self-correcting. Since investigators' procedures and measures are specified and open for inspection, they can learn from previous mistakes. This is especially true with regard to measurement problems in psychotherapy, and a number of recent reviewers of the area have put forward recommendations pertaining to the evaluation of treatment outcomes (Bergin and Lambert, 1978; Gottman and Markman, 1978; Strupp, 1978). These recommendations can be summarized as follows:

1. *The criteria for improvement should be individualized.* Since clients seek help because of a variety of maladaptive behaviors and diverse emotional problems, it is frequently impossible to set down a common therapeutic goal for all clients. A more precise method involves defining what constitutes improvement for each client and then tailoring measuring instruments to specifically evaluate the degree to which each client meets his or her goals.

One frequently used method for achieving individualized measurement is goal attainment scaling (Kiresuk and Sherman, 1968). In this procedure, a series of goals for the client is specified prior to treatment. Included with each goal is a graded set of criteria, ranging from least to most favorable, that will indicate how closely that aim of treatment was achieved. When proper care is taken to develop these criteria, a numerical score can be assigned to each goal attainment scale, thus permitting comparison of improvement scores across different subjects.

An example of such individualized evaluation can be drawn, let us say, from a treatment program generally aimed at improving interpersonal skills. Client A, being a rather shy, passive person may have as one goal the development of more outgoing, assertive behaviors. In contrast, client B, who is seeking treatment because of a generally brusque, aggressive style with others, has the goal of reducing assertiveness. These directions of behavioral change are distinctly different, yet each constitutes improvement. A single criterion measure of treatment effectiveness would hardly suffice in this example.

2. *Therapeutic changes occur in many areas of functioning, and therefore multiple measures should be used.* This recommendation is largely a reaction to the many early outcome studies that used only a single criterion of improvement (global rating by therapist, change in the frequency of one isolated behavior, etc.). Recent studies have shown that when many and diverse measures are used in an outcome study they do not correlate very highly with one another. Phrased another way, the results indicate that psychotherapy affects clients in different ways—with some clients showing vast improvement in, let us say, behavioral indices of change, and other clients showing maximal improvement in reducing feelings of anxiety or in developing an inner sense of mastery. Because of such diverse reactions to treatment, it is important for the investigator to gain as complete a picture as possible of the therapy outcomes. Such data are likely to aid future studies in identifying the client characteristics and the particular therapy procedures that result in specific types of changes, thus promoting the refinement and development of treatment programs.

3. *Measures that rely on clients' self-reports* (e.g., ratings of anxiety, symptom checklists, questionnaires regarding behaviors, personality inventories) are recommended, but call for several cautions. Since the items on such self-report instruments are usually very direct and obvious, there is ample opportunity for clients to give misleading answers. Clients may, for example, wish to impress the researcher and thus respond to questions in a *socially desirable* (but not necessarily accurate) manner. Similarly, clients may sense some pressure to fill out these reports in the way they think their therapist would like. Such *compliant* responding is likely to provide inflated estimates of treatment effectiveness when they occur at the close of therapy. Finally, when items ask clients to self-rate such general characteristics as "Are you an anxious person?" or "Do you have problems with losing your temper?" many respondents are unsure of how to interpret the question. Does the first item refer to being anxious all the time? How should one answer the second question if an occasional outburst of anger creates embarrassment at times? Such ambiguity often leads to inconsistent responding by clients because items may be interpreted in diverse ways. For this reason it has been recommended that self-report items be constructed with greater degrees of specificity, in the form, "How would you behave (or feel) in this particular situation, if this were happening?"

4. *Direct observations* of clients' maladaptive and adaptive behaviors perhaps offer the least ambiguous measures of treatment outcome, especially when records of several interrelated response systems are made. Here again, however, several problems are encountered that make such measures more difficult than might appear at first glance. First, the fact that observers and recorders of clients' behaviors are required introduces the possibility of human error. An individual observer, even when merely counting the occurrence of a discrete behavior, may operate with bias or inconsistency. The response being counted may be poorly defined or may overlap with other behaviors. The observer's personal interpretation of what constitutes the targeted behavior may be different from that intended by the researcher. Frequently the "meaning" of a behavior depends on the context in which it is occurring, thus requiring higher-level judgments by the observer. For these reasons several independent observers are usually required who are highly trained on the definitions and criteria of the behavioral categories being judged. These individuals have to demonstrate a high degree of consistency and agreement in their observations (interobserver reliability) before the recording system is considered trustworthy. When the recordings are to be made over relatively long periods of time, spot checks are recommended to ensure that a decay in reliability has not occurred.

Behavioral observations also involve an added problem known as *reactive effects*. When clients know or suspect that they are being observed, they may very possibly alter their behaviors. Their "public" reactions might be considerably different than those that would occur under naturalistic, "private" circumstances. One way to deal with this issue is to utilize unobtrusive measures, where individuals' attention to the recording process is minimized or where they are completely unaware that they are being observed. Such techniques, however, present both ethical and practical problems that may be difficult to surmount.

Using behavioral observations as part of an assessment battery also requires that adequate samples of the response systems under study be obtained. In practical terms this means that observation periods of reasonable length need to be programmed, along with the recordings taking place in settings that offer generalizability to clients' everyday lives.

5. Measures of the *broad social effects* of treatment are recommended in many circumstances. These measures, which assess naturally occurring life events before and after therapy, may provide some of the most practical demonstrations of treatment outcome. Treated alcoholics who now can maintain a life outside of skid row and can keep a steady job provide one such example. A reduction in the frequency of arrests and convictions among habitual delinquents is another. An increase in the academic achievement scores of hyperactive children is yet a third illustration. Naturally such derivative measures are subject to many other factors that are independent of therapy. For example, middle-class adolescents may be less likely than teenagers from working-class neighborhoods to have minor delinquent acts recorded by the local police. An alcoholic may be better able to hold a job during periods of labor shortage simply because employers are willing to tolerate absenteeism, and so forth. Social action measures therefore require careful analysis in order to correct for some of the nontreatment variables that may affect them.

6. It is evident that *human judgments* are an important part of most of the measures described in this section. Observers may have to rate clients' behaviors. Research assistants who administer tests have to score and interpret them. The researcher may have to make judgments about clients' self-reports. As indicated earlier, all such judgments leave room for bias, and one of the largest sources of bias are the research personnel themselves. They may harbor hopes that the results of the study will indicate, let us say, that treatment A will do better than treatment B. To ensure that such biasing cannot take place (even subconsciously) those personnel involved in measurement should not be aware of the treatment condition to which research clients are assigned.

It is apparent from this brief review of measurement that all is not clear-cut in assessing the effects of treatment. Technical problems of reliability and validity blend with conceptual issues of defining improvement. These in turn relate to questions of values and philosophy as to what constitutes mental health. Is the shy, penniless recluse who feels at peace with himself any better or worse off than the socially adept and well-to-do extrovert who suffers from self-doubt and lack of confidence? In developing goals and measures of treatment outcomes, researchers at some level have to wrestle with such questions. That's what makes it such an interesting profession.

In the practical realm of doing research on therapy effectiveness, a major task confronting investigators is to select the appropriate group of measures for their study. The particular measures that are chosen will, of course, depend on the nature of the problems and therapies being evaluated; however, most current-day studies attempt to use a combination of self-report, behavioral, and social action measures in order to provide a broad basis for assessment.

Experimental Designs

An experimental design is the way a research study is set up in order to answer the question under investigation. As stated earlier in this chapter, a variety of questions can be asked in evaluating psychotherapy; hence, there is no single, "best" experimental design. The investigator must use logic and care in designing the research so that the data permit a reasonably clear answer to the question under study.

Let us first look at the fundamental issues of experimental design and then consider some of the complicating factors as we proceed. Most researchers agree that the minimum ingredients for an adequate study of therapy effectiveness are the following: (1) a sample of subjects representing a defined clinical problem is divided into two groups, one to receive the treatment being evaluated and the other to receive no treatment; (2) the subgroups are essentially identical in composition, containing subjects who are matched for age, education, severity and chronicity of symptoms, motivation for therapy, and so forth; (3) a battery of appropriate measures is administered prior to treatment, immediately after treatment, and after a follow-up period (in order to evaluate the permanence of any treatment-related improvement); and (4) in order to demonstrate that improvement has occurred *as a result of the therapy*, the treated group has to show a statistically greater degree of improvement than the untreated group on the posttherapy and follow-up measures. This basic design is pictured in Fig. 11.1.

Now, we can ask whether this minimum design is adequate to answer our question. If the treated group displays substantial improvement relative to the untreated control group, is this enough evidence to conclude that the treatment procedures were effective? Most therapy researchers would answer no. They would argue that there are a number of explanations for these findings other than the effects of treatment. It is suggested, therefore, that additional controls are necessary in order to rule out these alternative interpretations. Let us take a look at some of these alternatives and how they might be dealt with.

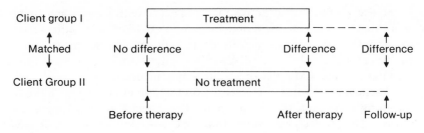

Points of measurement

Figure 11.1 Minimum features of an experimental design to evaluate the effectiveness of a therapy program.

Attention-placebo effects It could be argued that the reason for improvement in the treated group is not the therapy procedures themselves but rather the fact that these clients are receiving attention and are having general contact with a therapist. The improvement effect could therefore be equivalent to that observed in studies that evaluate the medical effects of drugs, that is, that some subjects improve even when they are given an inert placebo (e.g., a sugar pill). Such attention-placebo improvements have been frequently noted in psychological research (see Shapiro and Morris, 1978) and therefore need to be taken into account. This could be accomplished by adding another group of matched subjects to our design. Subjects in this attention-placebo control group would have regular contact with a therapist, to the same extent as the treated clients, only the meetings would be of a nontherapeutic, general nature. With the addition of this control group, our basic design can now be diagrammed as in Fig. 11.2.

In this figure we can note that the treated group is required to display greater improvement than both the attention-placebo and the no-treatment control groups before we can conclude that the therapy procedures were effective. An additional feature of this design is that an estimate can be made of the beneficial effects of attention-placebo factors alone by comparing groups II and III.

Comparison of treatments It can be argued that a more cost-efficient way of doing therapy research is to compare the effectiveness of several treatments in the same design. In practical terms this approach might involve an evaluation of some newly developed treatment procedure relative to one that has been traditionally used. Here again, no-treatment and attention-placebo controls are required. Thus in essence, this design, portrayed in Fig. 11.3, can serve as a vehicle for scientifically based improvements in treatment procedures. New therapies can be evaluated in comparison to untreated controls and in relation to standard therapy.

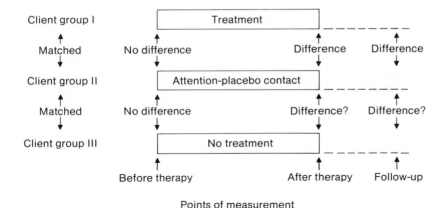

Figure 11.2 An expanded experimental design to evaluate the effectiveness of a therapy program.

Therapist effects As we get into the more complex designs involving the comparison of treatments, variables associated with therapists become progressively more important. Even in the rudimentary design seen in Fig. 11.1, therapist factors need to be considered. In this simple case, where the effectiveness of a treatment procedure is evaluated against a no-treatment group, we might expect to find no difference in improvement between the groups if the therapists who are administering the therapy are poorly trained or grossly inexperienced. Thus a treatment might be judged to be ineffective not because the procedures themselves are poor but because the researcher did not exercise care in seeing that they were properly administered.

In the more complicated research design portrayed in Fig. 11.3, such therapist factors can again create misleading results. By way of example, let us consider a study where the effectiveness of "new" therapy A is being compared to "traditional" therapy B. There are not many therapists around who are familiar with therapy A, so our researcher trains some advanced graduate students in these procedures. In contrast, the researcher has no trouble in finding many experienced therapists who are well-practiced in therapy B, since this is the standard treatment in the field. In now actually carrying out this research, we can see that the experimental design is deficient; that is, therapists in the two treatment groups are not equal in terms of experience. Any differences that are found between therapy A and therapy B may be due to the treatment techniques, *or* they may be due to differences in the level of training, experience, and general sophistication of the therapists.

Two solutions to this dilemma are suggested, and in carefully designed studies both are usually implemented: (1) the therapists assigned to each of the treatment groups should be matched in experience, level of training, personal

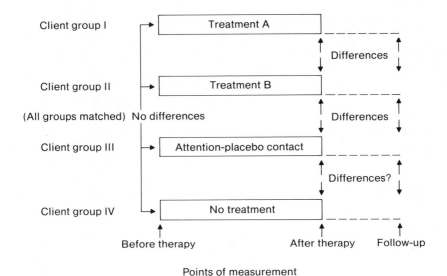

Figure 11.3 Design for comparing the relative effectiveness of two (or more) treatments.

commitment to the treatment, and such nonspecific factors as warmth, empathy, and interpersonal skills; (2) the administration of the treatment procedures themselves should be monitored (or spot checked) by the researcher to ensure that therapists are not deviating from the intended procedures.

Analyzing specific treatment processes In the foregoing sections we have reviewed the major elements of design in conducting therapy evaluation research. However, answering questions about the relative effectiveness of one treatment procedure over another does not tell the whole story. Important research can also be conducted that attempts to investigate the *therapy process* itself — as, for example, identifying critical components of treatment procedures, analyzing why some clients fail to improve, or even studying the factors that cause some clients to get worse. Such research can be immensely important in providing information for improving treatments and for making them safer for high-risk clients. In the following paragraphs several types of these process studies will be reviewed.

A frequently used method for evaluating the components of a particular therapy is called the *active ingredients* design. In a fairly simple form, we can take the example of a treatment composed of three components, as in a standard Wolpe counterconditioning procedure with phobic clients. One component consists of gradually exposing clients to progressively more fearful stimuli in their hierarchy of phobic stimuli. This may be called the "desensitization" component. A second element is the relaxation training that clients undergo. The third component is the actual counterconditioning procedure in which clients are exposed to items in the fear hierarchy coupled with their being in a relaxed state. A valid scientific question that can be asked in this situation is, Which of these components is the active therapeutic agent in producing improvement? If, for example, it were found that the desensitization component alone produced as much improvement as the more complex counterconditioning procedure, then the entire treatment package could be simplified and made more efficient. An experimental design to analyze the relative contributions of these components thus would involve several groups of matched phobic clients: one group receiving only the graduated exposure to the fear stimuli (desensitization group); a second group receiving only relaxation training; a third group receiving the full counterconditioning treatment; and the fourth and fifth groups representing attention-placebo and no-treatment controls.

A second major approach to the study of therapeutic process is called the *correlation design*. Here the investigator is usually interested in studying the relationship between two (or more) variables in a treatment situation. In most instances the emphasis in this type of design is to merely analyze the relationship, let us say, between variables A and B, not necessarily to determine whether A *causes* B. This correlational approach thus generally has more modest aims than the designs described earlier and frequently does not require the elaborate control groups and matching procedures involved in evaluation research. However, correlation methods serve the important function of empirically highlighting important variables that affect the treatment process.

By way of example, let us consider the investigator in a large, research-oriented clinic who is concerned about an unusually high dropout rate among clients who begin treatment. This researcher is particularly interested in the kinds of "personal chemistry" that take place between clients and therapists. The working hypothesis adopted by the investigator is that certain clients drop out of treatment because they do not sense a general personal rapport with their therapists. To pursue this idea, the researcher randomly selects one hundred client-therapist pairs and calculates an index of the degree to which each pair has common interests, educational attainment, and ethnic background. This index can now be statistically correlated with whether or not clients subsequently leave therapy prematurely, their degree of satisfaction with treatment, and of course, the degree of improvement shown (by independent criteria). Should this "commonality index" prove to be highly related to these measures, the researcher will have uncovered an important factor that can be useful in assigning clients to therapists in the future.

The last approach to be mentioned in the area of process studies is called the *time series* design. This type of design is particularly useful when conducting research involving small numbers of clients or even a single subject. Although studies involving such few subjects may not be generalizable to larger populations of clients, they can serve many useful purposes, such as pilot testing a new treatment, demonstrating the operation of a theoretically important procedure, or evaluating a therapy technique with a relatively rare disorder (where insufficient clients are available for the larger designs).

The time series methodology, in essence, first involves careful and continuous measurement of a particular symptom pattern for a relatively long period of time without the imposition of the treatment under study. Presumably the symptom will not change during this "control" measurement period. Thereafter, the treatment is introduced and assessment is made of the symptomatic changes that occur. Naturally, any improvement that takes place is not attributable to the treatment with complete assurance; however, there is a strong suggestion of a positive treatment effect in such a finding.

More complex variations of time series designs may involve (1) several repetitions of the treatment, interspersed with measurement periods in which the treatment is absent (reversal designs); or (2) introduction of the treatment at different times for different subjects, but with measurement taking place throughout the process (time-lagged designs). Such methods provide greater confidence in pinpointing the treatment itself as the agent of improvement, rather than some extraneous variable (Cook and Campbell, 1979).

Time series designs, which are appropriate for single-subject research, represent an important tool for practicing clinicians. These designs permit a reasonably careful evaluation of the effects of specific treatment interventions with an individual client. An important component of such ongoing assessments during therapy is the careful measurement of the target behaviors and symptoms that are under study. Using these methods clinicians have the opportunity to select and refine particular therapy techniques for each client in a systematic, empirical fashion.

Summary of design issues It is hoped that the reader has developed an understanding of notions involving experimental design from the foregoing material. It has only touched the surface of a very complex and fascinating area of science, and it has necessarily omitted important issues from the related discipline of statistics. For our purposes, however, the central concern for therapy research is that experimental controls and methods be devised so that treatments can be evaluated as fairly and as logically as the situation permits. The scientific method is understandably slow and expensive; yet clients who receive treatment have a right to expect therapists to use the most defensible and scientifically sound therapies that are available.

CURRENT STATUS OF THERAPY EVALUATION RESEARCH

Students who are interested in conducting psychotherapy research in the future need not fear that they will run out of researchable questions. There is a staggering amount of work yet to be done. As one reviews the evaluation research which has been published to date, it is clear that much of this work is either too general or methodologically unsound to permit any firm conclusions. The entire field seems to be making progress in terms of improved measures, designs, and asking relevant research questions, but the improvements are hardly faster than a snail's pace.

A number of reviews of the psychotherapy research literature have been published over the last decade, encompassing several hundred individual studies (Bergin, 1971; Luborsky, Singer, and Luborsky, 1975; Beutler, 1976; Goldstein and Stein, 1976; Smith and Glass, 1977; Bergin and Lambert, 1978). The conclusions drawn from these reviews may be summarized under the various kinds of questions asked in the research studies.

Does Psychotherapy Work?

Most reviewers agree on the main points with regard to this question. First, there is consensus that when the major forms of treatment (insight-oriented, behavioral, cognitive) are lumped together, they produce improvement rates among diverse nonpsychotic client groups that are better than the spontaneous recovery rate of untreated clients. Despite Eysenck's negative conclusions of several decades ago, the more recent and better-done studies indicate that, yes indeed, psychotherapy does work. The estimates of improvement rates for treated and untreated clients vary considerably from study to study, but in rough form the results suggest a spontaneous improvement rate of about 40 percent for clients not in therapy, while those receiving treatment show better than 65 percent.

These kinds of gross comparisons can be misleading, however, and it is likely that therapy may be generally even more effective than is implied in these figures. The improvements in treated clients occur over a much shorter period of time and are of substantially greater magnitude than those in the untreated clients. When we consider that those who do not receive treatment may show symptomatic improvement after two years, whereas treated clients show comparable (or greater) improvement after just a few months, we can appreciate the value of therapy. In addition, many reviewers suggest that there may be many subtle but important benefits of treatment, such as improved self-concept and generally better interpersonal relations, that are unmeasured in the research studies and therefore are not reflected in the overall percentage figures.

The comparison between treated and untreated clients is also misleading because there is good reason to believe that the improvement percentage assigned to untreated groups is inflated, that is, it is actually less than the 40 percent estimate. What is questioned here is whether it is appropriate to label these subjects as "untreated." Several national surveys (e.g., Gurin, Veroff, and Feld, 1960) found that a majority of persons who suffer psychological problems do not seek out professional psychotherapists for help. Rather, they go to clergymen, family physicians, teachers, friends, and so forth. Furthermore, these individuals report a relatively high degree of satisfaction with the help that was received. In this light, then, it appears that a good proportion of the research subjects who are listed as untreated are in reality actually receiving some form of psychological help, even though it is coming from nonprofessional "therapists." It therefore becomes very important, in conducting this type of research, to determine how many of the so-called untreated control subjects are actually receiving assistance from other sources.

The improvements that occur in "untreated" individuals (the spontaneous recovery phenomenon) draw comment from most reviewers from a somewhat different perspective as well. They suggest that the term *spontaneous* is an unfortunate one that has become ingrained in the field. It implies that improvement comes about merely through the passage of time, or that psychological maladjustments are self-correcting in some automatic fashion. Common sense dictates otherwise. It is far more likely that improvement occurs with "untreated" persons because something active and therapeutic is happening to them in the natural course of their lives. Hence, the task facing the therapy researcher becomes the broader one of trying to identify what these natural therapeutic events are and then attempting to incorporate them in formal treatment programs.

Is One School of Therapy More Effective Than Others?

If we take a balanced overview of the studies that have addressed this issue, the answer seems to be a qualified no. The research suggests that the major therapy approaches all produce significant improvement among a general population of clients (over that of untreated or placebo controls) *and* that no approach distinguishes itself as being generally better than the others. Thus, when comparing such major approaches as psychoanalytic, humanistic, behavioral, and cognitive therapies, research results do not recommend any one of them as an especially effective *overall* approach.

Reviewers are generally critical of the lack of precision in studies that attempt to compare schools of therapy. The major problem is that simply listing a therapist's theoretical preference does not provide enough information about what actually takes place in treatment. Therapists within the same "school" may vary considerably in the techniques that are used. Moreover, as detailed in earlier chapters, many of the historic distinctions between approaches are becoming very blurred in contemporary practice—particularly among behavioral, cognitive, and psychodynamic viewpoints (see for example, Chapter 8). This makes it notoriously difficult to set up research designs that compare "pure" treatments representing each school.

Which Specific Treatment Procedures Are Best for Which Type of Client?

Most reviewers of therapy research agree that this is the question that leads to the greatest payoff; that is, pinpointing the specific therapy interventions that are most beneficial for particular types of psychological problems is a major goal. The reviewers also bemoan the fact that not much research has been directed at this question, even though it has been recognized as a central one for over a decade.

Researchers from within the behavioral ranks seem to have taken the lead in this area of investigation. A small but growing literature is thus developing, and we can begin to see several diagnostic categories for which well-defined treatment procedures seem to be especially effective. Considerable attention has been devoted to the comparison of various procedures for treating clients with *specific phobias*. Well-controlled studies (e.g., Paul, 1966; Gelder, Marks, and Wolff, 1967; Gillan and Rachman, 1974) have demonstrated the superiority of a behavioral, counterconditioning procedure over psychodynamic treatment for this syndrome. This line of investigation has progressed to the point where variations of very specific behavioral techniques are being compared as to effectiveness, in efforts to refine the now widely accepted desensitization approach.

On a lesser scale, similar findings are emerging in the treatment of neurotic clients who display compulsive, ritualistic patterns. For example, Marks, Hodgson, and Rachman (1975) compared several behavioral procedures in various combinations (relaxation, modeling, response prevention) as to their effectiveness in reducing ritualistic patterns, and they found response prevention to be clearly superior. This procedure requires that the client temporarily inhibit the undesirable behavior in situations that normally elicit it. The client is thereby exposed (and presumably desensitized) to the fearful stimuli that prompt the ritualistic behavior. Thus this treatment can be viewed as a variant of counterconditioning techniques that have proved successful with phobias. The comparative research on compulsions has not progressed to the same point as that on phobias, however, and a great deal of further investigation is needed.

A number of studies have compared various therapy procedures in treating *sexual dysfunctions* (e.g., desensitization, personal counseling, psychoanalytic therapy, Masters and Johnson-type direct practice approach), and the evidence suggests that the behavioral practice treatment is superior (see Marks, 1978). This area of investigation is instructive in that specific symptoms (sexual malfunctions) frequently occur in the context of general marital problems, and hence a combination of treatments may be most beneficial. Crowe (1976) found, for example, that a specific, operant-behavioral program to improve interpersonal skills coupled with a Masters and Johnson behavioral approach to enhance sexual functions was the most effective treatment for couples experiencing marital and sexual discord.

The treatment of several child and adolescent disorders have also been investigated in a comparative fashion, and they also point to the superiority of one specific therapy program over others. *Bed-wetting* seems to be the most effectively treated with a Mowrer-type classical conditioning approach (DeLeon and Mandell, 1966; DeLeon and Sacks, 1972) (see also Chapter 6). *Self-injurious behaviors* among severely disturbed children seem best handled by aversive and time-out procedures from within the behavioral framework (see Bachman, 1972). *Delinquent patterns* have shown marked improvement in family-style foster-home settings in which a positive reinforcement and token-economy program form the core of treatment (Fixsen, Phillips, Phillips, and Wolf, 1972).

It should be noted that many of the studies in this section involve comparisons of very specific behavioral procedures with several more general therapies emanating from the psychodynamic camp. This highlights one of the problems inherent in doing research involving nonbehavioral therapies. In most cases procedures cannot be detailed to the same degree as behavioral techniques, and hence they suffer from a lack of specificity in these comparative studies. This is perhaps one of the central reasons why more research in this important sphere has not been done.

Therapist Variables

A considerable amount of research has been aimed at identifying therapist characteristics that promote positive (and negative) outcomes of treatment. It appears, however, that many of the findings in this area either conflict or fail to be replicated in further studies. Thus many of the conclusions to be drawn are merely tentative, and require careful follow-up. The work of Parloff, Waskow, and Wolfe (1978) and Bergin and Lambert (1978) in critically reviewing this research literature are important scientific advances.

First, it appears that the personal qualities of the therapist (apart from technical skills) are important. The characteristics of warmth, empathy, and genuineness seem to be fundamental to successful treatment, especially in long-term therapy. Researchers agree, however, that more complex "relationship" factors are probably involved and require further study. At the other extreme are a growing number of studies that point to "pathogenic" therapist qualities that may actually lead to client deterioration. Although these studies are far from definitive, it appears that therapists who are psychologically disturbed themselves may produce these negative effects. The mechanisms by which harm is transmitted may vary considerably, but such therapist patterns as fostering dependency, being aggressively interpretative, or exposing clients to severe anxiety seem to be major offenders. Naturally, the more disturbed the client is to begin with, the greater the risk of being damaged by such therapist malpractices.

The therapist's level of experience is also a factor in treatment outcome, although much research is still needed on this question. It appears that less experienced practitioners may make faulty decisions, pursue irrelevant side issues, or overlook some subtle factor, thereby impeding therapy. More critical are such factors as matching therapists' and clients' expectations about therapy and the compatibility of their personalities, values, and sociocultural backgrounds. Such compatible pairing makes intuitive sense when one considers the complex communications and emotions that occur in psychotherapy, and the developing research literature in this area is both exciting and important.

Research on therapist variables also has important implications for the selection and training of students in this area. What are the responsibilities of medical schools, graduate programs, paraprofessional training courses, and so on, to screen out students who may become "pathogenic" therapists? What sorts of training experiences are most effective in developing both technical competencies and enhancing personal "therapeutic" qualities? These and related questions represent additional research questions that will undoubtedly be addressed in the years to come.

Client Variables

A great deal of research has been conducted on the relationship between client characteristics and the outcome of psychotherapy. The results of this extensive body of literature are difficult to summarize because of the uneven quality of the investigations and the conflicting findings that are often obtained. However, several consistent patterns of results seem to stand out, and these touch on some critically important issues.

One of the paramount practical problems in psychotherapy is the drop-out rate, that is, the number of clients who decide to discontinue treatment prior to its completion. This many-sided problem, as we shall see, has repercussions for the entire profession. At its core is the issue, touched on earlier, of bringing about a proper pairing of client and therapist at the beginning of treatment. The issue is even larger than this, however, in that the "atmosphere" of clinics and treatment agencies (the setting, attitudes of personnel, routine procedures) must be conducive to clients' needs and sensitivities. Furthermore, clinic fees, hours, and location, to some degree, should be arranged to fit with clients' financial resources, work schedules, transportation facilities, and so forth.

Taking all these diverse variables into account, the research findings on client dropout rates are rather shocking (Garfield, 1971, 1978). Let us first review the overall statistics and then consider some of the specific factors.

The figures that will be presented are conservative estimates, and therefore the problems to be discussed may well be of even greater magnitude. Numerous large-scale surveys reveal that roughly 30 percent of clients who go through the intake process at clinics and are accepted for treatment fail to return for their first therapy appointment.

The problem becomes even more serious when we consider clients who actually begin treatment. Here the general finding is that about 40 percent of clients discontinue therapy before the sixth session; that is, clients themselves decide to drop out prior to the completion of treatment. This rough statistic has been obtained in a wide variety of settings (community clinics, private practice, university health services, veterans' facilities); hence it seems to be a general and pervasive phenomenon.

Taking a closer look at those who drop out of treatment, several general characteristics stand out. The most important factors are social class, educational level, and race. Clients on the lower end of the social class and educational dimensions are more likely to discontinue, as are black clients. It seems reasonably clear that typical treatment facilities do not meet these clients' needs and expectations about therapy, nor do they make these clients feel particularly welcome.

We can see the other side of the coin in the research literature on those clients who are accepted and rejected for treatment by mental health agencies (see also Chapter 4). Those who are accepted tend to be from higher socioeconomic levels, are better educated, more verbal, and more psychologically sophisticated, and tend to share the same frame of reference and "speak the same language" as the predominantly well-educated therapists in the clinics. The actual percentages of clients who are not accepted by agencies is difficult to determine. The few studies that have looked at this issue vary widely in their estimates, probably because clinics themselves differ so widely in their acceptance criteria. Lorenzen (1967) found, for example, that the figures vary between a 20 percent to 85 percent acceptance rate, depending on the nature of the clinic. For purposes of our discussion, let us for the moment accept the most generous estimate of 85 percent. This in effect means that 15 percent of applicants are denied individual psychotherapy, and as indicated earlier, these are likely to be individuals of relatively low socioeconomic and educational status.

The picture that begins to emerge from these findings is not a pleasant one. Vast segments of our society who are in need of therapy are not receiving it from professional sources. Many clients are denied treatment outright, and of those who are offered therapy, the majority decide to discontinue before it is completed. The immensity of the problem is highlighted in Table 11.1.

This analysis, based on conservative statistics, reveals that effective mental health services are reaching a disheartening small proportion of people in need. The picture may be even more dismal in that we do not know what proportion of individuals needing professional assistance seek help elsewhere to begin with and thus are not tallied in the research figures. One conclusion seems inevitable: mental health agencies, for one reason or another, are not meeting the needs of the communities they are supposed to serve.

These statistics also place the evaluation research described earlier in this chapter in a somewhat different perspective. When a comparative, outcome study asks whether therapy A does better than therapy B, the results of such an investigation are typically based *only on clients who complete treatment.* Dropouts are placed in a separate category and are usually forgotten in some small corner of the research report. This means, of course, that the comparison of the two treatments may be based on a very small proportion of clients who suffer from a particular maladjustment.

We can see from this discussion that research efforts to evaluate psychotherapy go beyond the simple question of whether or not it works. In a limited

Table 11.1
**What happens to potential clients? Conservative estimates of clinic acceptance rates
and client dropout rates**

Stage in treatment process	Percentage of clients lost	Percentage of potential clients remaining
Community in which X number of people need mental health services		X = 100%
Seek help from nonprofessional sources	?	100%
Apply to mental health agency and are not accepted	15%	85%
Accepted by clinic, but fail to keep first appointment	30%	55%
Start treatment, but drop out before sixth session	40%	15%
Clients remaining who receive treatment beyond six sessions		15%

sense we can say that it does work if we only consider "selected" clients who stay with a treatment program to its completion. In a broader sense, however, if we ask whether various therapy programs are meeting the needs of a community and of all clients who need and seek treatment, the answer is probably no. Moreover, those who fail to receive adequate therapy are likely to be the disadvantaged segments of the population.

Efforts to redress these critical problems of community mental health will probably be the major issue of the next decade.

SUMMARY

It is hoped that the reader has gained an appreciation of the complex and difficult tasks facing the therapy researcher. Numerous kinds of questions may be asked pertaining to psychotherapy effectiveness, and of course, a variety of experimental designs and measures are available with which to address these questions. With all this diversity, progress has been slow; in all honesty, no earth-shaking new discoveries have emerged from the research literature. What we have is a gradual and painstaking accumulation of knowledge about psychotherapy—a communal process involving many investigators that will undoubtedly continue for many decades in the future. Some of the important trends that will continue to challenge future researchers are the following:

1. Continued striving to ask more precise (and limited) research questions pertaining to the effectiveness of specific treatments for specific disorders.

2. Searching for new measures of therapy outcome that are both scientifically sound and also reflect the realities of clients' day-to-day patterns of adjustment.

3. Continued efforts to develop innovative and rigorous research designs that are practical in terms of the resources available to the average investigator (or agency).

4. Sharpening the descriptions of the therapy techniques being investigated, particularly among those growing out of psychodynamic theories.

5. Exploring the critical area of how to match therapist-client characteristics to bring about maximum therapeutic gain.

6. Vigorously studying the problems of high drop-out rates and developing ways to reduce them.

REFERENCES

Abramson, L. Y., Seligman, M.E.P., and Teasdale, J. D. Learned helplessness in humans: Critique and reformulation. *Journal of Abnormal Psychology*, 1978, *87*, 49-74.

Adler, A. *Practice and theory of individual psychology*. New York: Harcourt, Brace, 1927.

Albee, G. W. Does including psychotherapy in health insurance represent a subsidy to the rich from the poor? *American Psychologist*, 1977, *32*, 719-721.

Alexander, F. and French, T. M. *Psychoanalytic therapy*. New York: Ronald, 1946.

Allport, G. W. *Personality and social encounter*. Boston: Beacon Press, 1960.

American Psychiatric Association. *Diagnostic and statistical manual of mental disorders* (3rd ed.). Washington, D.C., 1980.

Ayllon, T., and Azrin, N. H. The measurement and reinforcement of behavior of psychotics. *Journal of Experimental Analysis of Behavior*, 1965, *8*, 357-383.

Bachman, J. A. Self-injurious behavior: A behavioral analysis. *Journal of Abnormal Psychology*, 1972, *80*, 211-224.

Bandura, A. *Aggression: A social learning analysis*. Englewood Cliffs, N.J.: Prentice-Hall, 1973.

Bandura, A. Self-efficacy: Towards a unifying theory of behavioral change. *Psychological Review*, 1977, *84*, 191-215.

Baum, O. E., Felzer, S. B., D'Zmura, T. L., and Shumaker, E. Psychotherapy, dropouts and lower socioeconomic patients. *American Journal of Orthopsychiatry*, 1966, *36*, 629-635.

Beck, A. T. *Cognitive therapy and the emotional disorders*. New York: International Universities Press, 1976.

Beck, A. T. *Depression: Clinical, experimental, and theoretical aspects.* New York: Hoeber, 1967.

Bergin, A. E. The evaluation of therapeutic outcomes. In A. E. Bergin and S. L. Garfield (eds.), *Handbook of psychotherapy and behavior change: An empirical analysis.* New York: Wiley, 1971.

Bergin, A. E., and Strupp, H. H. New directions in psychotherapy research. *Journal of Abnormal Psychology,* 1970, *75,* 13-26.

Bergin, A. E., and Garfield, S. L. *Handbook of psychotherapy and behavior change: An empirical analysis.* New York: Wiley, 1971.

Bergin, A. E., and Lambert, M. J. The evaluation of therapeutic outcomes. In S. L. Garfield and A. E. Bergin (eds.), *Handbook of psychotherapy and behavior change: An empirical analysis* (2nd ed.). New York: Wiley, 1978.

Bernard, V. W. Some principles of dynamic psychiatry in relation to poverty. *American Journal of Psychiatry,* 1965, *122,* 254-267.

Beutler, L. E. Psychotherapy: When what works with whom. Unpublished manuscript. Baylor College of Medicine, Houston, Texas, 1976.

Beutler, L. E., Pollack, S., and Jobe, A. On "accepting" patients vs. "accepting" therapists. Paper presented at the Ninth Annual Meeting of the Society for Psychotherapy Research, Madison, Wisconsin, 1977.

Bordin, E. S. *Psychological counseling.* New York: Appleton-Century-Crofts, 1955.

Bowlby, J. *Separation: Anxiety and anger. Psychology of attachment and loss series* (Vol. 3). New York: Basic Books, 1973.

Brigham, J. C. Ethnic stereotypes. *Psychological Bulletin,* 1971, *76,* 15-38.

Butcher, J. N., and Koss, M. P. Research on brief and crisis-oriented psychotherapies. In S. L. Garfield and A. E. Bergin (eds.), *Handbook of psychotherapy and behavior change: An empirical analysis* (2nd ed.). New York: Wiley, 1978.

Butcher, J. N., and Maudal, G. R. Crisis intervention. In I. B. Weiner (ed.), *Clinical methods in psychology,* New York: Wiley, 1976.

Camus, A. *Exile and the kingdom.* New York: Knopf, 1957.

Caplan, G. *An approach to community mental health.* New York: Grune and Stratton, 1961.

Caplan, G. *Principles of preventive psychiatry.* New York: Basic Books, 1964.

Carson, R. C., and Heine, R. W. Similarity and success in therapeutic dyads. *Journal of Consulting Psychology,* 1962, *26,* 38-43.

Cautela, J. R. Covert processes and behavior modification. *Journal of Nervous and Mental Disease,* 1973, *157,* 27-36.

Chafetz, M., and Demone, H. W. *In facts about alcohol and alcoholism. 1974* (DHEW Publication No. ADM 75-31).

Ciminero, A. R., Calhoun, K. S., and Adams, H. E. (eds.). *Handbook of behavioral assessment*. New York: Wiley-Interscience, 1977.

Cook, T. D., and Campbell, D. T. Quasi-experimentation: Design and analysis issues for field settings. Chicago: Rand McNally, 1979.

Cowen, E. L. Social and community intervention. In P. H. Mussen and M. R. Rosenzweig (eds.), *Annual review of psychology*. Palo Alto, Calif.: Annual Reviews, 1973.

Crowe, M. J. Evaluation of conjoint marital therapy. D.M. dissertation, University of Oxford, 1976.

Cummings, N. A. The anatomy of psychotherapy under national health insurance. *American Psychologist*, 1977, *32*, 711-718.

Dahlstrom, W. G., Welsh, G. S., and Dahlstrom, L. E. *An MMPI handbook. Vol. 2: Research developments and applications*. Minneapolis: University of Minnesota Press, 1975.

DeLeon, G., and Mandell, W. A comparison of conditioning and psychotherapy in the treatment of functional enuresis. *Journal of Clinical Psychology*, 1966, *22*, 326-330.

DeLeon, G., and Sacks, S. Conditioning functional enuresis: A four year follow-up. *Journal of Consulting and Clinical Psychology*, 1972, *39*, 299-300.

DiLoreto, A. O. *Comparative psychotherapy: An experimental analysis*. Chicago: Aldine-Atherton, 1971.

Ellis, A. *The essence of rational psychotherapy: A comprehensive approach to treatment*. New York: Institute for Rational Living, 1970.

Endler, N. S., and Magnusson, D. Toward an interactional psychology of personality. *Psychological Bulletin*, 1976, *83*, 956-974.

Erikson, E. H. *Childhood and society* (2nd ed.). New York: W. W. Norton, 1963.

Exner, J. E. Projective techniques. In I. B. Weiner (ed.), *Clinical methods in psychology*. New York: Wiley-Interscience, 1976.

Eysenck, H. J. The effects of psychotherapy: An experimental analysis. *Journal of Consulting Psychology*, 1952, *16*, 319-324.

Eysenck, H. J. *Handbook of abnormal psychology*. London: Pitman, 1961.

Fixsen, D. L., Phillips, E. L., Phillips, E. A., and Wolf, M. M. The teaching-family model of group home treatment. Paper presented at the meeting of the American Psychological Association, Honolulu, Hawaii, September, 1972.

Frankl, V. E. *The doctor and the soul* (2nd ed.). New York: Knopf, 1965.

Friedman, P. R. Legal regulation of applied behavior analysis in mental institutions and prisons. *Arizona Law Review*, 1975, *17*, 39-104.

Fromm, E. *Man for himself*. New York: Holt, Rinehart and Winston, 1947.

Garfield, S. L. Research on client variables in psychotherapy. In S. L. Garfield and A. E. Bergin (eds.), *Handbook of psychotherapy and behavior change: An empirical analysis* (2nd ed.). New York: Wiley, 1978.

Garfield, S. L., and Bergin, A. E. (eds.). *Handbook of psychotherapy and behavior change: An empirical analysis* (2nd ed.). New York: Wiley, 1978.

Gelder, M. G., Marks, I. M., and Wolff, H. Desensitization and psychotherapy in phobic states: a controlled enquiry. *British Journal of Psychiatry*, 1967, *113*, 53.

Gillan, P., and Rachman, S. An experimental investigation of behavior therapy in phobic patients. *British Journal of Psychiatry*, 1974, *124*, 392.

Glowgower, F., and Sloop, E. W. Two strategies of group training of parents as effective behavior modifiers. *Behavior Therapy*, 1976, *7*, 177-184.

Goldfried, M. R. Systematic desensitization as training in self-control. *Journal of Consulting and Clinical Psychology*, 1971, *37*, 228-234.

Goldfried, M. R., and Davison, G. C. *Clinical behavior therapy*. New York: Holt, Rinehart and Winston, 1976.

Goldman, G. D., and Milman, D. S. (eds.). *Psychoanalytic psychotherapy*. Reading, Mass.: Addison-Wesley, 1978.

Goldstein, A. P. *Structured learning therapy: Toward a psychotherapy for the poor*. New York: Academic Press, 1973.

Goldstein, A. P., and Stein, N. *Prescriptive psychotherapies*. New York: Pergamon Press, 1976.

Gottesman, I., and Shields, J. *Schizophrenia and genetics: A twin study vantage point*. New York: Academic Press, 1972.

Gottman, J. M., and Markman, H. J. Experimental designs in psychotherapy research. In S. L. Garfield and A. E. Bergin (eds.), *Handbook of psychotherapy and behavior change: An empirical analysis* (2nd ed.). New York: Wiley, 1978.

Green, B. L., Gleser, G. C., Stone, W. N., and Seifert, R. F. Relationships among diverse measures of psychotherapy outcomes. *Journal of Consulting and Clinical Psychology*, 1975, *43*, 689-699.

Gurin, G., Veroff, J., and Feld, S. *Americans view their mental health*. New York: Basic Books, 1960.

Gynther, M. D., and Gynther, R. A. Personality inventories. In I. B. Weiner (ed.), *Clinical methods in psychology*. New York: Wiley-Interscience, 1976.

Hafner, J., and Marks, I. M. Exposure in vivo of agoraphobics: the contributions of diazepam, group exposure and anxiety evocation. *Psychological Medicine*, 1976, *6*, 71-88.

Harlow, H. F. Age-mate or peer affectional system. In D. S. Lehrman, R. A. Hende, and E. Shaw (eds.). *Advances in the study of behavior* (Vol. 2). New York: Academic Press, 1969.

Harlow, M. K., and Harlow, H. F. Affection in primates. *Discovery*, 1966, *27*, 11-17.

Haynes v. *Harris*, 344 F. 2d 463 (8th Cir. 1965).

Heitler, J. B. Preparation of lower-class patients for expressive group psychotherapy. *Journal of Consulting and Clinical Psychology*, 1973, *41*, 251-260.

Heitler, J. B. Preparatory techniques in initiating expressive psychotherapy with lower-class, unsophisticated patients. *Psychological Bulletin*, 1976, *83*, 339-352.

Hiler, E. W. An analysis of patient-therapist compatibility. *Journal of Consulting Psychology*, 1958, *22*, 341-347.

Hollon, S., and Beck, A. T. Psychotherapy and drug therapy: Comparisons and combinations. In S. L. Garfield and A. E. Bergin (eds.), *Handbook of psychotherapy and behavior change: An empirical analysis* (2nd ed.). New York: Wiley, 1978.

Holroyd, J. C., and Brodsky, A. M. Psychologists' attitudes and practices regarding erotic and nonerotic physical contact with patients. *American Psychologist*, 1977, *32*, 843-849.

Ivey, A. E. *Microcounseling: Innovations in interviewing training.* Springfield, Ill.: Charles C. Thomas, 1971.

Jacobs, D., Charles, E., Jacob, T., Weinstein, H., and Mann, D. Preparation for treatment of the disadvantaged patient. Effects on disposition and outcome. *American Journal of Orthopsychiatry*, 1972, *42*, 666-674.

Jacobsen, E. *Progressive relaxation.* Chicago: University of Chicago Press, 1938.

Kadushin, C. *Why people go to psychiatrists.* New York: Atherton Press, 1969.

Kaimowitz v. *Michigan Department of Mental Health*, 42 *U.S. L. Week* 2063 (Mich. Cir. Ct., Wayne Cty., 1973).

Kanfer, F. H., and Phillips, J. S. *Learning foundations of behavior therapy.* New York: Wiley, 1970.

Kazdin, A. E. The application of operant techniques in treatment, rehabilitation and education. In S. L. Garfield and A. E. Bergin (eds.), *Handbook of psychotherapy and behavior change: An empirical analysis* (2nd ed.). New York: Wiley, 1978.

Kelly, G. A. *The psychology of personal constructs* (Vols. 1 and 2). New York: Norton, 1955.

Kesey, K. *One flew over the cuckoo's nest.* New York: New American Library, 1962.

Kiesler, D. J. Experimental designs in psychotherapy research. In A. E. Bergin and S. L. Garfield (eds.), *Handbook of psychotherapy and behavior change: An empirical analysis.* New York: Wiley, 1971.

Kiresuk, T. J., and Sherman, R. E. Goal attainment scaling: A general method for evaluating comprehensive community mental health programs. *Community Mental Health Journal*, 1968, *4*, 443-453.

Kleinmuntz, B. *Personality measurement: An introduction*. Homewood, Ill.: Dorsey Press, 1967.

Korchin, S. J. *Modern clinical psychology*. New York: Basic Books, 1976.

Korchin, S. J. Clinical psychology and minority problems. *American Psychologist*, 1980, *35*, 262-269.

Korner, I. N. Crisis reduction and the psychological consultant. In G. A. Specter and W. L. Claiborn (eds.), *Crisis intervention* (Vol. 2). New York: Behavioral Publications, 1973.

Lake v. *Cameron*, 364 F2d 657 (D.C. 1966).

Lazarus, R. S. *Psychological stress and the coping process*. New York: McGraw-Hill, 1966.

Levinson, D. J. *The seasons of a man's life*. New York: Knopf, 1978.

Lindsley, O. R. Free operant conditioning and psychotherapy. In J. Masserman (ed.), *Current psychiatric therapies*. New York: Grune and Stratton, 1963.

Lorenzen, I. J. Acceptance or rejection by psychiatric clinics. M. A. Essay, Columbia University, 1967,

Lorion, R. P. Research on psychotherapy and behavior change with the disadvantaged. In S. L. Garfield and A. E. Bergin (eds.), *Handbook of psychotherapy and behavior change: An empirical analysis* (2nd ed.). New York: Wiley, 1978.

Lovaas, O. I. A behavior therapy approach to the treatment of childhood schizophrenia. In J. Hill (ed.), *Minnesota Symposium on Child Psychology*. Minneapolis: University of Minnesota Press, 1967.

Luborsky, L., Singer, B., and Luborsky, L. Comparative studies of psychotherapies. *Archives of General Psychiatry*, 1975, *32*, 995-1008.

Magnusson, D., and Endler, N. S. (eds.). *Personality at the crossroads: Current issues in interactional psychology*. Hillsdale, N.J.: Erlbaum, 1977.

Mahoney, M. J. Personal science: A cognitive learning therapy. In A. Ellis and R. Grieger (eds.), *Handbook of rational psychotherapy*. New York: Springer, 1977.

Mahoney, M. J., and Arnkoff, D. Cognitive and self-control therapies. In S. L. Garfield and A. E. Bergin (eds.), *Handbook of psychotherapy and behavior change: An empirical analysis* (2nd ed.). New York: Wiley, 1978.

Maris, R., and Connor, H. E., Jr. Do crisis services work: A follow-up of a psychiatric outpatient sample. *Journal of Health and Social Behavior*, 1973, *14*, 311-322.

Marks, I. Behavioral psychotherapy of adult neurosis. In S. L. Garfield and A. E. Bergin (eds.), *Handbook of psychotherapy and behavior change: An empirical analysis* (2nd ed.). New York: Wiley, 1978.

Marks, I. M., Hodgson, R., and Rachman, S. Treatment of chronic obsessive-compulsive neurosis by in vivo exposure: a two year follow-up and issues in treatment. *British Journal of Psychiatry*, 1975, *127*, 349.

Martin, B. *Abnormal psychology: clinical and scientific perspectives*. New York: Holt, Rinehart and Winston, 1977.

Maslow, A. H. *Toward a psychology of being* (2nd ed.). Princeton, N.J.: Van Nostrand, 1968.

Matarazzo, R. G. Research on the teaching and learning of psychotherapeutic skills. In S. L. Garfield and A. E. Bergin (eds.), *Handbook of psychotherapy and behavior change: An empirical analysis* (2nd ed.). New York: Wiley, 1978.

May, R. (ed.). *Existential psychology*. New York: Random House, 1961.

McSweeny, A. J. Including psychotherapy in national health insurance: Insurance guidelines and other proposed solutions. *American Psychologist*, 1977, *32*, 722-730.

Miller, A. *Death of a salesman*. New York: Viking Press, 1949.

Miller, N. E. Learning of visceral and glandular responses. *Science*, 1969, *163*, 434-445.

Mischel, W. *Introduction to personality* (Rev. ed.). New York: Holt, Rinehart and Winston, 1976.

Mitchell, K. M., Bozarth, J. D., and Krauft, C. C. A reappraisal of the therapeutic effectiveness of accurate empathy, nonpossessive warmth, and genuineness. In A. S. Gurman and A. M. Razin (eds.), *Effective psychotherapy: A handbook of research*. New York: Pergamon Press, 1977.

Mowrer, O. H. Apparatus for the study and treatment of enuresis. *American Journal of Psychology*, 1938, *51*, 163-166.

Murray, E. J., and Jacobson, L. I. Cognition and learning in traditional and behavioral psychotherapy. In S. L. Garfield and A. E. Bergin (eds.), *Handbook of psychotherapy and behavior change: An empirical analysis*, (2nd ed.). New York: Wiley, 1978.

New York City Health and Hospital Corporation v. *Stein*, 335 N.Y.S.2d 461 (Sup. Ct. 1972).

Parloff, M. B., Waskow, I. E., and Wolfe, B. E. Research on therapist variables in relation to process and outcome. In S. L. Garfield and A. E. Bergin (eds.), *Handbook of psychotherapy and behavior change: An empirical analysis*, (2nd ed.). New York: Wiley, 1978.

Paul, G. L. *Insight vs. desensitization in psychotherapy*. Stanford, Ca.: Stanford University Press, 1966.

Pavlov, I. P. *Conditioned reflexes*. New York: Dover, 1960. (Originally published, 1927.)

Phares, E. J. *Clinical psychology: Concepts, methods, and profession*. Homewood, Ill., Dorsey Press, 1979.

Powers, E., and Witmer, H. *An experiment in the prevention of delinquency*. New York: Columbia University Press, 1951.

Rachman, S. *The effects of psychotherapy*. Oxford: Pergamon Press, 1971.

Report of the Research Task Force of the National Institute of Mental Health. *Research in the Service of Mental Health*. DHEW Publication No. (ADM) 75-236. Rockville, Md.: 1975.

Rogers, C. R. *Client-centered therapy*. Boston: Houghton Mifflin, 1951.

Rogers, C. R. A theory of therapy, personality, and interpersonal relationships as developed in the client-centered framework. In S. Koch (ed.), *Psychology: A study of a science* (Vol. 3). New York: McGraw-Hill, 1959.

Rogers, C. R. (ed.). *The therapeutic relationshp and its impact: A study of psychotherapy with schizophrenics*. Madison, Wis.: University of Wisconsin Press, 1967.

Rosenthal, T., and Bandura, A. Psychological modeling: Theory and practice. In S. L. Garfield and A. E. Bergin (eds.), *Handbook of psychotherapy and behavior change: An empirical analysis* (2nd ed.). New York: Wiley, 1978.

Ross, A. O. Behavior therapy with children. In S. L. Garfield and A. E. Bergin (eds.), *Handbook of psychotherapy and behavior change: An empirical analysis* (2nd ed.). New York: Wiley, 1978.

Rotter, J. B. *Social learning and clinical psychology*. Englewood Cliffs, N. J.: Prentice-Hall, 1954.

Rouse v. *Cameron*, 373 F.2d 451 (D.C. Cir. 1966).

Sawrey, J. M., and Telford, C. W. *Adjustment and Personality*. Boston: Allyn and Bacon, 1975.

Sears, R. R. Relation of early socialization experiences to self-concepts and gender roles in middle childhood. *Child Development*, 1970, *41*, 267-289.

Sechrest, L. Incremental validity: A recommendation. *Educational and Psychological Measurement*, 1963, *23*, 153-158.

Seligman, M. E. P. *Helplessness: On depression, development and death*. San Francisco: Freeman, 1975.

Selye, H. *The stress of life*. New York: McGraw-Hill, 1956.

Shapiro, A. K., and Morris, L. A. Placebo effects in medical and psychological therapies. In S. L. Garfield and A. E. Bergin (eds.), *Handbook of psychotherapy and behavior change: An empirical analysis* (2nd ed.). New York: Wiley, 1978.

Sheehy, G. *Passages: Predictable crises of adult life.* New York: Dutton, 1976.

Siegal, J. M. A brief review of the effects of race in clinical service interactions. *American Journal of Orthopsychiatry,* 1974, *44*, 555-562.

Sifneos, P. E. *Short-term psychotherapy and emotional crisis.* Cambridge, Mass.: Harvard University Press, 1972.

Skinner, B. F. *Science and human behavior.* New York: MacMillan, 1953.

Smith, M. L., and Glass, G. V. Meta-analysis of psychotherapy outcome studies. *American Psychologist,* 1977, *32*, 752-760.

Snyder, S. H. Dopamine and schizophrenia. In L. C. Wynne, R. L. Cromwell, and S. Matthysse (eds.), *The nature of schizophrenia: New approaches to research and treatment.* New York: Wiley, 1978.

Soloman, R. L., and Wynne, L. C. Traumatic avoidance learning: Acquisition in normal dogs. *Psychological Monographs,* 1953, *67*, No. 4, Whole No. 354.

Spielberger, C. D., Gorsuch, R. L., and Lushene, R. E. *The State-Trait Anxiety Inventory (STAI) Test Manual for Form X.* Palo Alto, Calif.: Consulting Psychologists Press, 1970.

Spivack, G., Platt, J. J., and Shure, M. D. *The problem-solving approach to adjustment.* San Francisco: Jossey-Bass, 1976.

Stampfl, T. G., and Levis, D. J. Essentials of implosive therapy: A learning-theory based psycho-dynamic behavioral therapy. *Journal of Abnormal Psychology,* 1967, *72,* 496-503.

Strupp, H. H. Psychotherapy research and practice: An overview. In S. L. Garfield and A. E. Bergin (eds.), *Handbook of psychotherapy and behavior change: An empirical analysis* (2nd ed.). New York: Wiley, 1978.

Strupp, H. H., Hadley, S. W., and Gomes-Schwartz, B. *Psychotherapy for better or worse: An analysis of the problem of negative effects.* New York: Jason Aronson, 1977.

Sundberg, N. D. *Assessment of persons.* Englewood Cliffs, N.J.: Prentice-Hall, 1977.

Thorndike, E. L. Reward and punishment in animal learning. *Comparative Psychology Monographs,* 1932, *8,* Whole No. 39.

Truax, C. B., and Carkhuff, R. R. *Toward effective counseling and psychotherapy: Training and practice.* Chicago: Aldine, 1976.

Truax, C. B., and Mitchell, K. M. Research on certain therapist interpersonal skills in relation to process and outcome. In A. E. Bergin and S. L. Garfield (eds.)., *Handbook of psychotherapy and behavior change: An empirical analysis.* New York: Wiley, 1971.

Warren, N., and Rice, L. Structuring and stabilizing of psychotherapy for low-prognosis clients. *Journal of Consulting and Clinical Psychology,* 1972, *39,* 173-181.

Watson, J. B., and Rayner, R. Conditioned emotional reactions. *Journal of Experimental Psychology*, 1920, *3*, 1-14.

Whitehorn, J. C., and Betz, B. J. A study of psychotherapeutic relationships between physicians and schizophrenic patients. *American Journal of Psychiatry*, 1954, *111*, 321-331.

Wolberg, L. R. *The technique of psychotherapy* (2nd ed.). New York: Grune and Stratton, 1967.

Wolpe, J. *Psychotherapy by reciprocal inhibition*. Stanford, Calif.: Stanford University Press, 1958.

Wrightsman, L. S. *Social psychology in the seventies*. Monterey, Calif.: Brooks/Cole, 1972.

Wyatt v. *Stickney*, 344 F. Supp 373, 344 F. Supp. 387 (M. D. Ala. 1972) affirmed sub nom. *Wyatt* v. Aderholt, 503 F. 2d 1305 (5th Cir. 1974).

Zelin, M. L. Validity of the MMPI scales for measuring twenty psychiatric dimensions. *Journal of Consulting and Clinical Psychology*, 1971, *37*, 286-290.

NAME INDEX

SUBJECT INDEX